Fluids and Electrolytes

with Clinical Applications
A Programmed Approach

8th Edition

Joyce LeFever Kee, MS, RN
Associate Professor Emerita
College of Health Sciences
University of Delaware
Newark, Delaware

Betty J. Paulanka, EdD, RN
Dean and Professor
College of Health Sciences
University of Delaware
Newark, Delaware

Carolee Polek, PhD, RN
Associate Professor of Nursing
College of Health Sciences
University of Delaware
Newark, Delaware

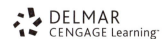

DELMAR
CENGAGE Learning·

Australia · Canada · Mexico · Singapore · Spain · United Kingdom · United States

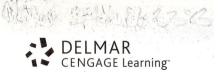
DELMAR
CENGAGE Learning

Fluids and Electrolytes with Clinical Applications: A Programmed Approach, 8th Edition
Joyce LeFever Kee, Betty J. Paulanka, and Carolee Polek

Vice President, Career and Professional Editorial: Dave Garza

Director of Learning Solutions: Matthew Kane

Executive Editor: Steven Helba

Managing Editor: Marah Bellegarde

Senior Product Manager: Juliet Steiner

Editorial Assistant: Meaghan O'Brien

Vice President, Career and Professional Marketing: Jennifer McAvey

Marketing Director: Wendy Mapstone

Marketing Manager: Michele McTighe

Marketing Coordinator: Scott Chrysler

Production Director: Carolyn Miller

Production Manager: Andrew Crouth

Content Project Manager: Andrea Majot

Senior Art Director: Jack Pendleton

For product information and technology assistance, contact us at **Professional & Career Group Customer Support, 1-800-648-7450**
For permission to use material from this text or product, submit all requests online at **cengage.com/permissions.**
Further permissions questions can be e-mailed to **permissionrequest@cengage.com**.

Library of Congress Control Number: 2008931928

ISBN-13: 978-1-4354-5367-8

ISBN-10: 1-4354-5367-0

Delmar
5 Maxwell Drive
Clifton Park, NY 12065-2919
USA

Cengage Learning is a leading provider of customized learning solutions with office locations around the globe, including Singapore, the United Kingdom, Australia, Mexico, Brazil, and Japan. Locate your local office at: **international.cengage.com/region**

Cengage Learning products are represented in Canada by Nelson Education, Ltd.

For your life long learning solutions, visit **delmar.cengage.com**

Visit our corporate website at **cengage.com**.

Notice to the Reader

Publisher does not warrant or guarantee any of the products described herein or perform any independent analysis in connection with any of the product information contained herein. Publisher does not assume, and expressly disclaims, any obligation to obtain and include information other than that provided to it by the manufacturer. The reader is expressly warned to consider and adopt all safety precautions that might be indicated by the activities described herein and to avoid all potential hazards. By following the instructions contained herein, the reader willingly assumes all risks in connection with such instructions. The publisher makes no representations or warranties of any kind, including but not limited to, the warranties of fitness for particular purpose or merchantability, nor are any such representations implied with respect to the material set forth herein, and the publisher takes no responsibility with respect to such material. The publisher shall not be liable for any special, consequential, or exemplary damages resulting, in whole or part, from the readers' use of, or reliance upon, this material.

Printed in United States of America
2 3 4 5 X X 11 10 09

Dedication

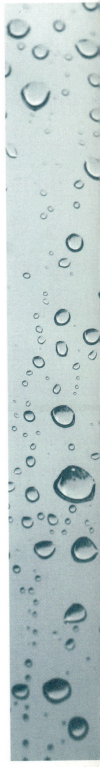

To
The Faculty, Staff, and Alumni of the School of Nursing in the University of Delaware's College of Health Sciences for their commitment to excellence in nursing education.

To
Joyce Kee for her continued commitment to nursing publications and support for faculty scholarship through authorship in her books.

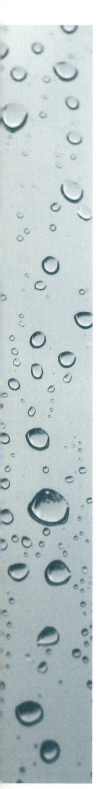

Contents

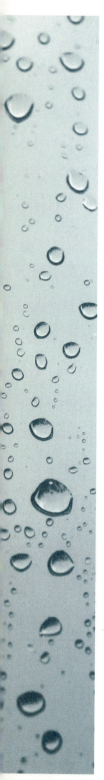

Preface

Nurses and health care professionals are involved continually in the assessment of fluid and electrolyte imbalance. Medical advances and new treatment modalities have increased the importance of a strong background in the physiologic concepts associated with these imbalances. Additionally, the expanded role of nurses in the community requires them to function more autonomously in assisting patients to control fluid and electrolyte imbalances. Every seriously or chronically ill person is likely to develop one or more of these imbalances, and the very young and the very old are especially vulnerable to changes in fluid and electrolyte balance. Even those who are only moderately ill are at high risk for these imbalances. Multiple health care providers are responsible for maintaining homeostasis of fluid and electrolyte balance when caring for patients. After completing this book, the learner should understand more fully the effects of fluid, electrolyte, and acid-base balance and imbalance on the body as they occur in many clinical health problems across the life span.

New to This Edition

The eighth edition of this programmed text, *Fluids and Electrolytes with Clinical Applications*, has been completely updated to meet the current assessment, management, and clinical interventions recommended for fluid, electrolyte, and acid-base imbalances related to common, recurring clinical health problems. The chapters include learning outcomes, introduction, pathophysiology, etiology, clinical manifestations, clinical management, clinical applications, clinical considerations, case studies, and nursing diagnoses with clinical interventions, appropriate rationale, and evaluation outcomes. This new edition also includes:

- Increased emphasis on evaluation and outcomes for each chapter helps to clarify expected outcomes and identify best practices.
- Extensive revisions have been made throughout the book. Case studies have eliminated patient names to emphasize new HIPPA regulations and promote a model of patient privacy when discussing clinical patients and situations. In addition, Web sites have been added at the end of many chapters as another resource for learning fluid and electrolyte content.

● Chapter 12 has been completely rewritten to simplify concepts related to *Acid-Base Imbalances.*

● Chapter 18, *Gastrointestinal (GI) Surgery with Fluid and Electrolyte Imbalances*, has been expanded to include content on bariatric surgery.

● The content related to COPD in Chapter 20 has been completely revised and updated.

● The glossary has been expanded and updated with new and revised definitions.

● The *References/Bibliography* has been completely updated with many new sources of reference.

● Three new appendices have been added; a table of common lab studies for fluid and electrolyte imbalances, a table of *Foods Rich in Potassium, Sodium, Calcium, Magnesium, Chloride, and Phosphorus*, and a copy of the Joint Commission's recommendations for abbreviations.

● Many of the numerous tables and figures have been updated to current standards for accurate references to pertinent information.

The content of this book has been geared to three levels of learning among the healthcare professions. First, it is intended for beginning students who have had some background in the biological sciences or who have completed an anatomy and physiology course. Second, it is for students who have a sufficient background in the biological sciences, chemistry, and physics but who need to learn about specific clinical health problems that cause fluid and electrolyte imbalances. Many of these students might wish to review the entire text to reinforce their previous knowledge and/or practice their skills in providing accurate nursing assessments and interventions. Finally, this book is intended to aid graduate nurses who wish to review and improve their knowledge of fluid and electrolyte changes in order to assess their patients' needs and enhance the quality of patient care. Summary charts have been included as quick reference sources for working professional.

What Is a Programmed Approach?

The programmed approach is a self-instructional method of learning that helps the instructor to use class time more efficiently, and enables students to work at their own pace while learning the principles, concepts, and application of fluids and electrolytes.

Throughout, an asterisk (*) on an answer line indicates a multiple-word answer. The meanings for the following symbols are: ↑ increased, ↓ decreased, > greater than, < less than. A dagger (†) in tables indicates the most common signs and symptoms. A glossary covers words and terms used throughout the text. It should be useful to the student who had minimal preparation in the biological sciences.

Joyce LeFever Kee, MS, RN
Betty J. Paulanka, EdD, RN
Carolee Polek, PhD, RN

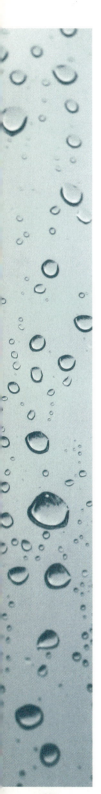

Acknowledgments

For the eighth edition, we wish to extend our deepest appreciation to Faculty Ingrid Pretzer-Aboff, Judy Herrman, Carolee Polek, William Rose, Kathy Schell, Gail Wade, Erlinda Wheeler and Alumni and Linda Laskowski Jones in the College of Health Sciences at the University of Delaware for their contributions and assistance.

We especially wish to thank Barbara Vogt in the Dean's Office of the College of Health Sciences at the University of Delaware for her work in coordinating correspondence and typing materials.

We also offer our thanks to our editors Steven Helba and Juliet Steiner at Delmar, Cengage Learning for their helpful suggestions and assistance with this revision.

Joyce LeFever Kee
Betty J. Paulanka
Carolee Polek

Contributors and Consultants

Pretzer-Aboff, RN
Associate Professor
College of Health Sciences
University of Delaware
Newark, Delaware

Judith Herrman, PhD, RN, ANP
Associate Professor/Undergraduate
  Clinical Coordinator
College of Health Sciences
University of Delaware
Newark, Delaware

Linda Laskowski-Jones, RN, MS, CCRN, CEN
Vice President: Trauma, Emergency
  Medicine and Aero Medical Services
Christiana Care Health Systems
Wilmington, Delaware

William C. Rose, PhD
Assistant Professor
College of Health Sciences
University of Delaware
Newark, Delaware

Kathleen Schell, DNSc, RN
Assistant Professor
College of Health Sciences
University of Delaware
Newark, Delaware

Gail Wade, DNSc, RN
Associate Professor
College of Health Sciences
University of Delaware
Newark, Delaware

Erlinda Wheeler, DNS, RN
Associate Professor
College of Health Sciences
University of Delaware
Newark, Delaware

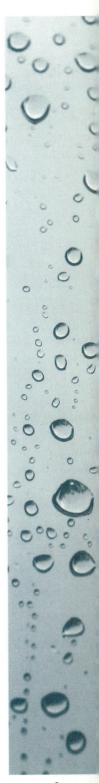

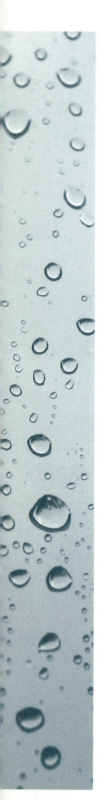

Reviewers

Deb Aucoin-Ratcliff, RN, DNP
American River College
Sacramento, California

Vicki Bingham, PhD, RN
Chair of Academic Programs and
    Assistant Professor of Nursing
School of Nursing
Delta State University
Cleveland, Mississippi

Doreen DeAngelis, MSN, RN
Nursing Instructor
Penn State Fayette, The Eberly Campus
Uniontown, Pennsylvania

Deborah J. Marshall, MSN, RN
Associate Professor, Nursing
Palm Beach Community College
Lake Worth, Florida

Deborah A. Raines, PhD, RN
Professor
Christine E. Lynn College of Nursing
Florida Atlantic University
Boca Raton, Florida

Barbara Scheirer RN, MSN
Assistant Professor
School of Nursing
Grambling State University
Grambling, Louisiana

Diann S. Slade, MSN, RN
Instructor
College of Pharmacy, Nursing, and
    Allied Health Sciences
Howard University
Washington, D.C.

Helpful Suggestions from the Authors

To the Student

Many students believe that the subject of fluids and electrolytes is very difficult to comprehend. This programmed book provides you with important data on fluids and electrolytes from various points of view. If you apply this material to clinical problems and previous and present experiences, it is not so difficult to understand and retain.

By taking easy steps provided in this book, you can proceed through the chapters more quickly than you might expect. This book is written using a self-instruction format that allows you to proceed at your own pace. Each step is a learning process. A better quality of learning occurs when you either complete a chapter at a time or spend a minimum of two hours at one sitting. Never end the study period without at least completing all questions related to a single topic.

It is helpful to begin each study session with the final questions from the previous material; this enables you to check your retention of material that was presented previously. The case study reviews in each chapter give immediate reinforcement of the data learned. The assessment factors, nursing diagnoses, and interventions should be useful when applying fluid, electrolyte, and acid-base concepts in various clinical settings. The clinical assessment tool is useful for determining fluid, electrolyte, and acid-base balance and imbalance. A glossary is included to assist you with words and terms used throughout the text.

Study each diagram and table before proceeding to the questions. If you make mistakes in the program, you need not be concerned so long as you rectify the mistakes. This learning modality and the content in this book should increase your knowledge and understanding of fluids and electrolytes. This model of learning can be a great asset for applying this knowledge to your clinical practicum experiences.

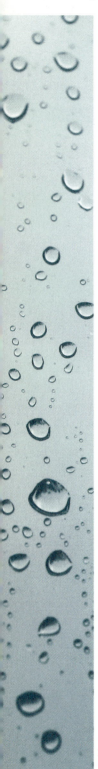

To the Instructor

Class time is frequently spent on reviewing material or presenting new material that can easily be given through programmed (learning) instruction. This method of instruction enables the instructor to minimize the time spent in lecture on fluids and electrolytes, thus devoting more time to clinical discussions and/or a seminar format to enhance the students' understanding of fluid and electrolyte imbalance by active class participation.

You may find it helpful to cover the material in this book by one of three ways: (1) assigning the students a chapter at a time, (2) assigning a unit for the students to complete by a certain date, or (3) assigning the students a given length of time to complete the entire text and having them present material using their clinical experiences.

Joyce LeFever Kee
Betty J. Paulanka
Carolee Polek

BODY FLUID AND ITS FUNCTION

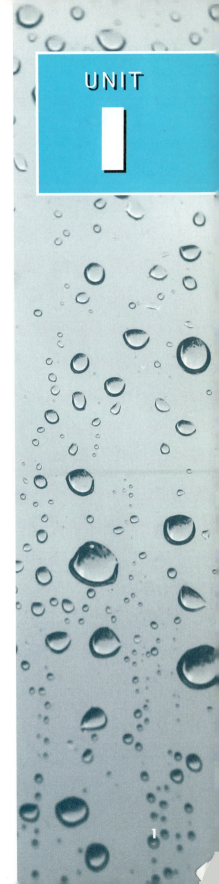

● LEARNING OUTCOMES

Upon completion of this unit, the reader will be able to:

- Compare the percentage of water found in the body of the average adult, newborn infant, and embryo.
- Identify the three compartments (spaces) where water is distributed in the body.
- Identify the two classifications of body fluids and their percentages.
- Describe five functions of body fluids.
- Define homeostasis in terms of its role in maintaining body fluid equilibrium.
- Describe how the body loses and maintains body fluid.
- Define the following homeostatic mechanisms: osmotic pressure, oncotic pressure, semipermeable membranes, selectively permeable membranes, osmol, and osmolality.
- Describe the effects of the above homeostatic mechanisms on the movement of body fluid.
- Describe four measurable pressures that determine the flow of fluid between the vessels and tissues in terms of their effects on the exchange of fluid.
- Describe the concept of a pressure gradient.
- Explain the significance in colloid osmotic (oncotic) and hydrostatic pressure gradients.
- Discuss the body's regulators of fluid balance.
- Describe isotonic (iso-osmolar), hypotonic (hypo-osmolar), and hypertonic (hyperosmolar) solutions in terms of their effects on body cells.
- Discuss the relationship between milligrams and milliequivalents and the significance of this relationship in the body.

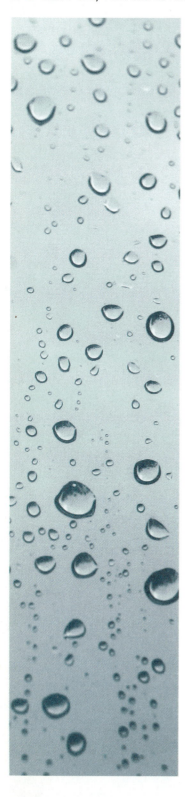

- Develop select nursing diagnoses appropriate for patients experiencing fluid imbalances.
- Describe the effects of selected fluid changes on the observable symptoms of patients in your clinical area.

● INTRODUCTION

The human body is a complex machine that contains hundreds of bones and the most sophisticated interaction of systems of any structure on earth. Yet, the substance that is basic to the very existence of the body is the simplest substance known—water. In fact, it makes up almost two-thirds of an adult's body weight.

The body is not static; it is alive, and solid particles within its framework are able to move into and out of cells and systems, and even into and out of the body, only because there is water.

The basis of all fluids is water, and as long as the quantity and composition of body fluids are within the normal range, we just take it for granted and enjoy being healthy. But if the water content of the body for some reason departs from this range, the whole delicate balance of body systems is disrupted, and disease can find an easy target.

An asterisk (*) on an answer line indicates a multiple-word answer. The meanings for the following symbols are: ↑ increased, ↓ decreased, > greater than, < less than.

Body Fluid, Its Function and Movement

● INTRODUCTION

The greatest single constituent of the body is water. Body water movement and distribution are influenced by fluid intake, fluid pressures, and osmolality of the body fluid.

In this chapter, distribution of body fluids, fluid compartments, functions of body fluid, intake and output for homeostasis, definitions, fluid pressures, regulators of body fluid, and osmolality of body fluid and solutions are discussed. Also included are a case study review, assessment factors, diagnoses, interventions, and evaluation/outcome process.

ANSWER COLUMN

1.

The greatest single constituent of the body is water, which represents about 60% of the total body weight in the average adult, 45–55% of the older adult, 70–80% of a newborn infant, and 97% of the early human embryo.

 Label the following drawings with the proper percentage of water to body weight.

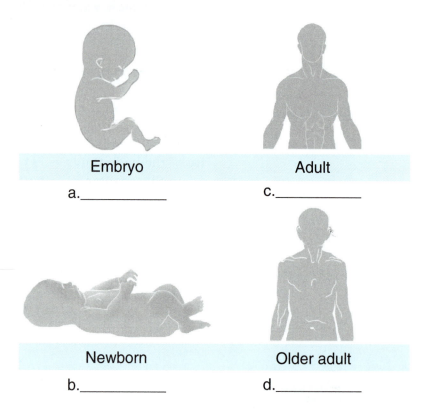

Embryo

a._____

Adult

c._____

Newborn

b._____

Older adult

d._____

1. a. 97%; b. 70–80%; c. 60%;
d. 45–55%

2.

Which has the highest percentage of water in relation to body weight (adult, newborn infant, embryo, older adult)? _____
Which has the lowest? _____

2. embryo, older adult

3. Infants have a larger body surface area in relation to their weight, so extra water may act as a cushion against injury.

4. person weighing 125 pounds (lean)

5. a. cell; b. tissue space; c. blood vessel

3.

Speculate why the early human embryo and the infant have a higher proportion of water to body weight than the adult.

*_____

_____

4.

The percentage of body water varies with the amount of body fat. Because body fat is essentially free of water, the leaner the individual, the greater the proportion of water in total body weight. Water is retained in muscle.

Who has more water as body weight, a person weighing 225 pounds or a lean person weighing 125 pounds? _____

● FLUID COMPARTMENTS

5.

Body water is distributed among three types of "compartments": cells, blood vessels, and tissue spaces between blood vessels and cells that are separated by membranes.

Label the three compartments where body water (fluid) is found.

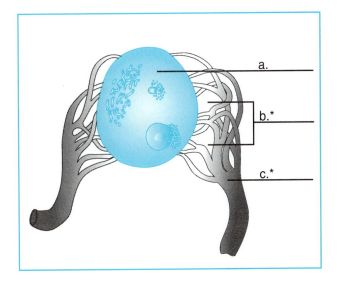

a.

b.*

c.*

6.

The term for the water (fluid) in each type of "compartment" is as follows:

    1. In the cell—*intracellular* fluid or *cellular* fluid

    2. In the blood vessels—*intravascular* fluid

    3. In tissue spaces between blood vessels and cells—*interstitial* fluid

Label the diagram with the proper terms for body water in each of the three compartments.

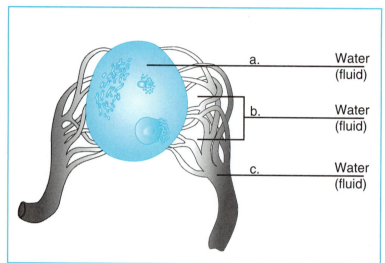

a. _____ Water (fluid)

b. _____ Water (fluid)

c. _____ Water (fluid)

6. a. intracellular or cellular
    b. interstitial;
    c. intravascular

7.

Fluid within the cell is classified as intracellular fluid, whereas intravascular fluid and interstitial fluid are classified as extracellular fluid.

    The area within the cell is called the _____ space, whereas the tissue spaces between blood vessels and cells and the area within blood vessels are known as the _____ space.

7. intracellular;
    extracellular

8.

Approximately two-thirds of the body fluid is contained in the intracellular compartment.

    We have already said that the total body weight in the adult body is _____ % water; therefore, intracellular fluid must represent _____ % of the total body weight, and extracellular fluid represents _____ % of the total body weight.

8. 60; 40; 20

9. interstitial fluid

9.

If one-fourth of the extracellular fluid is intravascular fluid, then three-fourths of extracellular fluid is *_____.

10.

Therefore, extracellular fluid represents _____ % of the total body weight. Interstitial fluid represents _____ % of total body weight and intravascular fluid represents _____ % of total body weight.

10. 20; 15; 5

● FUNCTIONS OF BODY WATER

The body is unable to maintain a healthy state without water. Five main functions of body water are listed in Table 1-1.

Table 1-1	Functions of Body Water
• Transportation of nutrients, electrolytes, and oxygen to the cells • Excretion of waste products • Regulation of body temperature • Lubrication of joints and membranes • Medium for food digestion	

11.

Name three of the five main functions of body water:

a. *_____

b. *_____

c. *_____

11. Select three from the five functions listed in Table 1-1.

● INTAKE AND OUTPUT FOR HOMEOSTASIS

12.

We already have learned that the percentage of body fluid varies with age and percentage of body fat. Then the proportion of intracellular and extracellular fluid in a person with more body fat would be (greater/lesser) _____ in proportion to body weight. (Refer to page 5, item 4.)

12. lesser

13. It maintains equilibrium to the physical and chemical properties of body fluid.

14. deficit

15. a. decrease; b. increasing

16. liquid, food, and oxidation of food

17. lungs, skin, urine, and feces

18. equilibrium or homeostasis

13.

Homeostasis is a term used to describe the state of equilibrium of the internal environment. In relation to body fluids, homeostasis is the process of maintaining equilibrium or stability in relation to the physical and chemical properties of body fluid.

   Explain the relationship of homeostasis to body fluid.

* _____

_____

14.

The body normally maintains a state of equilibrium between the amount of water taken in and the amount of water lost. The volume of body water is regulated primarily by the kidneys. When body water is insufficient and the kidneys are functioning normally, urine volume diminishes and the individual becomes thirsty. Therefore, the patient drinks more water to correct the fluid (excess/deficit) _____.

15.

When we drink an excessive amount of water, our urinary output increases.

   a. If you did not drink any fluids or if the body loses excessive water, the urinary volume should (increase/decrease) _____.

   b. If there were an excess of water in the body, the urinary volume would adapt by (increasing/decreasing) _____.

16.

The three normal sources of body water intake are *_____

_____.

Refer to Figure 1-1.

17.

The four avenues for daily water loss are *_____

_____.

Refer to Figure 1-1.

18.

If your water intake amounted to 2500 mL for the day and your water output was 2500 mL, your body has maintained a state of _____ of body fluid.

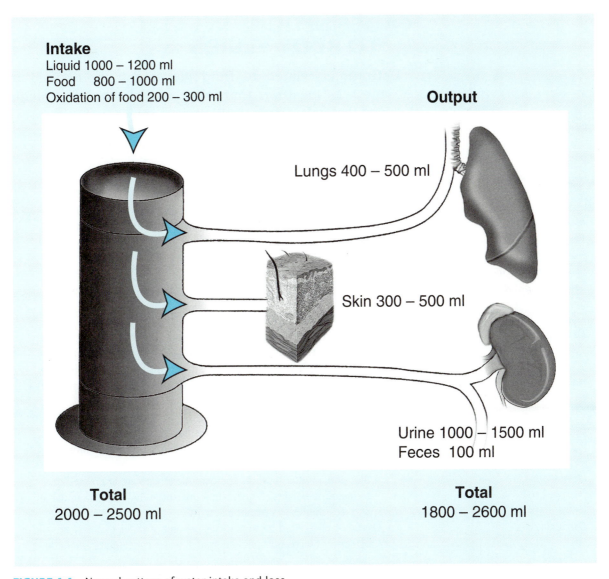

Intake
Liquid 1000 – 1200 ml
Food   800 – 1000 ml
Oxidation of food 200 – 300 ml

Output

Lungs 400 – 500 ml

Skin 300 – 500 ml

Urine 1000 – 1500 ml
Feces 100 ml

Total
2000 – 2500 ml

Total
1800 – 2600 ml

FIGURE 1-1   Normal pattern of water intake and loss.

19. When the summer atmospheric temperature is high, water loss via skin and lungs increases.

19.
Evaporation of water from the skin, as we perspire, is a protective mechanism against overheating the body. It acts as a cooling system, keeping the body at a normal temperature. The rate of water loss and gain is different in summer and winter. Describe why you think this occurs. *_____

DEFINITIONS RELATED TO BODY FLUIDS

Definitions related to fluid movement are defined in Table 1-2. Questions that follow explain the physiologic terms that affect body fluid movement.

Table 1-2	Definitions Related to Fluid Functions and Movement
Membrane	A layer of tissue covering a surface or organ or separating spaces
Permeability	The capability of a substance, molecule, or ion to diffuse through a membrane
Semipermeable membrane	An artificial membrane such as a cellophane membrane
Selectively permeable membrane	Permeability of the human membranes
Solvent	A liquid with a substance in solution
Solute	A substance dissolved in a solution
Osmosis	The passage of a solvent through a membrane from a solution of lesser solute concentration to one of greater solute concentration *Note*: Osmosis may be expressed in terms of water concentration instead of solute concentration. Water molecules pass from an area of higher water concentration (fewer solutes) to an area of lower water concentration
Diffusion	The movement of molecules such as gas from an area of higher concentration to an area of lesser concentration. Large molecules move less rapidly than small molecules
Osmol	A unit of osmotic pressure. The osmotic effects are expressed in terms of osmolality. A milliosmol (mOsm) is 1/1000th of an osmol and determines the osmotic activity
Osmolality	Osmotic pull exerted by all particles per unit of water, expressed as osmols or milliosmols per kilogram of water concentrate and body fluids
Osmolarity	Osmotic pull exerted by all particles per unit of solution, expressed as osmols or milliosmols per liter of solution
Ion	A particle carrying a positive or negative charge
Plasma	Blood minus the blood cells (composed mainly of water)
Serum	Plasma minus fibrogen (obtained after coagulation of blood)
Tonicity	The effect of fluid on cellular volume concentration of IV solution

20.

Diffusion is the movement of molecules/solutes across a selectively permeable membrane along its own pathway, irrespective of all other molecules. Large molecules move *less* rapidly than small molecules. Molecules move faster from an area of higher concentration to an area of lower concentration.

Diffusion is the *_____

across a selectively permeable membrane. Small molecules move (faster than/slower than) *_____ large molecules.

Molecules/solutes tend to move faster from *_____

_____ to *_____.

20. movement of molecules/solutes; faster than; an area of higher concentration; an area of lower concentration

21.

Body water loss by diffusion through the skin that is immeasurable and independent of sweat gland activity is called *insensible perspiration.*

When sweat gland activity occurs and water appears on the skin, this is called *sensible perspiration.*

In a relatively comfortable temperature would insensible perspiration or sensible perspiration occur? _____

Why? *_____

_____

21. insensible; Heat and activity cause sufficient sweat gland activity. With comfortable temperature, normal loss occurs through insensible perspiration; thus water diffuses via skin and evaporates quickly.

22.

Explain the difference between a solvent and a solute.

Solvent *_____

Solute *_____

22. a liquid with a substance in solution; a substance dissolved in solution

23.

In an effort to establish equilibrium, water in the body moves from a lesser solute concentration (fewer solute particles per unit of solvent) to a greater solute concentration (more solute particles per unit of solvent) through a *_____ membrane.

23. selectively permeable or human

24.

Osmotic pressure is the pressure or force that develops when two solutions of different strengths or concentrations are separated by a selectively permeable membrane.

To establish osmotic equilibrium, water moves from the (lesser/greater) _____ solute concentration to the (lesser/greater) _____ solute concentration.

24. lesser; greater; osmotic pressure

The force that draws water across a selectively permeable membrane is called *_____.

● FLUID PRESSURES (STARLING'S LAW)

25.

Extracellular fluid (ECF) shifts between the intravascular space (blood vessels) and the interstitial space (tissues) to maintain a fluid balance within the ECF compartment.

Four fluid pressures regulate the flow of fluid between the intravascular and interstitial spaces in order to maintain fluid homeostasis or equilibrium.

25. intravascular; interstitial; homeostasis or equilibrium

ECF flows back and forth between the _____ space and the _____ space to maintain _____.

26.

E. H. Starling formulated the Law of Capillaries, which states that equilibrium exists at the capillary membrane when the amount of fluid leaving circulation and the amount of fluid returning to circulation are exactly equal.

There are four measurable pressures that determine the flow of fluid between the intravascular and interstitial spaces. These are the colloid osmotic (oncotic) pressures and the hydrostatic pressures that occur in both the vessels and the tissue spaces.

26. capillary membrane

According to Starling, equilibrium exists at the *_____.

27.

Three new terms to define:

Colloid: a nondiffusible substance; a solute suspended in solution

Hydrostatic: pressure exerted by a stationary liquid

Oncotic pressure: osmotic pressure of a colloid (protein) in body fluid

28. the hydrostatic pressure; the colloid osmotic pressure (oncotic pressure)

28.

The measurable pressures influencing body fluid flow within the ECF compartment that are present in both the blood vessels and tissue fluid are *_____ and *_____.

29. capillary

30. artery; vein

31. venular end

32. 6 mm Hg

33. colloid osmotic pressure gradient; hydrostatic pressure gradient

29.

The colloid osmotic pressure and the hydrostatic pressure of the blood and tissues influence the movement of fluid through the _____ membrane.

30.

Do you know the meanings of the arterioles and venules? If not: *Arterioles:* minute arteries that lead into a capillary bed *Venules:* minute veins that lead from the capillary bed Which is larger, the arteriole or the artery? _____ The venule or the vein? _____

31.

Fluid exchange occurs only across the walls of capillaries and not across the walls of arterioles or venules. Therefore, fluid moves into the interstitial space at the arteriolar end of the capillary and out of the interstitial space into the capillary at the *_____ of the capillary.

32.

Fluid flows only when there is a difference in pressure at the two ends of the system. This difference in pressure between two points is known as the *pressure gradient.*

If the pressure at one end was 32 mm Hg (millimeters of mercury) and at the other end was 26 mm Hg, the pressure gradient is *_____.

33.

The plasma in the capillaries has hydrostatic pressure and colloid osmotic pressure. The tissue fluids have hydrostatic pressure and colloid osmotic pressure.

The difference in pressure between the plasma colloid osmotic pressure and the tissue colloid osmotic pressure is known as the *_____.

The difference in pressure between the plasma hydrostatic pressure and the tissue hydrostatic pressure is known as the *_____

It is this difference in pressure that makes the fluid flow between and among compartments.

34.

The plasma colloid osmotic pressure is 28 mm Hg and the tissue colloid osmotic pressure is 4 mm Hg. Refer to Figure 1-2. The colloid osmotic pressure gradient would be *_____.

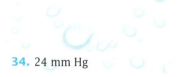

34. 24 mm Hg

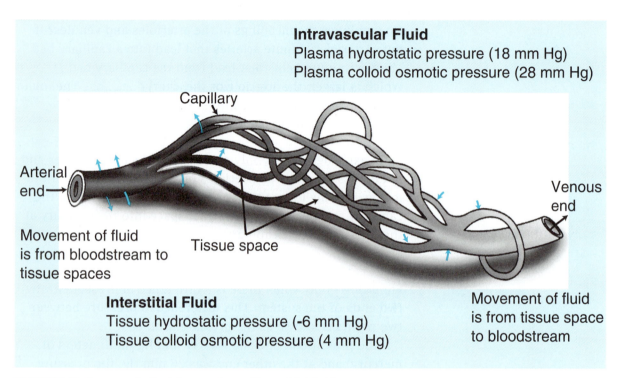

Intravascular Fluid
Plasma hydrostatic pressure (18 mm Hg)
Plasma colloid osmotic pressure (28 mm Hg)

Capillary

Arterial end→

Venous end

Movement of fluid is from bloodstream to tissue spaces

Tissue space

Interstitial Fluid
Tissue hydrostatic pressure (-6 mm Hg)
Tissue colloid osmotic pressure (4 mm Hg)

Movement of fluid is from tissue space to bloodstream

FIGURE 1-2 Pressures in the intravascular and interstitial fluids.

35.

The hydrostatic fluid pressure is 18 mm Hg in the capillary, and the hydrostatic tissue pressure is –6 mm Hg; therefore, the hydrostatic pressure gradient is *_____. Refer to Figure 1-2.

35. 24 mm Hg

36.

The hydrostatic pressure gradient across the capillary membrane (24 mm Hg) is equal to the colloid osmotic pressure gradient across the membrane (24 mm Hg). Thus, the two pressures are _____.

36. equal or same pressure

37. The plasma hydrostatic pressure is higher than the tissue pressure; plasma osmotic pressure is higher than tissue pressure.

38. is; Fluid stays in the tissues, causing accumulation and tissue swelling; insufficient

39. Starling; Plasma and tissue colloid osmotic and hydrostatic pressures regulate the flow of blood constituents between the interstitial and intravascular compartments.

40. Vulnerable to fluid loss (deficit) and dehydration

37.

The plasma hydrostatic pressure gradient tends to move fluid out of the capillary. Why? *_____ Refer to Figure 1-2 if reply is unknown.

The colloid osmotic pressure gradient tends to move fluid into the capillary. Why? *_____

38.

The balance between the two forces keeps the blood volume constant for circulation. In this way fluid does not accumulate in the intravascular or the interstitial compartments.

Without the colloid osmotic forces, fluid (is/is not) _____ lost from circulation. Explain. *_____

_____

The blood volume is (sufficient/insufficient) _____ to maintain circulation.

39.

Name the man who formulated the Law of Capillaries. _____ Define this law in your own words. *_____

_____

● REGULATORS OF FLUID BALANCE

40.

Thirst, electrolytes, protein and albumin, hormones, lymphatics, skin, and kidneys are the major regulators that maintain body fluid balance. Thirst alerts the person that there is a fluid loss, thus stimulating the person to increase his or her oral intake.

When there is a body fluid deficit, the thirst mechanism alerts the person that there is a fluid need.

The thirst mechanism in the medulla may not respond effectively to fluid loss in the older adult and young child. Therefore, these groups of individuals are *_____.

A discussion regarding regulators of fluid balance follows. Refer to Table 1-3.

Table 1-3	Regulators of Fluid Balance
Regulators	**Actions**
Thirst	An indicator of fluid need.
Electrolytes and Nonelectrolytes	
Sodium	Sodium promotes water retention. With a water deficit, less sodium is excreted via kidneys; thus more water is retained.
Protein, albumin	Protein and albumin promote body fluid retention. These nondiffusible substances increase the colloid osmotic (oncotic) pressure in favor of fluid retention.
Hormones and Enzymes	
Antidiuretic hormone (ADH)	ADH is produced by the hypothalamus and stored in the posterior pituitary gland (neurohypophysis). ADH is secreted when there is an ECF volume deficit or an increased osmolality (increased solutes). ADH promotes water reabsorption from the distal tubules of the kidneys.
Aldosterone	Aldosterone, a hormone, is secreted from the adrenal cortex. It promotes sodium, chloride, and water reabsorption from the renal tubules.
Renin	Decreased renal blood flow increases the release of renin, an enzyme, from the juxtaglomerular cells of the kidneys. Renin promotes peripheral vasoconstriction and the release of aldosterone (sodium and water retention).
Body Tissues and Organs	
Lymphatics	Plasma protein that shifts to the tissue spaces cannot be reabsorbed into the blood vessels. Thus, the lymphatic system promotes the return of water and protein from the interstitial spaces to the vascular spaces.
Skin	Skin excretes approximately 300–500 ml of water daily through normal perspiration.
Lungs	Lungs excrete approximately 400–500 ml of water daily through normal breathing.
Kidneys	The kidneys excrete 1000–1500 ml of body water daily. The amount of water excretion may vary according to the balance between fluid intake and fluid loss.

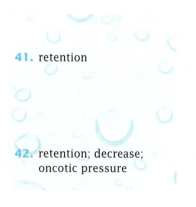

41. retention

42. retention; decrease;
oncotic pressure

41.
The electrolyte, sodium, promotes the (retention/excretion) _____ of body water.

42.
Protein and albumin help in promoting the (retention/excretion) _____ of body fluid (water). A decrease in protein can (increase/decrease) _____ the colloid osmotic pressure. Another name for colloid osmotic pressure is *_____.

43. ADH (antidiuretic hormone); aldosterone

44. An increased excretion of water from the kidney tubules.

45. It absorbs water from the kidney tubules; to dilute the solute

46. ADH; a. ADH would not be released; b. More water would be excreted from the body.

47. It becomes diluted; reduces

48. By drinking water or other liquids when thirsty.

43.

The two major hormones that influence fluid balance are _____ and _____.

44.

The antidiuretic hormone (ADH), increases the permeability of the cells of the kidney tubules to water, thus allowing more water to be reabsorbed. With a decrease in the production of ADH, what would occur? *_____

_____

45.

The posterior pituitary gland is influenced by the solute (sodium, protein, glucose) concentration of the plasma. If there is an increase in the amount of solute in the plasma, the posterior pituitary gland releases the hormone, ADH, which holds water in the body.
Explain how. *_____

    For what reason should there be more water? *_____

_____

46.

A small increase of solute concentration in the plasma above the normal amount is sufficient to stimulate the posterior pituitary gland to release _____.

    Name two things that occur when there is less solute concentration in the plasma.

    a. *_____

    b. *_____

47.

When you drink a lot of fluids, what happens to the solute concentration of your plasma? *_____

    The posterior pituitary then (releases/reduces) _____ ADH.

48.

When the solute concentration increases, the thirst mechanism is stimulated and the individual ingests water.

    Based on the above statement how can homeostasis be maintained? *_____

_____

49.

Aldosterone promotes (water/sodium) _____ retention.
   An increase in aldosterone release can be due to fluid
volume (loss/excess) _____ and stress.

49. sodium; loss

50.

An ECF deficit causes the release of two (2) hormones called
*_____.

50. ADH and aldosterone

51.

Increased renin (enzyme) secretion is a response to *_____
_____.
   How does renin affect fluid balance? *_____
_____

51. decreased renal blood
flow; It promotes
aldosterone secretion.

52.

The response of the lymphatic system to the maintenance of
fluid balance is *_____
_____.

52. to promote the return of
ECF and protein from the
interstitial to the
vascular spaces

● OSMOLALITY

53.

Osmolality is determined by the number of dissolved particles
(sodium, urea (BUN), and glucose) per kilogram of water.
Sodium is the largest contributor of particles to osmolality.
BUN is the final product of protein metabolism excreted in the
kidney, the other two major particle groups that contribute to
osmolality are *_____
_____.
   These dissolved particles exert an osmotic pull or pressure.

53. urea and glucose

54.

An *osmol* is a unit of osmotic pressure. The osmotic effects
are expressed in terms of osmolality. A *milliosmol* (mOsm) is
1/1000th of an osmol and will determine the osmotic activity.
Refer to Table 1-2 for definitions of osmol and osmolality. The
basic unit used to express the force exerted by the
concentration of solute or dissolved particles is a(n) _____.

The osmotic effect of a solute concentration in water is expressed as _____, a property that depends on the number of osmols or milliosmols contained in a solution.

54. osmol; osmolality

55.
Osmolality of fluid may be determined in serum and intravenous solutions. In serum, sodium, urea (BUN), and glucose are the most plentiful solutes and are the major contributors of serum osmolality. Sodium is most abundant in (extracellular/intracellular) _____ fluid and is available with most laboratory test results.

55. extracellular

56.
The normal serum osmolality range is 280–295 mOsm/kg (milliosmols per kilogram). A serum osmolality of 288 mOsm/kg would represent (hypo/iso/hyper) _____ osmolality.

56. iso-osmolality

57.
Match the serum osmolality concentrations on the left with the type of osmolality:

_____ 1. 299 mOsm/kg   a. Hypo-osmolality
_____ 2. 292 mOsm/kg   b. Iso-osmolality
_____ 3. 274 mOsm/kg   c. Hyperosmolality
_____ 4. 305 mOsm/kg
_____ 5. 269 mOsm/kg

57. 1. c; 2. b; 3. a; 4. c; 5. a

58.
The terms *osmolality* and *tonicity* have been used interchangeably; though similar, they are different. Osmolality is the concentration of body fluids and tonicity is often associated with the concentration of IV solutions. Increased osmolality (hyperosmolality) can result in impermeable solutes such as sodium and from permeant solutes such as urea (blood urea nitrogen). Hypertonicity results from an increase of impermeant solutes such as sodium but *not* of permeant solutes such as urea (BUN).
    A high sodium level can cause (hypertonicity/hyperosmolality) _____. High BUN and sodium levels can cause (hypertonicity/hyperosmolality/both) _____.

58. hypertonicity; hyperosmolality

59.

The osmolality of an intravenous solution can be hypo-osmolar or hypotonic, iso-osmolar or isotonic, and hyperosmolar or hypertonic. The osmolality of the intravenous (IV) solution is determined by the average serum osmolality, which is 240–340 mOsm/L. The normal range for the osmolality of a solution is +50 mOsm or –50 mOsm of 290 mOsm.

The concentration of IV solutions is referred to as hypotonic, isotonic, and hypertonic.

The average osmolality of IV solution is 240 to _____ mOsm/L.

59. 340

60.

Plasma (from vascular fluid) is considered to be a(n) (hypo-osmolar/iso-osmolar/hyperosmolar) _____ fluid.

The osmolality of solutions is compared to *_____.

60. iso-osmolar; plasma osmolality or serum osmolality

61.

Match the types of solutions on the left with their solute concentrations:

_____ 1. Isotonic   a. Higher solute concentration than plasma

_____ 2. Hypotonic   b. Same solute concentration as plasma

_____ 3. Hypertonic   c. Lower solute concentration than plasma

61. 1. b; 2. c; 3. a

62.

An IV solution having less than 240 mOsm is considered _____, and a solution having more than 340 mOsm is considered _____.

62. hypotonic; hypertonic

63.

The following is a list of milliosmol values of IV fluids (solution). Classify them as isotonic, hypotonic, or hypertonic.

Milliosmol Values (mOsm)	Type of Osmolality
220	_____
75	_____
350	_____
310	_____
560	_____

63. hypotonic; hypotonic; hypertonic; isotonic; hypertonic

64.

64. osmosis; Cells shrink and become smaller in size; dehydration

Extracellular hyperosmolar fluid has a greater osmotic pressure than the cell; thus, intracellular water moves out of the cells and into the extracellular hyperosmolar (hypertonic) fluid by the process of _____.

　　When cells lose water, what happens to their form and size? *_____. Cellular (hydration/dehydration) _____ results.

65.

65. plasma; isotonic

A liter of 5% dextrose in water (D_5W) is 250 mOsm, and a liter of 0.9% sodium chloride or normal saline is 310 mOsm, having somewhat the same osmotic pressure as _____.

　　These solutions are (isotonic/hypotonic/hypertonic) _____.

66.

66. 560; hypertonic

The sum of 5% dextrose in normal saline equals _____ mOsm. This solution is a(n) _____ solution.

● MILLIGRAMS VERSUS MILLIEQUIVALENTS

67.

67. osmotic; *Milligrams:* the weight of ions.; *Milliequivalents:* the chemical activity of ions.

In studying serum chemistry alterations and concentrations, one is concerned with how much the ions or chemical particles weigh. The weight of ions and chemical particles is measured in milligrams percent (mg%), which is the same as mg/100 ml or milligrams per deciliter (mg/dl). The number of electrically charged ions is measured in milliequivalents per liter (1000 ml), or mEq/L.

　　The term *milliequivalent* involves the chemical activity of elements, whereas milliosmol involves the _____ activity of the solution.

　　How do milligrams and milliequivalents differ? *_____

68.

Milliequivalents provide a better method of measuring the concentration of ions in the serum than milligrams.

68. weight

69. 15 females and 15 males; Otherwise, you would have an unequal number of males and females, for not every individual weighs exactly 100 pounds.

70. milliequivalents

Milligrams measure the _____ of ions and give no information concerning the number of ions or the electrical charges of the ions.

69.

The following is a simple analogy to compare milligrams and milliequivalents.

If you were having a party and wanted to invite equal numbers of males and females, which would be more accurate—inviting 1500 pounds of females and 1500 pounds of males or inviting 15 females and 15 males? *_____.
Why? *_____

_____.

70.

From the example in question 69, which would be more accurate in determining the serum chemistry of chemical particles or ions in the body—milliequivalents or milligrams? _____.

You will find both measurements used in this book and in your clinical settings for determining changes in our serum chemistry. Therefore, when referring to ions, milliequivalents will be used in this book. The mEq is the most commonly used unit of measure for electrolytes in the United States.

● CLINICAL APPLICATIONS

71.

There are several diseases that affect the plasma colloid osmotic pressure due to the loss of serum protein.

Memorize these five important definitions:

Protein: a nitrogenous compound, essential to all living organisms
Plasma protein: relates to albumin, globulin, and fibrinogen
Serum protein: relates to albumin and globulin
Serum albumin: a simple protein; constitutes about 50% of the blood protein
Serum globulin: a group of simple protein

Patients with diagnoses of kidney and liver diseases or malnutrition lose serum protein. What are the two groups of simple proteins found in the serum?

*_____

71. albumin and globulin

72.

The main function of serum albumin is to maintain the colloid osmotic pressure of blood.

Without colloid osmotic pressure, what would happen to the fluid in the tissues? *_____

_____

72. Fluid would accumulate in the tissues (interstitial spaces) and swelling would occur. This is known as edema.

73. Possible answers include:
a. Report abnormal serum laboratory findings immediately.;
b. Observe and report physical findings of swelling or edema.;
c. Keep an accurate record of fluid intake and output.

73.

Identify three nursing responsibilities you think are important when caring for patients with diseases that cause abnormal serum albumin and serum globulin levels.

a. *_____

b. *_____

c. *_____

74.

Edema, or swelling, occurs when there is fluid retention. Dehydration occurs with excess fluid removal or loss.

If the osmolality of intravascular fluid is greater than the osmolality of intracellular fluid, the cells would (lose/gain) _____ water.

(Edema/Dehydration) _____ would occur to the cells.

74. lose; Dehydration

75.

With any internal venous obstruction, such as inflammation, there is an increased venous hydrostatic pressure. This in turn inhibits the fluid moving out of the tissues, causing the tissues to *_____

_____.

75. retain/accumulate fluid and swell (edema)

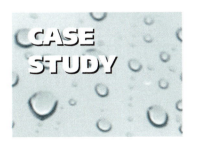

CASE STUDY

REVIEW

A young male had been vomiting for several days. His urine output decreased. He was given 1 liter of 5% dextrose in water and then 1 liter of 5% dextrose in normal saline (0.9% NaCl).

ANSWER COLUMN

1. 60; 40; 20

2. He is losing body fluid from vomiting and a lack of fluid intake.

3. liquid, food, and oxidation of food; lungs, skin, urine, and feces

4. more

5. isotonic

6. hypotonic

7. 240–340; hypotonic

8. hypotonic

1. In his adult stage, his body water represents ——— % of his total body weight. What percentage of his total body weight is in the intracellular compartment? ——— % What percent of water is in the extracellular compartment? ——— %

2. Explain why his urine output is decreased. *——————
——————————————————

3. The three primary sources for water intake are *———
——————————————————.
The four primary mechanisms for daily water loss (output) are *——————————————————
——————————————————.

4. Vomiting caused the patient to lose body fluids and caused a decrease in urine output. The solute concentration was increased. As a result of an increased solute concentration, the posterior pituitary gland releases (more/less) ——— ADH.

5. The patient received 1 liter of 5% dextrose in water, which has a similar osmolality as plasma. When administering D_5W, dextrose is metabolized quickly, leaving water. A solution with osmolality similar to that of plasma is considered to be (an isotonic/hypotonic/hypertonic) ———.

6. The second liter he received was 5% dextrose in normal saline. This solution is a(n) ——— solution.

7. The normal range of osmolality of plasma is ——— mOsm. A solution with less than 240 mOsm is considered ———.

8. One-half of normal saline (0.45% NaCl) solution has 155 mOsm/L. What is this type of solution? ———.
The patient developed edema of the lower extremities. Laboratory results revealed a lower than normal serum protein.

9. Starling's Law of Capillaries

10. a. difference in pressure between two points in a fluid; b. nondiffusible substances; c. simple protein

11. tissues

12. protein and albumin

13. a. capillaries; surrounding tissues (interstitial spaces); b. tissues; capillary

14. edema

15. Fluid accumulates in the tissue, causing swelling (edema).

9. Factors regulating the movement of body constituents between the interstitial and intravascular compartments are stated by *_____.

10. Define the following four terms.
a. *Pressure gradient* *_____
b. *Colloids* *_____
c. *Albumin* *_____

11. Pressure gradients are responsible for the exchange of fluid between the capillaries and the _____.

12. The amount of colloid osmotic pressure that develops depends on the concentration of nondiffusible substances such as *_____.

13. The direction of the movement of fluid depends on the results of the opposing forces.
a. The hydrostatic pressure is greater than the colloid osmotic pressure at the arterial end of the capillary; thus the fluid moves out of the _____ and into the *_____.
b. The osmotic pressure is greater than the hydrostatic pressure at the venous end of the capillary; thus the fluid moves out of the _____ and reenters the _____.

14. The decrease in his serum protein level could account for his (edema/dehydration) _____.

15. He has a venous obstruction due to varicosities. This causes an increase in venous hydrostatic pressure, preventing fluid from moving out of tissues and into the circulation. Explain what happens to the fluid. *_____
_____

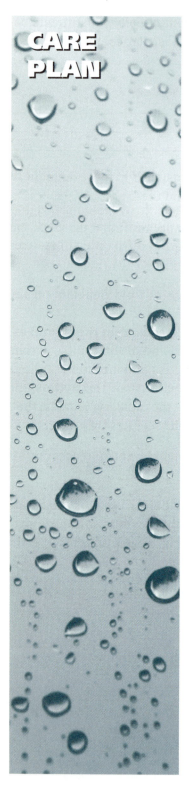

CARE PLAN

PATIENT MANAGEMENT: DEFICIENT FLUID VOLUME AND EXCESS FLUID VOLUME

Assessment Factors

● Assess the intake and output status of the patient. Fluid intake and urine output are normally in proportion to each other.

● Recognize that infants and lean individuals have a higher proportion of body water than other adults, older adults, and people with increased body fat.

● Assess excess fluid loss from the skin and lungs. Diaphoresis (excess sweating) and tachypnea (rapid breathing) cause excess body water loss through the skin and lungs.

● Obtain baseline vital signs. Baseline vital signs are used for comparison with subsequent vital signs.

● Assess for fluid balance by checking the patient's serum osmolality with the laboratory test results. A serum osmolality >295 mOsm/kg can indicate hemoconcentration due to fluid loss. A serum osmolality <280 mOsm/kg can indicate hemodilution due to fluid excess.

Nursing Diagnosis

● Deficient fluid volume related to body fluid imbalance.
● Excess fluid volume related to body fluid imbalance.

Interventions and Rationale

1. Monitor vital signs. Report abnormal vital signs or significant changes from baseline measurements.

2. Monitor intake and output. Report urine output of less than 600 ml/day and less than 30 ml/hr.

3. Monitor weight daily. Note any changes.

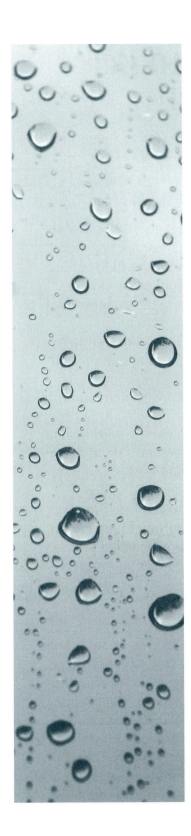

4. Check the osmolality of IV solutions daily. Know that IV solutions with osmolality between 240 and 340 mOsm/L are isotonic and are similar to plasma. Remember that a solution of 5% dextrose in water is 250 mOsm and a normal saline solution (0.9% sodium chloride) is 310 mOsm; both are isotonic solutions. Continuous use of hypotonic (0.45% sodium chloride) and hypertonic (10% dextrose in water, $D_{10}W$): IV solutions may cause a fluid imbalance. However, remember that dextrose is metabolized rapidly; with D_5W, the solution eventually becomes hypotonic. D_5/NSS (normal saline solution) is hypertonic but becomes isotonic after dextrose is metabolized. With the continuous use of dextrose in normal saline solutions, hyperosmolality occurs.

5. Monitor the fluid status of the patient: check laboratory studies to determine the serum osmolality.

6. Monitor the serum albumin and serum protein levels of patients with malnutrition, liver disease (such as cirrhosis of the liver), and kidney disease. Low serum albumin and serum protein levels decrease the colloid osmotic (oncotic) pressure; thus fluid remains in the tissue spaces (edema). While diuretics are helpful in decreasing edema, they can also markedly decrease the circulating fluid volume.

Evaluation/Outcome

1. Maintain intake and output approximately equal to one another.

2. Determine that the serum osmolality level has remained within normal range.

3. Evaluate daily the types of intravenous solutions prescribed to ensure that these solutions are within a normotonicity.

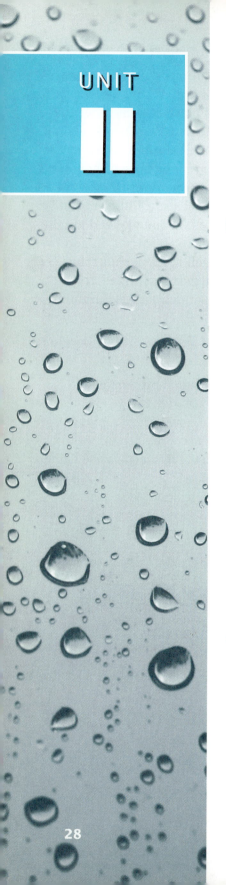

FLUIDS AND THEIR INFLUENCE ON THE BODY

LEARNING OUTCOMES

Upon completion of this unit, the reader will be able to:
- Describe the physiologic factors leading to extracellular fluid volume deficit, extracellular fluid volume excess, and intracellular fluid volume excess.
- State the difference between a hyperosmolar fluid deficit and an iso-osmolar fluid deficit.
- Compare the extracellular fluid volume shift in hypovolemia with the extracellular fluid volume shift in hypervolemia.
- Identify assessments associated with dehydration, edema, and water intoxication.
- Develop selected nursing diagnoses appropriate for patients with clinical manifestations of extracellular fluid volume deficits and excess and intracellular fluid volume excess.
- Identify selected interventions to alleviate the symptoms of dehydration, edema, and water intoxication.
- Identify selected outcomes appropriate to the management of dehydration, edema, and water intoxication.

INTRODUCTION

Many disease entities have some degree of fluid and electrolyte imbalance. Much of the imbalance is the result of fluid loss, fluid excess, and/or fluid volume shift. Four major fluid imbalances—extracellular fluid volume deficit (ECFVD), extracellular fluid volume excess (ECFVE), extracellular fluid volume shift (ECFVS), and intracellular fluid volume excess (ICFVE)—are discussed in four separate chapters with regard to pathophysiology, etiology, clinical manifestations (signs and symptoms), clinical applications, clinical management, and clinical consideration. Assessment factors, nursing diagnoses, interventions, and evaluations are listed along with the case reviews related to patients with fluid imbalances.

The health care provider computes and orders fluid replacement; however, the nurse should understand reasons for various types of fluid imbalances and should assess physical changes that may occur before and during clinical management. Refer to Chapter 1 for background information related to body fluids and their concentration and function.

An asterisk (*) on an answer line indicates a multiple-word answer. The meanings for the following symbols are: ↑ increased, ↓ decreased, > greater than, and < less than.

Table U2-1 Clinical Problems Associated with Fluid Imbalances

Clinical Problems	ECFVD	ECFVE	ECFVS	ICFVE
Gastrointestinal				
Vomiting and diarrhea	+			
GI fistula	+			
GI suctioning	+			
Increased salt intake	+			
Intestinal obstruction	+		+	
Perforated ulcer	+		+	
Excessive hypotonic fluids oral and intravenous				+
Renal				
Renal failure		+		
Renal disease		+		
Cardiac				
Heart failure		+		
Miscellaneous				
Brain tumor/injury				+
Fever	+			
Profused diaphoresis	+			
SIADH (syndrome of inappropriate antidiuretic hormone)		Initially +		+
Burns	+	+	+	
Diabetic ketoacidosis	+			
Ascites (cirrhosis)		+	+	
Venous obstruction		+		
Sprain			+	
Massive trauma	+		+	
Drugs				
Cortisone group of drugs		+		

Extracellular Fluid Volume Deficit (ECFVD)

🔵 INTRODUCTION

Extracellular fluid volume deficit (ECFVD) is a loss of body fluid from the interstitial (tissue) and intravascular (vascular-vessel) spaces. With a severe ECF loss and an increase in serum osmolality (more solutes than water), there is an intracellular (cellular-cells) fluid loss. If the loss of water and loss of solutes are equal, then intracellular fluid loss is unlikely to occur.

Dehydration means a lack of water. Dehydration may occur due to ECF loss. It may also result from a decrease in fluid intake. The term fluid volume deficit should not be used interchangeably with the term dehydration.

ANSWER COLUMN

1. interstitial and
intravascular

2. may not

3. intracellular or cellular

4. loss of body water; ECF
loss

5. 280–295 mOsm/kg
(milliosmols per
kilogram)

6. less; hypo-osmolar or
hypotonic

7. more; hyperosmolar or
hypertonic

1.

As discussed in Chapter 1, extracellular fluid (ECF) represents
20% of total body weight. One-fourth of this extracellular fluid
is intravascular fluid and three-fourths is interstitial fluid.
Extracellular fluid loss results primarily from the loss of body
fluid in the _____ and _____ spaces.

2.

Severe loss of ECF (may/may not) _____ cause
fluid loss from the cells.

3.

An increase in osmolality (more solutes than water) along with
a severe loss of ECF, results in _____ fluid loss.

4.

Dehydration is another name used to describe *_____.
Dehydration may be due to *_____.

● **PATHOPHYSIOLOGY**

5.

The concentration of body fluids or plasma/serum osmolality
is determined by the number of particles or solutes in relation
to the volume of body water (refer to Chapter 1 for a
description of osmolality).

   The normal range of plasma/serum osmolality is *_____
_____

6.

If the serum osmolality is less than 280 mOsm/kg, there are
(more/less) _____ solutes/particles in proportion
to the volume of body water. This body fluid is described as
(hypo-osmolar/iso-osmolar/hyperosmolar) _____.

7.

If the serum osmolality is greater than 295 mOsm/kg, there are
(more/less) _____ solutes in proportion to body
water; the fluid imbalance is known as _____.

8.

8. iso-osmolar or isotonic

A loss of the electrolyte sodium is usually accompanied by a simultaneous fluid loss. With a loss of sodium, ECF is usually decreased or moves from the ECF to the ICF (intracellular fluid) compartment.

When fluid and sodium are lost in equal amounts, the type of fluid deficit (FVD) that usually occurs is (iso-osmolar/hyperosmolar) _____.

9.

When the amount of water lost is in excess of the amount of sodium lost, the serum sodium level is (elevated/decreased) _____.

9. elevated; hyperosmolar

This type of fluid deficit is called (hypo-osmolar/iso-osmolar/hyperosmolar) _____ fluid volume deficit.

10.

Plasma/serum osmolality increases with the retention of sodium or the loss of water. This causes water to be drawn from the cells. With the elevation of serum sodium, the ECF becomes (hyperosmolar/hypo-osmolar) _____, which results in a(an) (increase/decrease) _____ in plasma/serum osmolality. This change in serum osmolality causes a withdrawal of fluid from the _____ compartment.

10. hyperosmolar; increase; cell or intracellular

11.

Hyperosmolar ECF causes intracellular (dehydration/hydration) _____.

Explain. *_____

11. dehydration; The hyperosmolar ECF pulls ICF from the cells by osmosis.

12.

With an iso-osmolar fluid volume loss, the loss of water and solute is (equal/varied) _____. The plasma/serum osmolality is (increased/decreased/unchanged) _____.

12. equal; unchanged

13.

An iso-osmolar fluid volume loss is not classified as dehydration, although dehydration can occur with this type of fluid loss.

A hyperosmolar fluid volume loss is referred to as _____. Explain.

*_____

13. dehydration; Moderate to severe fluid volume losses can cause symptoms of dehydration.

14.

Compensatory mechanisms such as an increased heart rate and blood pressure attempt to maintain the fluid volume necessary for vital organs to receive adequate perfusion.

When more than one-third of the body fluid is lost, what might occur? * _____

_____

14. Vascular collapse or shock or inadequate organ perfusion.

● ETIOLOGY

The causes of hyperosmolar and iso-osmolar fluid volume deficits differ. Both types of fluid volume deficits (FVD) may be caused by vomiting and diarrhea; however, in most cases, the severity of vomiting and diarrhea indicates the type of ECFVDs. Table 2-1 discusses the types and causes with rationale for ECFVDs. Refer to Table 2-1 as needed.

15.

Usually with severe vomiting and diarrhea, the loss of water is greater than the loss of sodium. This type of fluid loss causes
* _____.

15. hyperosmolar fluid volume deficit

16.

With "equal" proportional loss of fluid and solutes due to mild or moderate vomiting or diarrhea, what type of fluid volume deficit might occur? _____

With severe body fluid and solute loss due to severe vomiting and/or diarrhea, what type of fluid volume deficit might occur? _____

16. iso-osmolar; hyperosmolar

17.

Match the type of ECFVD with its possible cause. (See Table 2-1)
   a. iso-osmolar fluid volume deficit
   b. hyperosmolar fluid volume deficit
   _____ 1. Hemorrhage
   _____ 2. Diabetic ketoacidosis
   _____ 3. Increased salt and protein intake
   _____ 4. Burns
   _____ 5. GI suctioning
   _____ 6. Inadequate fluid intake
   _____ 7. Profuse diaphoresis and/or fever

17. 1. a; 2. b; 3. b; 4. a; 5. a; 6. b; 7. a

Table 2-1	Causes of Extracellular Fluid Volume Deficits
Types and Causes	**Rationale**
Hyperosmolar Fluid Volume Deficit	
Inadequate fluid intake	A decrease in water intake results in an increase in the number of solutes in body fluid. The body fluid becomes hyperosmolar.
Increased solute intake (salt, sugar, protein)	An increase in solute intake increases the solute concentration in body fluid; the body fluids can become hyperosmolar with a normal or decreased fluid intake.
Severe vomiting and diarrhea	Results in a loss of body water greater than the loss of solutes such as electrolytes, resulting in hyperosmolar body fluid.
Diabetes ketoacidosis	An increase in glucose and ketone bodies can result in body fluids becoming more hyperosmolar, thus causing diuresis. The resulting fluid loss is greater than the solute loss (sugar and ketones).
Sweating	Water loss is usually greater than sodium loss.
Iso-osmolar Fluid Volume Deficit	
Vomiting and diarrhea	Usually result in fluid losses that are in proportion to electrolyte (sodium, potassium, chloride, bicarbonate) losses.
Gastrointestinal (GI) fistula or draining abscess and GI suctioning	The GI tract is rich in electrolytes. With a loss of GI secretions, fluid and electrolytes are lost in somewhat equal proportions.
Fever, environmental temperature, and profuse diaphoresis	Results in fluid and sodium losses via the skin. With profuse sweating, the sodium is usually lost in proportions equal to water losses. Depending upon the severity of the sweating and fever, symptoms of mild, moderate, or marked fluid loss may be observed.
Hemorrhage	Excess blood loss is fluid and solute loss from the vascular fluid. If hemorrhage occurs rapidly, fluid shifts to compensate for blood losses can be inadequate.
Burns	Burns cause body fluid with solutes to shift from the vascular fluid to the burned site and surrounding interstitial space (tissues). This may result in an inadequate circulating fluid volume.
Ascites	Fluid and solutes (protein, electrolytes, etc.) shift to the peritoneal space, causing ascites (third-space fluid). A decrease in circulating fluid volume may result.
Intestinal obstruction	Fluid accumulates at the intestinal obstruction site (third-space fluid), thus decreasing the vascular fluid volume.

18.

Indicate which situations are representative of iso-osmolar or hyperosmolar fluid volume deficits.

    a. Iso-osmolar

    b. Hyperosmolar

_____ 1. There is a proportional loss of both body fluids and solutes.

_____ 2. The loss of body fluids is greater than the loss of solutes.

_____ 3. A serum osmolality of 282 mOsm/kg occurring with ECFVD may indicate which type of fluid loss?

_____ 4. A serum osmolality of 305 mOsm/kg occurring with ECFVD may indicate which type of fluid loss?

18. 1. a; 2. b; 3. a; 4. b

● CLINICAL MANIFESTATIONS

The clinical manifestations (signs and symptoms) of dehydration are listed in Table 2-2. The table describes the degrees of ECF loss, percentage of body weight loss, symptoms, and body water deficit by liter for a man weighing 150 pounds.

    Study Table 2-2 carefully; be able to name the degrees of dehydration, the symptoms, the percentage of body weight loss, and an estimation of body fluid loss in liters. Hopefully, you will be able to recognize and identify degrees of dehydration that can occur to patients during your clinical experience. Refer back to Table 2-2 as you find necessary.

19.

Thirst is a symptom that occurs with mild, marked, and severe fluid loss. Lack of water intake is usually the contributing cause of mild dehydration.

    How can mild dehydration be corrected? * _____

_____

19. By increasing water (fluid) intake.

20.

With mild dehydration, the percentage of body weight loss is _____ %, which is equivalent to _____ liter(s) of body fluid loss.

20. 2; 1–2

Table 2-2		Degrees of Dehydration	
Degrees of Dehydration	**Percentage of Body Weight Loss (%)**	**Symptoms**	**Body Water Deficit by Liter**
Mild dehydration	2	1. Thirst	1–2
Marked dehydration	5	1. Marked thirst	3–5
		2. Dry mucous membranes	
		3. Dryness and wrinkling of skin— poor skin turgor	
		4. Hand veins: slow filling with hand lowered	
		5. Temperature—low-grade elevation, e.g., 99°F (37.2°C)	
		6. Tachycardia (pulse greater than 100) as blood volume drops	
		7. Respiration >28	
		8. Systolic BP 10–15 mm Hg ↓ in standing position	
		9. Urine volume <30 ml/hr	
		10. Specific gravity >1.025	
		11. Body weight loss	
		12. Hct ↑, Hgb ↑, BUN ↑	
		13. Acid-base equilibrium toward greater acidity	
Severe dehydration	8	1. Same symptoms as marked dehydration, plus:	5–10
		2. Flushed skin	
		3. Systolic BP <60 mm Hg	
		4. Behavioral changes, e.g., restlessness, irritability, disorientation, and delirium	
Fatal dehydration	20–30 total body water loss can prove fatal	1. Anuria	
		2. Coma leading to death	

Abbreviations: BP, blood pressure; Hg, mercury; Hct, hematocrit; Hgb, hemoglobin; BUN, blood urea nitrogen.

21. dehydrated or mildly dehydrated

21.

In the older adult, the thirst mechanism in the medulla does not alert the older adult that there is a water deficit. Therefore, the older adult may become *_____ without experiencing the symptom of thirst.

22.

Common symptoms of marked ECF loss include decreased skin turgor, dry mucous membranes, increased pulse rate, weight loss, and decreased urine output.

What percentage of weight loss is associated with marked dehydration? _____. This weight loss is equivalent to _____ liter(s) of body water loss.

22. 5%; 3–5

23.

The percentage of body weight loss is a guide for *_____ _____ therapy.

23. replacement fluid or intravenous (IV) fluid

24.

With marked and severe body fluid loss, the hematocrit, hemoglobin, and BUN (blood urea nitrogen — a byproduct of protein metabolism) may be (increased/decreased) _____. Why? *_____ _____

24. increased; Because of the increased number of solutes such as BUN and red blood cells or hemoconcentration.

25.

The red blood cell count, hemoglobin, hematocrit, and plasma/serum protein may be elevated as a result of hemoconcentration (increased blood cells and decreased vascular fluid).

Hemoconcentration occurs with dehydration. Why? *_____ _____

25. With body fluid loss, red blood cell count is increased, along with other solutes.

26.

With marked dehydration, increased urine concentration usually results. The specific gravity (SpGr) may be (increased/decreased)_____, such as SpGr (<1.010/>1.025) _____. The urine output is (increased/decreased) _____.

26. increased; >1.025; decreased

27.

Indicate which symptoms are associated with *severe* dehydration.

( ) a. Bradycardia

( ) b. Tachycardia as blood volume drops

( ) c. Temperature 99.6°F

( ) d. Urine volume is increased

( ) e. Specific gravity of urine of 1.025 and higher

( ) f. Skin flushed

( ) g. Irritability

( ) h. Restlessness and disorientation

( ) i. Specific gravity of urine lower than 1.010

( ) j. Marked thirst

What percentage of fluid loss is associated with severe dehydration? _____

27. b, c, e, f, g, h, j; 8%

● CLINICAL APPLICATIONS

28.

During early dehydration, the serum osmolality may not show any significant changes. As dehydration continues, fluid is lost in greater quantities from the extracellular space than from the intracellular fluid (ICF) space. This results in an ECF (excess/deficit) _____.

28. deficit

29.

When dehydration is severe, the serum osmolality increases, causing water to leave the cells.

A severe ECF deficit can lead to an ICF (excess/deficit) _____.

29. deficit

30.

When there is a marked or severe fluid volume loss, hypovoemia occurs. The prefix *hypo* indicates *_____. Volemia comes from the Latin word *volumen,* meaning "volume."

Hypovolemia is a diminished volume of circulating blood or vascular fluid. It is frequently referred to as a decrease in blood volume.

30. loss, less, deficit, or diminished

31.

The health professional can make a quick assessment of dehydration, or hypovolemia, by checking the peripheral veins in the hand. First hold the hand above heart level for a short time and then lower the hand below heart level. The peripheral veins in the hand below heart level should be engorged (swollen with fluids) within 5–10 seconds with a normal blood volume and circulating blood flow.

If the peripheral veins do not engorge in 10 seconds, this may be indicative of _____ _____.

31. dehydration or hypovolemia (low blood volume)

32.

Body weight is an important tool for assessing fluid imbalance. Two and two-tenths (2.2) pounds of body weight loss or gain is equivalent to 1 liter of water loss or gain.

Intake and output give the approximate amount of body fluid intake and output. What provides the more accurate assessment of fluid balance (body weight, intake and output balance)? *_____

32. body weight

33.

Vital signs provide another tool for assessing hypovolemia or loss of body fluid. With fluid loss due to dehydration, what physiologic symptoms occur with the following vital measurements?
Temperature *_____
Pulse *_____
Respirations *_____
Blood pressure *_____
Urine volume *_____

33. temperature: low-grade elevation; pulse: tachycardia (rate over 100); respirations: increased; systolic blood pressure: <10–15 mm Hg (standing position); urine volume: decreased or small amount and highly concentrated; (Kidney damage can occur if the systolic blood pressure is less than 60 for several hours.)

● **CLINICAL MANAGEMENT**

In replacing body water loss, the total fluid deficit is estimated according to the percentage of body weight loss. The health care professional computes the fluid replacement for the patient. The following is only an example. Many health care professionals use this method for replacement of fluid loss.

A male patient admitted to the hospital, had a weight loss of 10 pounds due to dehydration. His weight had originally been 154 pounds, or 70 kg (kilograms). To determine the percentage of body weight loss, divide the weight loss by the original weight; therefore, 10 ÷ 154 = 0.06, or 6%. To determine the total fluid loss, multiply the percentage of body weight loss by kilograms of body weight; therefore, 0.06 × 70 kg = 4.2 liters.

34.

Clinically, he has (mild/marked/severe) dehydration.

_____.

34. marked

35.

To determine the percentage of body weight loss, *_____

_____.

To determine the total fluid loss, *_____

_____.

35. divide the weight loss by the original weight; multiply the percentage of body weight loss by kilograms of body weight

36.

One-third of body water deficit is from ECF (extracellular fluid), and two-thirds of body water deficit is from ICF (intracellular fluid) (Chapter 1). To determine replacement therapy for the first day, you would multiply:

(a) $\frac{1}{3}$ × 4.2 L = 1.4 L (ECF replacement)

Replacement fluid needed for ECF is _____ liter(s), or _____ ml.

(b) $\frac{2}{3}$ × 4.2 L = 2.8 L (ICF replacement)

Replacement fluid needed for ICF is _____ liter(s), or _____ ml.

(c) 2.5 L, or 2500 ml, is added to replace the current day's losses (constant daily amount)

The total fluid replacement for the first day is _____ liter(s), or _____ ml (sum of ECF and ICF and current day's losses).

36. a. 1.4; 1400; b. 2.8; 2800; c. 6.7; 6700

37.

One-third of the water deficit is from the *_____, and two-thirds of the water deficit is from the *_____.

37. extracellular fluid; intracellular (cellular) fluid

38. ECF

38.

The sodium (Na) deficit is the amount contained in the ECF loss of 1.4 liters. Sodium is the main cation of (ECF/ICF)

_____.

   Normally there is a loss of sodium when there is a loss of ECF. However, the serum sodium level may be elevated if the fluid loss is greater than the sodium loss.

39.

The potassium (K) deficit is the amount contained in the ICF loss of 2.8 liters. Potassium is the main cation of (ECF/ICF)

_____.

   Usually when there is cellular fluid loss, there is potassium loss. However, the serum potassium level may be elevated when potassium leaves the cells and accumulates in the ECF. When diuresis occurs, the serum potassium (elevates/decreases)

_____.

39. ICF; decreases

40. Because of acidosis, the body bicarbonate is decreased. Chloride would combine with the hydrogen ion and increase acidosis, by creating hydrochloric acid (HCl). The formula would be $H_2O + NaCl = HCl + NaOH$.

40.

In severe dehydration, cellular breakdown usually occurs and acid metabolites such as lactic acid are released from the cells; thus, metabolic acidosis results. The serum CO_2 and the arterial bicarbonate (HCO_3) levels are decreased. Why do you think this happens? *_____

_____

   Bicarbonate is usually added to a liter or two of IV fluids to neutralize the body's acidotic state. Constant use of saline (NaCl) is not indicated. Explain why. *_____

_____

41.

As potassium is being restored to the cells (when there is a potassium deficit), fluid flows into the cells with potassium replacement. Cellular fluid is then (decreased/increased)

_____; thus, the cells become (hydrated/dehydrated) _____.

   Refer to Table 2-3 for suggested solution replacement needed to correct dehydration/extracellular fluid deficits.

41. increased; hydrated

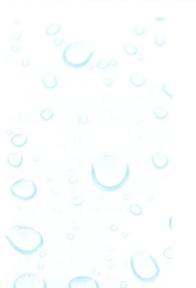

Table 2-3	Suggested Solution Replacement for ECF Deficit

1. Lactated Ringer's, 1500 ml, to replace ECF losses (varies according to the serum potassium and calcium levels).
2. Normal saline solution (0.9% NaCl solution), 500 ml.
3. Five percent dextrose in water (D_5W), 4700 ml, to replace the water deficit and increase urine output.
4. Potassium chloride, 40–80 mEq, may be divided into 3 liters to replace potassium loss. The serum potassium level must be closely monitored.
5. Bicarbonate as needed if an acidotic state exists.
6. Blood administered when volume loss is due to blood loss.

42. Eighty to 90% of potassium is excreted via kidneys. Poor urinary output leads to potassium excess, so urine output should be 250 ml per 8 hours.

42.

When potassium is being administered intravenously, explain your assessment concerns and the appropriate rationale related to the patient's urinary output? *_____

_____

43. assess degree of dehydration and replace fluid volume loss

43.

In correcting dehydration, two goals are to *_____

_____.

44.

Mild dehydration is frequently treated with dextrose, water, and small amounts of electrolytes.

Dextrose 5% in water (D_5W) is frequently given first followed by a solution of low electrolyte content such as *_____

_____.

(These solutions could be given in reverse, according to the patient's condition and health care professional's choice.)

When administering D_5W, dextrose is metabolized quickly, leaving _____.

44. lactated Ringer's solution or $D_5/\frac{1}{2}$ NSS (5% dextrose in 0.45% normal saline solution); water

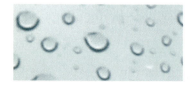

● CLINICAL CONSIDERATIONS

1. Thirst is an early symptom of ECFVD, or dehydration. Encourage fluid intake.

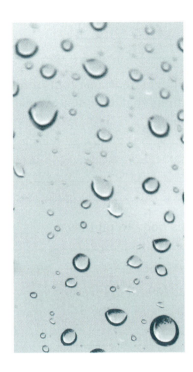

2. The serum osmolality is one method to detect dehydration. A serum osmolality of >300 mOsm/kg indicates dehydration.

3. Decreased skin turgor, dry mucous membranes, an increased pulse rate, a systolic blood pressure (while standing) <10–15 mm Hg of the regular BP, and/or decreased urine output are some signs and symptoms of dehydration.

4. A quick assessment of hypovolemia or dehydration can be accomplished by checking the peripheral veins in the hand. First hold the hand above heart level for 10 seconds and then lower the hand below the heart level. The peripheral veins in the hand below the heart level become engorged within 5–10 seconds with a normal blood volume.

5. Lactated Ringer's and 5% dextrose in $\frac{1}{3}$ or $\frac{1}{2}$ normal saline are solutions are helpful for treating ECFVD.

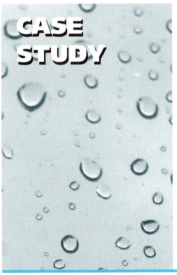

CASE STUDY

REVIEW

A 55-year-old male has been vomiting persistently for 3 days. On admission, he weighed 153 pounds. His original weight was 165 pounds (75 kg). The nurse assessed his fluid state and noted that his mucous membranes and skin were dry. His temperature was 99.4°F (37.5°C), pulse 112, respirations 32, blood pressure 110/88, and urine output in 8 hours 125 ml with a specific gravity of 1.036. Electrolyte findings were serum K, 3.5 mEq/L; Na, 154 mEq/L; and Cl, 102 mEq/L. His hematocrit and BUN were elevated.

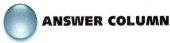

ANSWER COLUMN

1. hyperosmolar dehydration; Serum sodium is elevated with the fluid loss.

1. Name this type of dehydration (fluid volume loss).
   * _____ Explain the rationale for your selection.
   _____
   _____

2. hypovolemia

3. a. dry mucous membrane and dry skin; b. vital signs—temperature slightly elevated, tachycardia, respiration increased, systolic blood pressure ↓; c. elevated sodium level; d. Hct and BUN increased; Others— weight loss, urinary output ↓

4. 12 ÷ 165 = 0.07 × 100 = 7%

5. marked

6. 75 kg × 0.07 = 5.25 L loss

7. elevated Hct and BUN

8. water depletion

9. decreased; With dehydration, K leaves cells.

2. Another name for dehydration is *_____
_____

3. The nurse assesses his body fluid state. Name four of his symptoms and laboratory findings that are suggestive of the fluid imbalance (dehydration).
a. *_____
b. *_____
c. *_____
d. *_____

4. Determine the percentage of his body weight loss.
*_____
_____

5. Clinically, this patient has (mild/marked/severe) _____ dehydration.

6. His total fluid loss is *_____.
(Work space is provided.)

7. What two laboratory results were indicative of dehydration other than the electrolytes? *_____

8. Hypernatremia (increased sodium level) frequently results from *_____.

9. His serum potassium level of 3.5 mEq/L is considered low average. Do you think his cellular potassium is (increased/decreased) _____? Explain your rationale.
_____
_____

10. decreased; With hydration, K moves from the ECF back into cells; thus, serum K is lowered.

11. lactated Ringer's

10. If he is hydrated without potassium added, the nurse should expect his serum potassium to be (increased/decreased) _____.
    Why? * _____
    _____

11. What intravenous solution resembles the electrolyte concentration of plasma? * _____

CARE PLAN

PATIENT MANAGEMENT: EXTRACELLULAR FLUID VOLUME DEFICIT (ECFVD)

Assessment Factors

● Complete a patient history identifying factors that may cause a fluid volume deficit (FVD), such as vomiting, diarrhea, limited fluid intake, diabetes mellitus or diabetes insipidus, large draining wound, or diuretic therapy.

● Assess the skin for poor skin turgor by pinching the skin (pinched skin that remains pinched or returns slowly to its normal skin surface is indicative of poor skin turgor), dry mucous membranes, and/or dry cracked lips or tongue.

● Check vital signs: pulse rate, respiration, and blood pressure. When the blood volume decreases, the heart compensates for the fluid loss by increasing the heart rate. When the fluid volume continues to decrease, the systolic blood pressure begins to fall. Check the blood pressure first, while the patient is sitting and, then, if the patient is able to stand without difficulty, check blood pressure while standing (a fall of 10–15 mm Hg in systolic pressure may indicate marked dehydration). A narrow pulse pressure of less than 20 mm Hg can indicate severe hypovolemia. Pulse pressure is the difference between the systolic and diastolic blood pressure.

● Check the urine output for volume and concentration. A decrease in urine output may be due to a lack of fluid intake or excess body fluid loss such as from vomiting, GI suctioning, profuse diaphoresis, hemorrhage, and diabetic ketoacidosis.

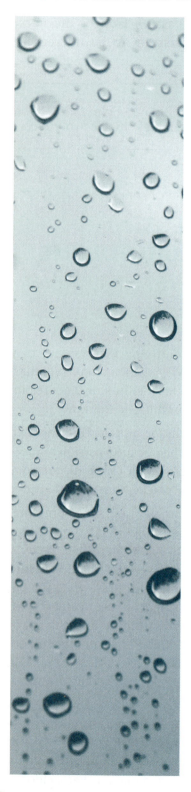

- Monitor weight gain/loss to assist in accurate fluid replacement.

- Assess hand and/or neck vein filling. A decrease in venous filling (in the vessels of the hand) when the hand is below the heart level and in the jugular vein when the patient is in a low Fowler's position may suggest a fluid volume deficit.

- Check laboratory findings such as BUN, hematocrit, and hemoglobin. Record and report abnormal findings.

Nursing Diagnosis 1

Deficient fluid volume: dehydration related to inadequate fluid intake, vomiting, diarrhea, hemorrhage, or third-space fluid loss (burns or ascites).

Interventions and Rationale

1. Monitor vital signs every 4 hours depending upon the severity of the fluid loss. Compare the vital signs to the patient's baseline vital signs. Check the blood pressure in lying, sitting, and standing positions.

2. Provide fluid intake hourly using fluids patient prefers and those indicated by electrolyte deficits. If intravenous (IV) method is used for fluid replacement, monitor IV flow rate. Guard against overhydration and infiltration of the IV fluids.

3. Monitor skin turgor, mucous membranes, and lips and tongue for changes: improvement or deterioration.

4. Weigh daily or as indicated. Remember 2.2 pounds (1 kg) loss is equivalent to 1 liter (1000 ml) of fluid loss.

Nursing Diagnosis 2

Risk for impaired tissue integrity related to a fluid deficit.

Interventions and Rationale

1. Use preventive measures to preserve skin and mucous membrane integrity. The patient's position should be changed on a regular schedule.

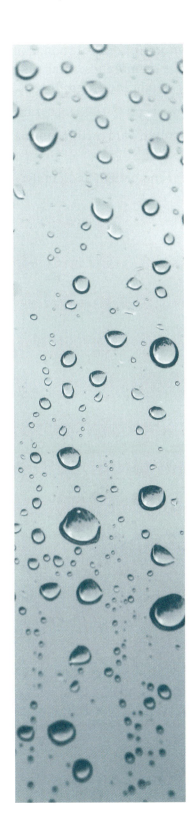

2. Apply lotion to increase circulation to the bony prominences.

3. Check skin turgor. Note skin color and temperature.

Nursing Diagnosis 3

Impaired oral mucous membranes related to dehydration.

Interventions and Rationale

1. Provide oral hygiene several times a day. Inspect mouth for sores, lesions, or bleeding. Avoid use of drying agents such as lemon and glycerine swabs or certain mouthwashes.

2. Apply water-soluble lubricant to the lips to prevent cracking and promote healing.

3. Promote adequate fluid replacement.

4. Avoid irritants (foods, fluids, temperature, etc).

Nursing Diagnosis 4

Ineffective tissue perfusion, renal, related to decreased renal blood flow and poor urine output secondary to ECFVD, hypovolemia, or dehydration.

Interventions and Rationale

1. Monitor urinary output. Report if urine output is less than 30 ml/hr or 250 ml/8 hr. Absence of urine output for 5–12 hours may indicate renal insufficiency due to decreased renal blood perfusion.

2. Note presence of pain on urination.

3. Monitor; report abnormal laboratory findings such as elevated BUN and elevated serum creatinine. Measure the specific gravity of urine every shift.

4. Weigh patient daily, at the same time in the morning.

Evaluation/Outcomes

1. Confirm that the cause of ECFVD has been controlled or eliminated.

2. Evaluate the effects of clinical management for ECFVD to see if the fluid deficit is lessened.

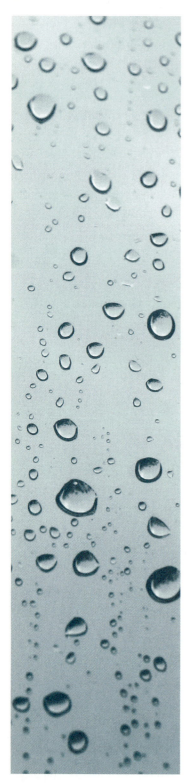

3. Remain free of signs and symptoms of dehydration; skin turgor improved, moist mucous membranes, vital signs within normal range, and body weight increased.

4. Urine output is within normal range (600–1500 ml/24 hr).

5. Determine if the serum electrolytes are within normal range.

6. Determine support measures for the patient and family.

Extracellular Fluid Volume Excess (ECFVE)

INTRODUCTION

Extracellular fluid volume excess (ECFVE) is increased fluid in the interstitial (tissues) and intravascular (vascular or vessel) spaces. Usually it relates to the excess fluid in tissues of the extremities (peripheral edema) or lung tissues (pulmonary edema). Generalized body edema is called anasarca.

ANSWER COLUMN

1. excess fluid volume in circulating blood volume

2. hypervolemia, overhydration, edema, and fluid overload

3. interstitial spaces of the ECF compartment or in serous cavities

4. hemodilution; decreased

1.

Hypervolemia and *overhydration* are interchangeable terms for ECFVE and edema.

Hypervolemia means *_____.

Hypervolemia and overhydration contribute to fluid excess in tissue spaces, or edema.

Fluid overload is another term for overhydration and hypervolemia.

2.

Edema is the abnormal retention of fluid in the interstitial spaces of the ECF compartment or in serous cavities. Frequently, edema results from sodium retention in the body, causing a retention of water and an increase in extracellular fluid volume. Four terms used for ECFVE are *_____

_____.

3.

Edema is the abnormal retention of fluid in the *_____

_____.

● PATHOPHYSIOLOGY

4.

When sodium and water are retained in the same proportion, the fluid is referred to as iso-osmolar fluid volume excess. Total body sodium is increased but concentration is unchanged because there is retention of sodium, chloride, and water. Usually the sodium level is within the normal range. This is most likely due to (hemoconcentration/hemodilution)

_____.

If only free water is retained, the excess is referred to as hypo-osmolar fluid volume excess. Serum sodium levels would be (increased/decreased) _____ due to the increase of free water.

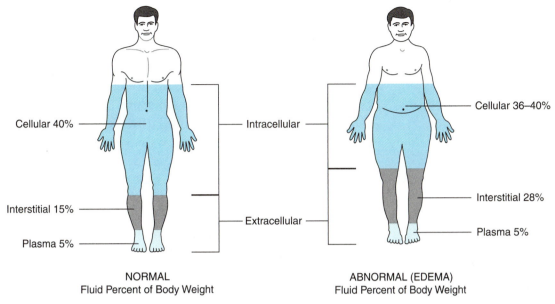

Cellular 40%

Intracellular

Cellular 36–40%

Interstitial 15%

Extracellular

Interstitial 28%

Plasma 5%

Plasma 5%

NORMAL
Fluid Percent of Body Weight

ABNORMAL (EDEMA)
Fluid Percent of Body Weight

FIGURE 3-1 Body fluid compartments and edema. These figures demonstrate the makeup of normal body fluid versus abnormal body fluid, such as with edema. As you recall from Chapter 1, 60% of the adult body weight is water; 40% of that is intracellular or cellular water, and 20% is extracellular water. Of the extracellular fluid, 15% is interstitial fluid and 5% is intravascular fluid or plasma. Note that with edema there is an increase of fluid in the interstitial space, which is between tissues and cells. The intracellular fluid may be decreased in extreme cases.

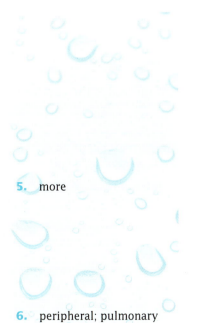

5.

Normally there is an exchange of fluid between the intravascular and interstitial spaces to maintain fluid balance in the ECF compartment.

The hydrostatic pressure in the arteries pushes fluid into the tissue spaces, and oncotic pressure in the arteries, which are made up of protein and albumin, holds fluid in the vessels. When there is fluid volume excess, the fluid pressure is greater than the oncotic pressure; therefore, (more/less) _____ fluid is pushed into the tissue spaces.

5. more

6.

In fluid volume excess, when standing for long periods of time, excess fluid in the lower extremities can occur, known as (peripheral/pulmonary) _____edema. The excess fluid that crosses the alveolar-capillary membrane of the lungs is known as (peripheral/pulmonary) _____ edema.

6. peripheral; pulmonary

7.

Edema in the extremities (peripheral edema) may result from inadequate heart, liver, or kidney function. If these are not adequately functioning, blood can back up into the venous system causing increased pressure in the vessels. This will result in an increased capillary pressure, which forces more fluids into the tissue spaces, primarily the extremities.

   If the kidneys cannot excrete excess vascular fluid, what might happen? *_____

_____.

7. peripheral edema, or fluid is pushed into the tissue spaces

8.

Excess vascular fluid may lead to (peripheral edema/pulmonary edema/or both) *_____.

8. peripheral and pulmonary edema (both)

● ETIOLOGY

Edema is commonly associated with excess extracellular body fluid or excess fluid due to fluid overload or overhydration.

   Physiologic factors leading to edema may be caused by various clinical conditions such as heart failure, kidney failure, cirrhosis of the liver, steroid excess, and allergic reactions. Table 3-1 lists the physiologic factors for edema, the rationale, and the clinical conditions associated with each physiologic factor.

9.

Blood backed up in the venous system increases the capillary pressure, forcing more fluid into *_____

_____.

   The clinical conditions in which edema may occur as a result of an increase of plasma hydrostatic pressure are:

   a. *_____
   b. *_____
   c. *_____
   d. *_____

9. the tissue spaces (interstitial spaces); a. heart failure; b. kidney failure; c. venous obstruction; d. pressure on the veins such as from casts or bandages that are too tight

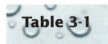

Table 3-1   **Physiologic Factors Leading to Edema**

Physiologic Factors	Rationale	Clinical Conditions
Plasma hydrostatic pressure in the capillaries	↑ Increased Blood dammed in the venous system can cause "back" pressure in capillaries, thus raising capillary pressure. Increased capillary pressure forces more fluid into tissue areas, thus producing edema.	1. Heart failure with increased venous pressure. 2. Kidney failure resulting in sodium and water retention. 3. Venous obstruction leading to varicose veins. 4. Pressure on veins because of swelling, constricting bandages, tight casts, tumors, pregnancy.
Plasma colloid osmotic pressure	↓ Decreased Decreased plasma colloid osmotic pressure results from diminished plasma protein concentration. Decreased protein content may cause water to flow from plasma into tissue spaces, thus causing edema.	1. Malnutrition due to lack of protein in diet. 2. Chronic diarrhea resulting in loss of protein. 3. Burns leading to loss of fluid containing protein through denuded skin. 4. Kidney disease, particularly nephrosis. 5. Cirrhosis of liver resulting in decreased production of plasma protein. 6. Loss of plasma proteins through urine.
Capillary permeability	↑ Increased Increased permeability of capillary membrane will allow plasma proteins to leak out of capillaries into interstitial space more rapidly than lymphatics can return them to circulation. Increased capillary permeability is a predisposing factor to edema.	1. Bacterial inflammation causes increased porosity. 2. Allergic reactions. 3. Burns causing damage to capillaries. 4. Acute kidney disease, e.g., nephritis.

(continues)

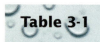

Table 3-1   **Physiologic Factors Leading to Edema—*continued***

Physiologic Factors	Rationale	Clinical Conditions
Sodium retention	↑ Increased Kidneys regulate the level of sodium ions in extracellular fluid. Kidney function depends on adequate blood flow. Inadequate blood flow, presence of excess aldosterone or glucocorticosteroids, and diseased kidneys are predisposing factors to edema since they cause sodium chloride and water retention.	1. Heart failure causing inadequate circulation of blood. 2. Renal failure—inadequate circulation of blood through kidneys. 3. Increased production of adreno-cortical hormones—aldosterone, cortisone, and hydrocortisone—will cause retention of sodium. 4. Cirrhosis of liver. A diseased liver cannot destroy excess production of aldosterone. 5. Trauma resulting from fractures, burns, and surgery.
Lymphatic drainage	↓ Decreased Blockage of lymphatics prevents the return of proteins to circulation. Obstructed lymph flow is said to be high in protein content. With inadequate return of proteins to circulation, plasma colloid osmotic pressure is decreased, thus causing edema.	1. Lymphatic obstruction, e.g., cancer of lymphatic system. 2. Surgical removal of lymph nodes. 3. Elephantiasis, the parasitic invasion of lymph channel, resulting in fibrous tissue growing in nodes, obstructing lymph flow. 4. Obesity because of inadequate supporting structures for lymphatics in lower extremities. Muscles are considered the supporting structures.

10.

A decrease in plasma protein results in a(n) (increase/decrease) _____ in the plasma colloid osmotic (oncotic) pressure. This causes water to move from the vessels into the
*_____.

Name at least four clinical conditions in which edema occurs as a result of decreased plasma/serum colloid osmotic (oncotic) pressure *_____

_____

10. decrease; tissue spaces; malnutrition, burns, kidney disease, heart failure, and liver disease (all clinical conditions due to loss or lack of protein intake)

11. capillaries; the tissue spaces (interstitial spaces); bacterial inflammation, allergic reactions, acute kidney disease such as nephritis, and burns

12. retention; heart failure, renal failure, adreno cortical hormones such as cortisone, cirrhosis of the liver, and trauma

13. protein; the intravascular space; the tissue spaces; cancer of the lymphatic system, removal of the lymph nodes, obesity, and elephantiasis

14. lung tissues

11.

An increase in the capillary membrane permeability allows plasma proteins to escape from _____, causing more water to move into *_____. Name at least three situations in which edema occurs as a result of increased capillary permeability.

*_____

12.

The kidneys regulate the gain/loss of sodium, chloride, and water via the renin-angiotensin-aldosterone system. An inadequate blood flow, the presence of excess aldosterone, or diseased kidneys result in sodium (excretion/retention)

_____.

  Name at least three clinical conditions that can cause sodium retention. _____

13.

Obstruction of the lymph flow prevents the return of proteins to the circulation. The obstructed lymph fluid is high in _____ content.

  A decrease in protein content in the plasma causes the water to move from *_____ into *_____.

  Name at least three clinical conditions that cause a decrease in lymphatic drainage. *_____

_____

14.

Edema of the lungs, often called *pulmonary edema*, can occur in patients with limited cardiac or renal reserve. When the heart is not able to function adequately and the kidneys cannot excrete a sufficient amount of urine, the fluid backs up into the pulmonary circulatory system.

  When the hydrostatic pressure of the blood in the pulmonary capillaries rises to equal or is greater than the plasma colloid osmotic pressure, the water moves from vessels into the *_____, leading to pulmonary edema.

15.

Giving excessive amounts of intravenous infusions to a person with pulmonary edema may cause the blood volume to increase. This increased blood volume is called _____.

Intravenous infusions should be regulated so that the rate of flow is not in excess of the urinary _____.

15. hypervolemia; output

● CLINICAL MANIFESTATIONS

There are numerous clinical manifestations of ECFVE as they relate to pulmonary edema and peripheral edema.

16.

When the fluid volume excess (overhydration/hypervolemia) causes a "backup" of fluid that seeps into the lung tissue, *_____ results.

16. pulmonary edema

17.

An early symptom of ECFVE is a constant, irritating, nonproductive cough. This is a sign of *_____
_____.

17. overhydration or hypervolemia or fluid volume excess or early pulmonary edema

Table 3-2 lists the clinical signs and symptoms of ECFVE related to pulmonary and peripheral edema. Laboratory test results influenced by ECFVE are included. Rationale for each sign and symptom and potential abnormal laboratory results are listed.

18.

One of the first clinical symptoms of ECFVE excess (hypervolemia or overhydration) is a *_____
_____.

18. constant, irritating, nonproductive cough

19.

Identify which of the following are signs and symptoms of pulmonary edema.
____ a. Dyspnea
____ b. Neck vein engorgement (distenden or swollen with fluids)
____ c. Hand vein engorgement (distenden or swollen with fluids)
____ d. Pitting edema in the extremities
____ e. Tight, smooth, shiny skin over edematous site
____ f. Moist crackles in lung

19. a,b,c,f

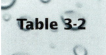

Table 3-2	Clinical Manifestations of ECFVE—Hypervolemia, Overhydration, Edema
Signs and Symptoms	**Rationale**
Pulmonary Edema	
Constant, irritating, nonproductive cough	An irritating cough is frequently the first clinical symptom of hypervolemia. It is caused by fluid "backed up" into the lungs (fluid is in the alveoli).
Dyspnea (difficulty in breathing)	Breathing is labored and difficult due to fluid congestion in lungs.
Neck vein engorgement	Jugular vein remains engorged when the patient is in semi-Fowler's or sitting position.
Sublingual vein engorgement	Engorged veins under the tongue may indicate hypervolemia.
Hand vein engorgement	Peripheral veins in the hand remain engorged with hand elevated above heart level for 10 seconds.
Moist crackles in lung	Lungs are congested with fluid. Moist crackles in lung can be heard with the stethoscope.
Bounding pulse	A full, bounding pulse may be present with hypervolemia. The pulse rate may increase.
Cyanosis	Can be a late symptom of pulmonary edema as a result of impaired gas exchange caused by fluid in the alveolar space.
Peripheral Edema	
Pitting edema in extremities	Peripheral edema present in the morning may result from inadequate heart, liver, or kidney function. A positive test of pitting edema is a finger indentation on the edematous area.
Tight, smooth, shiny skin over edematous area	Excess fluid in the peripheral tissues may cause the skin to be tight, smooth, and shiny.
Pallor, cool skin at edematous area	Excess fluid causes a decrease in circulation. The skin becomes pale, shiny, and cool.
Puffy eyelids (periorbital edema)	Swollen eyelids occur with generalized edema.
Weight gain evidenced as generalized edema or anasarca	A gain of 2.2 pounds is equivalent to a gain of 1 liter of body water.
Laboratory Tests	
Decreased serum osmolality	Excess fluid dilutes solute concentration; thus serum osmolality is below 280 mOsm/kg.
Decreased serum protein and albumin, BUN, Hgb, Hct	Serum protein, albumin, BUN, and Hgb and Hct levels can be decreased due to excess fluid volume (hemodilution).
Increased CVP (central venous pressure)	An increase in CVP measurement of more than 12–15 cm H_2O is indicative of hypervolemia, evidenced as an increase in the fluid pressure.

20. Pulmonary edema causes poor or inadequate ventilation.

20.

In pulmonary edema, the alveoli (air sacs) are filled with fluid. Explain the effect this fluid has on ventilation throughout the lung tissue. *_____

_____

21. extracellular fluid volume excess or hypervolemia

21.

When the jugular vein remains engorged (distended or swollen with fluids) after a person is put in a semi-Fowler's position (45° elevated), what type of fluid imbalance might this indicate? *_____

_____.

22. hypervolemia or overhydration; Hypervolemia is assessed with the hand above the heart level for vein engorgement and hypovolemia is assessed with the hand below the heart level for flat vein or no engorgement.

22.

A quick assessment for hypervolemia, or overhydration, can be done by checking the peripheral veins in the hand. Instruct the patient to hold a hand above the heart level. If the peripheral veins of the hand remain engorged after 10 seconds, this can be an indication of _____.

Explain how peripheral vein assessment for hypervolemia differs from peripheral vein assessment for hypovolemia.
*_____

_____.

23. moist crackles

23.

The nurse can assess the lungs for evidence of hypervolemia by listening for *_____ with a stethoscope.

24. late

24.

Cyanosis is a(n) (early/late) _____ symptom of pulmonary edema due to hypervolemia.

25.

The influence of gravity has an effect on the distribution of fluid in the edematous person. In a lying position, there is a more equal distribution of edema, whereas in an upright position the edema is more prevalent in the lower extremities. This is called *dependent edema.*

The eyelids of a person with generalized edema may be swollen in the morning, but by afternoon, with increased activity and gravity, the swelling is (more/less)

25. less

_____ marked.

26. ankles and feet; eyes or sacrum and buttocks, or more equally distributed

27. dependent edema

28. Dependent edema should not be present after the patient has been in a prone (lying face down) or supine (lying face up) position for the night. If edema is present in the morning it is most likely due to cardiac, renal, or liver disease and can be called *nondependent edema* (to differentiate between edema due to gravity versus edema due to cardiac, renal, or liver dysfunction; it can also be called *refractory edema* when edema does not respond to diuretics).

29. 1 (one)

30. hypervolemia; hypovolemia or dehydration

31. protein; It increases plasma colloid osmotic pressure and thus pulls fluid out of the tissues.

26.
With patients who are up and about, the peripheral edema is frequently found in the (ankles and feet/sacrum and buttocks) * _____. For those who are bedridden, edema fluid is most likely found in the * _____.

27.
The type of edema associated with gravity and the person's body position is called * _____.

28.
Explain why a nurse should assess for edema in the ankles and feet early in the morning. * _____
_____
_____

29.
Another tool for assessing edema and hypervolemia is body weight.
  If the patient has edema and has gained 2.2 pounds, this weight gain is equivalent to _____ liter(s) of water.

30.
When hemoglobin and hematocrit measurements have been in a normal range and suddenly decrease, not due to hemorrhage or loss of blood supply, the change in fluid imbalance is (hypovolemia/hypervolemia) _____.
  If the hemoglobin and hematocrit increase, the fluid imbalance might be indicative of _____.

● CLINICAL APPLICATIONS

31.
Many edematous persons are malnourished due to a loss of proteins or electrolytes. Unless contraindicated, the nurse should encourage the edematous patient to eat foods high in _____. Why? * _____
_____

32. The edema fluid is trapped in the interstitial space (tissue) and is not circulating such as ascites and peripheral edema.

33. decubiti (bedsores); tissue breakdown or constant pressure on the edematous tissues

34. frequent change of body position such as every 2 hours

35. will not; Salt (sodium) has a water-retaining effect and without the sodium the water would not increase the edema. However, caution should be taken with giving excess amounts of water.

36. water

37. diuretics, digoxin (digitalis preparation), and diet (low sodium)

32.
Edematous persons may suffer from decreased vascular volume. Explain why? *_____

33.
The tissues of an edematous person are said to be more vulnerable to injury, resulting in tissue breakdown.
   A bedridden person with edema of the sacrum and buttocks is apt to develop _____ due to *_____
_____.

34.
Identify a nursing intervention to prevent decubiti in the edematous person. *_____

● CLINICAL MANAGEMENT

35.
When edema is present, a diet that includes salt and water intake often increases the fluid retention.
   Water intake alone probably (will/will not) _____ increase the edema. Why? *_____
_____

36.
Drugs, such as diuretics, assist in decreasing fluid volume excess (FVE) by promoting sodium and water excretion. Examples include thiazide diuretics such as hydrochlorothiazide (Hydro DIURIL) and loop, or high-ceiling, diuretics such as furosemide (Lasix).
   Decreasing fluid pressure in the vascular system assists fluid in flowing back from the tissue spaces into the vessels in order to be excreted. This process is called "diuresing."
   Diuretics aid in the excretion of body sodium and
_____.

37.
In cardiac insufficiency, the digitalis medication, digoxin, may be needed to improve heart function and circulation.
   The three D's are frequently prescribed for the clinical management of ECFVE. They are *_____.

38.

Increasing protein intake in a malnourished person should (increase/decrease) _____ the oncotic pressure in the vessels, thus pulling water out of the tissues.

38. increase

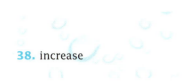

⬤ CLINICAL CONSIDERATIONS

1. ECFVE, overhydration or hypervolemia, usually relates to excess fluid in tissues of the extremities (peripheral edema) or lungs (pulmonary edema).

2. Body water retention (edema) usually results from sodium retention. If only free water is retained, the excess is referred to as hypo-osmolar fluid volume excess.

3. A constant, irritating, nonproductive cough is frequently the first clinical symptom of hypervolemia. It is caused by excess fluid "backed up" into the lungs.

4. For quick assessment of ECFVE, check for hand vein engorgement. If the peripheral veins in the hand remain engorged when the hand is elevated above the heart level for 10 seconds, ECFVE or hypervolemia is present.

5. Moist crackles in the lung usually indicate that the lungs are congested with fluid.

6. Peripheral edema present in the morning may result from inadequate heart, liver, or kidney function. Peripheral edema in the evening may be due to fluid stasis, dependent edema. Peripheral edema should be assessed in the morning before the patient gets out of bed.

7. A weight gain of 2.2 pounds is equivalent to the retention of 1 liter of body water.

8. Excess fluid dilutes solute concentration in the vascular space. A serum osmolality of <280 mOsm/kg indicates an ECFVE.

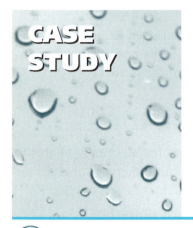

CASE STUDY

REVIEW

A 72-year-old female was admitted to the hospital with complaints of shortness of breath, coughing, and swollen ankles and feet. Her blood pressure was 190/110, pulse 96, and respirations 28 and labored. Her hemoglobin and hematocrit were slightly low. She has a history of a "heart condition" and hypertension.

ANSWER COLUMN

1. extracellular fluid volume excess or edema; edema; hypervolemia; overhydration

2. constant, irritating, nonproductive cough
3. increased hydrostatic pressure, decreased colloidal osmotic pressure, increased capillary permeability, increased sodium retention, and decreased lymphatic drainage
4. increased hydrostatic pressure and increased sodium retention

5. nondependent; inadequate heart, kidney, or liver function

6. extracellular fluid volume excess, or hypervolemia

1. The nurse assesses the patient's physical state. Her shortness of breath, coughing, and swollen ankles and feet may be indicative of *_____. Other names for extracellular fluid volume excess include _____, _____, and _____.

2. An early symptom of extracellular fluid volume excess or hypervolemia is a *_____ _____.

3. The five main physiologic factors that lead to edema are *_____ _____.

4. The two physiologic factors that may have caused her edema are *_____.

5. The nurse assesses the patient's ankles and feet in the morning to differentiate between dependent and nondependent edema. If her ankles and feet remain swollen before she arises in the morning, the edema is described as _____ edema. The cause of this type of edema is *_____.

6. The nurse assesses the patient's peripheral veins. Her veins are still engorged after holding her hand above the heart level for 10 seconds. This can be indicative of *_____ _____.

7. pulmonary; observe the jugular veins for engorgement when she is in semi-Fowler's position and assess chest sounds for moist crackles

8. inadequate heart and kidney function

9. 2; 2000

10. hypervolemia; dilution of red blood cells (RBCs) with a decrease in RBCs and an increase in water

11. decubiti; change body position such as every 2 hours

12. anasarca

7. Her shortness of breath or dyspnea and coughing may be due to _____ edema. Identify two assessment factors to assist the nurse in determining the type of edema present. *_____

_____

8. Identify two causes of pulmonary edema. *_____

9. She gained 5 pounds in 2 days. This weight gain would be approximately _____ liter(s) of body water gain, which is equal to _____ ml of body water.

10. Her hemoglobin and hematocrit have been normal. At present, they are decreased, which may indicate _____. Why? *_____

_____

11. If she developed generalized edema and was bedridden, what skin complication might result? _____ Identify a nursing intervention that can be taken to prevent this complication? *_____

12. Identify the name for generalized edema. _____

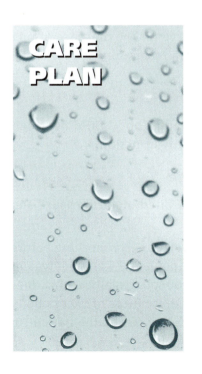

CARE PLAN

PATIENT MANAGEMENT: EXTRACELLULAR FLUID VOLUME EXCESS (ECFVE)

Assessment Factors

● Complete a patient history to identify health problems that may contribute to the development of ECFVE. Examples of such health problems may include a recurring heart problem such as heart failure; kidney or liver disease; infection; or malnutrition. Ask if there has been a recent weight gain.

● Obtain a dietary history that emphasizes sodium, protein, and water intake.

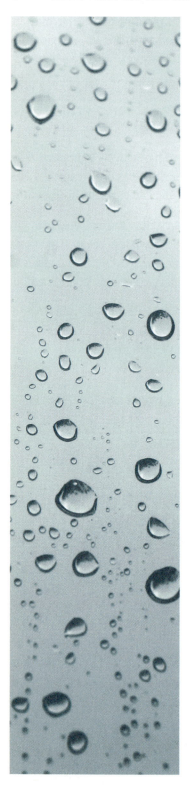

● Assess vital signs. Obtain baseline data that can be compared with past and future vital signs. Assess for a bounding pulse.

● Assess for signs and symptoms of hypervolemia (overhydration) such as constant and irritating cough, difficulty in breathing, neck and hand vein engorgement, chest crackles, and abnormal laboratory results such as a decreased hematocrit and hemoglobin level that had previously been normal. Serum sodium levels may or may not be elevated.

● Make a quick assessment of hypervolemia by checking the peripheral veins in the hand: first lowering the hand and then raising the hand above the heart level. Overhydration is present if the peripheral veins remain engorged after 10 seconds.

● Assess extremities for peripheral edema. Check for pitting edema in the lower extremities in the morning before the patient arises. Nondependent edema or refractory edema may be due to cardiac, renal, or liver dysfunction. Dependent edema (edema caused by gravity) is usually not present in the morning.

● Assess urine output. Decreased urinary output may be a sign of body fluid retention and/or renal dysfunction.

● Assess pulmonary status. Observe for the presence of pulmonary congestion or changes in respiratory status.

Nursing Diagnosis 1

Excess fluid volume: edema related to body fluid overload secondary to heart, renal, or liver dysfunction.

Interventions and Rationale

1. Monitor vital signs. Report elevated blood pressure and bounding pulse.

2. Monitor weight daily. Check weight every morning before breakfast. A weight gain of 2.2 pounds (1 kg) is equivalent to 1 liter or quart of water (1000 ml). Usually edema does not occur unless there is 3 or more liters of excess body fluids. Restrict fluids as necessary. Teach the patient to monitor intake, output, and weight.

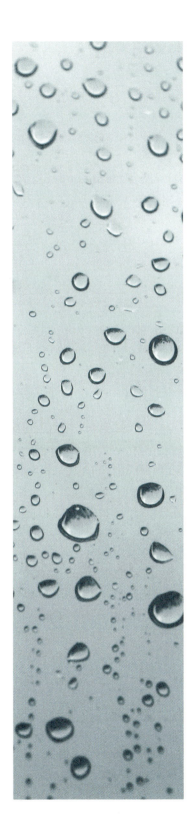

3. Observe for the presence of edema daily. Check for pitting edema in the extremities every morning. Press one or two fingers on the edematous area, and if indentation is present for 15 seconds or more, the degree of pitting edema should be recorded according to the length of time it takes for the indentation to disappear (+1 to +4). Monitor all IV fluids carefully.

4. Monitor diet. Teach appropriate food selections. Instruct the patient to avoid using excess salt on foods [salt (sodium) holds water and increases the edematous condition]. Teach the patient to avoid over-the-counter drugs without first checking with a nurse or physician.

5. Encourage the patient with a liver disorders such as cirrhosis to eat foods rich in protein. Protein increases the plasma/serum oncotic (colloid osmotic) pressure, thus pulling fluids from the tissue spaces and decreasing edema.

6. Encourage rest periods to support diuresis.

Nursing Diagnosis 2

Ineffective breathing patterns related to increased capillary permeability causing fluid overload in the lung tissue (pulmonary edema).

Interventions and Rationale

1. Monitor breathing patterns. Assess rate and depth of respiration. Evaluate chest sounds and chest excursion. Note changes and location of adventitious sounds.

2. Observe for changes in skin color and nasal flaring. Note any coughing. Report any progression of symptoms to physician.

3. Use semi-Fowler's position for those with dyspnea or orthopnea.

Nursing Diagnosis 3

Risk for impaired tissue integrity related to edematous tissues (peripheral edema).

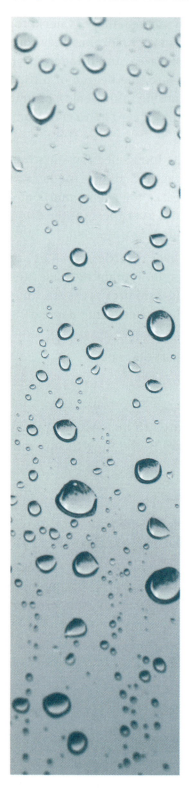

Interventions and Rationale

1. Monitor patient's mobility. Turn edematous patients frequently to prevent decubiti. Edematous persons are prone to tissue breakdown.

2. Identify and record changes in skin surfaces regarding color, temperature, and skin turgor.

3. Ambulate the patient to improve circulation and enhance fluid reabsorption from the tissue spaces to the vascular space.

4. Monitor laboratory results pertinent to electrolyte status and fluid balance. Report changes.

Nursing Diagnosis 4

Ineffective tissue perfusion related to hypervolemia as manifested by peripheral (tissue) edema.

Interventions and Rationale

1. Monitor fluid intake. Water and sodium restrictions may be necessary.

2. Monitor urine output. Urine output should be >30 ml/hr or >250 ml/8 hr. Large amounts of urine output can indicate a decrease in urine retention.

3. Administer diuretics as ordered. Assess fluid balance.

4. Check serum electrolyte values while patients is receiving diuretics. The more potent diuretics excrete both sodium and the important electrolyte potassium. Encourage foods high in potassium; potassium supplements may be necessary. Urine output should be closely monitored when potassium is given.

Evaluation/Outcomes

1. Confirm that the cause of ECFVE has been controlled or eliminated.

2. Evaluate the effects of clinical management for ECFVE. Pulmonary edema and/or peripheral edema are absent or decreased because of clinical management.

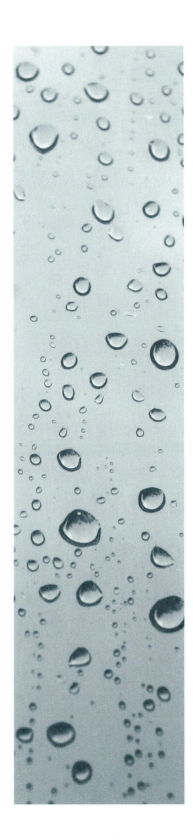

3. Remain free of signs and symptoms of overhydration/ hypervolemia. Dyspnea, neck vein engorgement, moist crackles in the lungs, and peripheral edema are absent.

4. Urine output is increased; vital signs are normal.

5. Patent airway and improved breath sounds.

6. Determine that the serum electrolytes are within normal range.

7. Maintain a support system for patient.

Extracellular Fluid Volume Shift (ECFVS)

 INTRODUCTION

In the ECF compartment, fluid volume with electrolytes and protein shifts from the intravascular
to the interstitial spaces. This fluid is referred to as
third-space fluid. The fluid is nonfunctional and is
considered to be physiologically useless. Later, third-
space fluid shifts back from the interstitial space to
the intravascular space.

ANSWER COLUMN

1.

Extracellular fluid is constantly shifting between the intravascular and interstitial spaces for the purpose of maintaining fluid balance.

1. third-space fluid, or "third spacing"

When abnormal amounts of fluid shift into the tissue spaces and remain there, it is called *_____.

PATHOPHYSIOLOGY

Refer to the Pathophysiology section in Chapters 2 (ECFVD) and 3 (ECFVE).

2.

Excess fluid in the tissue spaces, or third-space fluid, is nonfunctional and is considered *_____ _____.

2. physiologically useless

ETIOLOGY

3.

Clinical causes could be as simple as a blister or sprain or as serious as massive injuries, burns, ascites (an accumulation of serous fluid in the peritoneal cavity), abdominal surgery, a perforated peptic ulcer, intestinal obstruction, malnutrition, or liver dysfunction.

3. Hypovolemia, or fluid loss from the vascular space. If severe, shock can develop.

When massive amounts of fluid shift to the tissues and remain there, what happens to the state of vascular fluids? *_____ _____

4.

Minor causes of third-space fluid may be _____ and _____.

4. blisters; sprains; burns, trauma (massive injuries), and ascites (also, abdominal surgery, intestinal obstruction, perforated ulcer, malnutrition, or liver dysfunction)

Identify three severe health problems that can cause third-space fluid. *_____

5.

Burns and abdominal surgery are common causes of third-space fluid. With these two conditions, there are two phases of fluid shift.

In the first or loss phase, fluid is shifting from the intravascular space to the interstitial space. With a burn injury (partial or full thickness), fluid loss occurs at the surface of the burned area and surrounding tissues. Fluid from the vascular space "pours" into the burned site and remains for approximately 3 to 5 days.

In the second or reabsorption phase, fluid shifts from the *_____ to the *_____.

5. interstitial space (tissue and injured area); intravascular space

● CLINICAL MANIFESTATIONS

In a fluid shift due to tissue injury, it takes approximately 24 to 48 hours for the fluid to leave the blood vessels and accumulate in the injured tissue spaces. Edema may or may not be visible.

6.

When fluid shifts out of the vessels, changes in the vital signs occur that are similar to shock-like symptoms. These vital signs are similar to those of fluid volume deficit—marked dehydration. Indicate whether the following vital signs increase or decrease in such fluid shifts.

* _____ Pulse rate
* _____ Respiration
* _____ Systolic blood pressure

6. increased pulse rate; increased respiration; decreased systolic blood pressure (depends on the severity of fluid loss to the injured site)

7.

Three to five days after an injury causing tissue destruction, fluid shifts from the injured site to *_____.

7. blood vessels or intravascular space

8.

If the kidneys cannot excrete the excess fluid from the vascular space (blood vessels) that resulted from the fluid shift, what type of fluid imbalance might occur? _____

_____

8. hypervolemia or ECFVE

9. constant, irritating, nonproductive cough; dyspnea; and moist crackles (also hand and neck vein engorgement and full bounding pulse)

10. The edema from the burn is in the interstitial space, not in the circulation. Shock is due to the low circulating blood volume from "third spacing" of fluids and massive edema from the injury.

11. hypovolemia

12. less; Large quantities of fluid shift back into the vascular space and too much intravenous fluid may cause a fluid overload.

9.

Name three clinical signs and symptoms of hypervolemia.

* _____

_____

● CLINICAL APPLICATIONS

10.

The first 48 hours after a major burn injury is characterized by burn shock and massive edema (FVE) at the site of the burn (fluid accumulation). The fluid accumulates in the interstitial space. The next phase begins with the reversal of the shock state and is characterized by diuresis (fluid remobilization). This is when the edema begins to resolve as the fluid shifts back into the intravascular space.

An 18-year-old male was medevaced to the burn center after a firecracker exploded in his right hand. He arrived two hours after the injury. His right hand is missing two fingers, and his right arm is edemateous. The patient's vital signs indicate that he is in shock (low blood pressure, increased heart rate).

The burn patient may suffer from decreased intravascular volume (FVD), causing him to be at risk for shock. Explain why?

* _____

● CLINICAL MANAGEMENT

11.

An assessment must be completed in order to determine the cause of the third-space fluid. In the case of full thickness burns when severe tissue destruction results, the fluid shift may be so severe that (hypervolemia/hypovolemia) _____ occurs.

12.

The overall objective of clinical management for ECFVS is to maintain fluid balances. During the first phase of a fluid shift to the burn tissue site, intravenous infusion in the amount of two to three times the urine output may be necessary to maintain the circulating fluid volume.

During the second phase of fluid shift, (more/less) _____ IV fluids would be needed. Why? * _____

_____

13. increases; Urine excretion increases, with sufficient kidney function, to prevent fluid overload.

13.
During the second phase of the fluid shift, the urine output (increases/decreases) _____.
Explain. *_____

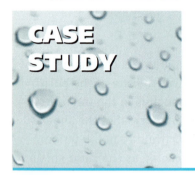

CASE STUDY

REVIEW

A midde-aged male was admitted with massive tissue injuries. His vital signs were blood pressure (BP) 98/54, pulse (P) 102, respiration (R) 32. Urine output was <30 ml/hr.

ANSWER COLUMN

1. ECFVD or hypovolemia

1. His vital signs could indicate what type of fluid imbalance? _____

2. third-space fluid or third spacing

2. When an abnormal amount of fluid shifts into the injured tissue space and remains there, the fluid in that space is called *_____.

3. massive tissue injury; With massive tissue injury, abnormal amounts of fluid shift to the injured site.

3. The cause for of his fluid shift is *_____.
Explain. *_____
_____

Clinical management for this patient included the administration of 4000 ml of 5% dextrose in $\frac{1}{2}$ normal saline (0.45% NaCl) solution and 5% dextrose in water. His vital signs after a few days were BP 114/64, P 92, and R 30.

4. to correct fluid loss from vascular space to tissue space

4. Why was he given a large amount of intravenous fluids?
*_____

Three days after he received daily large amounts of IV fluids, he developed a constant, irritating cough, mild dyspnea, and neck and hand vein engorgements.

5. ECFVE or overhydration or hypervolemia; John is receiving large amounts of IV solutions and at the same time the fluid is shifting back into the vascular space from the injured tissue area.
6. Intravenous fluids administration should be greatly reduced or discontinued.
7. phase 1, fluid in the intravascular space shifts to the injured site, and phase 2, fluid shifts from the injured area to the vascular space
8. sprain and blister

5. What type of fluid imbalance is he exhibiting? _____ Explain. *_____
_____

6. What corrective measures for this imbalance should be taken? *_____

7. What are the two phases of ECFV shift? *_____
_____

8. Two examples of minor causes for third-space fluid are
*_____
_____.

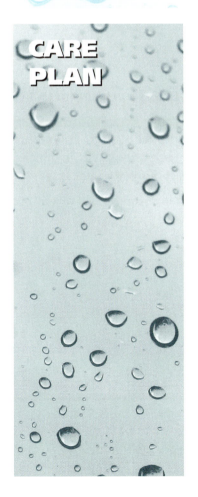

CARE PLAN

PATIENT MANAGEMENT: EXTRACELLULAR FLUID VOLUME SHIFT (ECFVS)

Assessment Factors

● Complete a patient history identifying factors that may cause a fluid volume shift: massive injury, burns, ascites, abdominal surgery, intestinal obstruction.

● Assess vital signs: pulse rate, respiration, and blood pressure. When intravascular volume decreases, the heart compensates for the fluid loss by increasing the heart rate.

● Assess urine output for volume and concentration. Decrease in urine output may be due to lack of fluid intake or excess body fluid loss.

● Monitor weight gain/loss to assist in accurate fluid replacement.

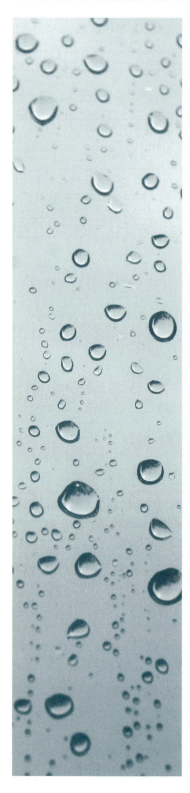

Nursing Diagnosis

Excess fluid volume: edema related to body fluid overload
Deficient fluid volume: third-space fluid loss

Interventions and Rationale

1. Monitor vital signs every 4 hours depending on the severity of the fluid shift. Compare to the patient's baseline.

2. Monitor urinary output. Report if urine output is less than 30 ml/hr or 250 ml/8 hrs. Absence of urine output for 5–12 hours may indicate renal insufficiency due to decreased renal blood perfusion.

3. Assess fluid intake and output hourly. Guard against overhydration.

4. Weigh daily or as indicated. Remember that loss of 2.2 pounds (1 kg) is equivalent to 1 liter (1000 ml of fluid loss).

Evaluation/Outcome

1. Confirm that the cause of the ECFVS has been controlled or eliminated.

2. Remain free of signs and symptoms of fluid volume excess or fluid volume deficit: vital signs within normal range and body weight returns to normal range.

3. Urine output is within normal range (600–1200 ml/24 hr).

[Intracellular F]luid [Volume Excess] (ICFVE)

[IN]TRODUCTION

[Intrace]llular fluid volume excess (ICFVE) is when [fluids] shift into the intracellular space resulting in [exce]ss of intracellular fluid. This can be caused [by e]xcess intake of water or an undue retention [of wate]r. The result can be hypo-osmolality, hy-[ponatre]mia, or both.

ANSWER COLUMN

1. hypo-osmolar

2. water intoxication; decreased

3. osmosis

4. (intra) cellular fluid overload or cellular edema

5. cerebral edema or cellular fluid overload

1.

Intracellular fluid volume excess (ICFVE), also referred to as *water intoxication*, results from an excess of water or decrease in solutes in the intravascular system. With an ICFVE there is an excess of fluid in the intracellular compartment. Fluid in the blood vessels is (hypo-osmolar/iso-osmolar/hyperosmolar) _____ when there is an ICFVE.

2.

Another name for ICFVE is *_____. As a result of this fluid imbalance, the serum osmolality is (increased/decreased) _____.

● PATHOPHYSIOLOGY

Hypo-osmolar fluid (decreased solute concentration in the circulating vascular fluid) moves by the process of osmosis from the areas of lesser solute concentration to the areas of greater concentration. The intracellular fluid (cells) is iso-osmolar, so the hypo-osmolar fluid from the vascular space moves into the cells, thus causing the cells to swell.

3.

Fluid shifts from the areas of lesser solute concentration to the areas of greater solute concentration due to the process of (diffusion/osmosis) _____.

4.

Excess fluid that may accumulate in the cells can cause *_____ _____.

5.

In an ICFVE, the cerebral cells are usually the first cells involved in the fluid shift from the vascular to the cellular space.

What might happen if there are large amounts of fluid shifting into the cerebral cells? *_____ _____.

6.

An excess secretion of the antidiuretic hormone (ADH) causes fluid to be reabsorbed from the renal tubules. This can result in what type of vascular fluid? _____

7.

Edema may result from an excess of _____, whereas water intoxication results from an excess of _____.

With edema, there is excessive fluid in the *_____ compartment, whereas with water intoxication there is excess fluid in the *_____ compartment.

8.

Water intoxication (is/is not) _____ the same as edema. Generally, edema is the accumulation of fluid in the interstitial spaces. With water intoxication, the excess hypo-osmolar fluid (increases/lowers) _____ serum osmolality.

As the result of the hypo-osmolar fluid in the vascular space, water moves into the cells, causing the cells to (shrink/swell) _____.

● ETIOLOGY

Intracellular fluid volume excess is not as common as ECFVD and ECFVE, but if untreated, it can cause serious health problems.

Common causes of water intoxication are the intake of water-free solutes and the administration of hypo-osmolar intravenous fluids such as 0.45% sodium chloride ($\frac{1}{2}$ normal saline solution) and 5% dextrose in water (D_5W). Dextrose 5% in water is an iso-tonic IV solution; however, the dextrose is metabolized quickly, leaving water or a hypo-tonic solution.

9.

The two most common types of fluid imbalance are
*_____. The acronym ICFVE stands for
*_____.

---

6. hypo-osmolar

7. sodium; water; extracellular fluid; intracellular fluid

8. is not; lowers; swell

9. ECFVD and ECFVE; intracellular fluid volume excess

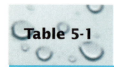

Table 5-1	Causes of Intracellular Fluid Volume Excess: Water Intoxication	
Conditions	**Causes**	**Rationale**
Excessive water intake	Excessive plain water intake	Water intake with few or no solutes dilutes the vascular fluid.
	Continuous use of IV hypo-tonic solutions (0.45% saline, D$_5$W)	Overuse of hypo-tonic solutions can cause hypo-osmolar vascular fluid. Dextrose is metabolized rapidly, leaving water.
	Psychogenic polydipsia	Compulsive drinking of plain water can result in water intoxication.
Solute deficit	Diet low in electrolytes and protein	Decrease in electrolytes and protein may cause hypo-osmolar vascular fluids.
	Irrigation of nasogastric tube with water (not saline)	GI tract is rich in electrolytes. Plain water can wash out the electrolytes.
	Plain water enema	Plain water can wash out the electrolytes.
Excess ADH secretion	Stress, surgery, drugs (narcotics, anesthesia), pain, and tumors (brain, lung)	Overproduction of ADH is known as secretion (syndrome) of inappropriate antidiuretic hormone (SIADH), which causes mass amounts of water reabsorption by the kidneys and results in hypo-osmolar fluids.
	Brain injury or tumor	Cerebral cell injury may increase ADH production, causing excessive water reabsorption.
Kidney dysfunction	Renal impairment	Kidney dysfunction can decrease water excretion.
Abnormal laboratory tests	Decreased serum sodium level and decreased serum osmolality	Because of hemodilution, the solutes in the vascular fluid are decreased in proportion to water.

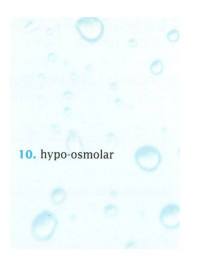

10. hypo-osmolar

10.

There are four major conditions that may cause plain ICFVE:
 a. Excessive plain water intake
 b. Solute deficit (electrolytes and protein)
 c. Increased secretion of antidiuretic hormone (ADH)
 d. Kidney dysfunction (inability to excrete excess water)
 These conditions may cause an increase in (hypo-osmolar/hyperosmolar) _____ fluid in the vascular space (vessels).

Table 5-1 lists four major conditions and laboratory tests to assess for ICFVE, their causes, and rationale. Study Table 5-1 carefully and refer to it as needed.

11. excess plain water intake, solute deficit or lack of electrolytes and protein, increased secretion of inappropriate ADH (SIADH), and kidney dysfunction or renal impairment

12. dextrose is metabolized rapidly, leaving water solution. When D$_5$W is used continuously without other solutes, hypo-osmolar fluid results.

13. more; stress and surgery [also drugs (narcotics) and pain]

14. water intoxication from water taken without solutes; dysfunction

15. low or decreased or <280 mOsm/kg; decreased

16. headache, nausea and vomiting, excessive perspiration, and weight gain

11.

Name four major conditions that might cause water intoxication.
*_____

_____

12.

The iso-tonic IV solution D$_5$W becomes a hypo-tonic solution when *_____

_____

13.

Overproduction of ADH or SIADH causes (more/less)
_____ water reabsorption from the tubules of the kidneys.

   Two causes of excess secretion of ADH are *_____

_____.

14.

If the circulation through the kidneys is impaired and there is an excessive amount of plain water intake, the fluid imbalance most likely to occur is *_____.

   Impairment of the renal circulation can occur due to arteriosclerosis. If the kidneys do not receive sufficient blood circulation, kidney (function/dysfunction) _____ can result.

15.

If there is a water excess, the serum osmolality is most likely
*_____, and the serum sodium level is most likely
_____.

● CLINICAL MANIFESTATIONS

The clinical signs and symptoms and rationale of water intoxication or ICFVE are explained in Table 5-2. Refer to Table 5-2 as necessary.

16.

Identify four early symptoms of water intoxication. *_____

_____

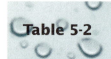

Table 5-2

Clinical Signs and Symptoms of Intracellular Fluid Volume Excess—Water Intoxication

Type of Symptoms	Signs and Symptoms	Rationale
Early	Headache Nausea and vomiting Excessive perspiration Acute weight gain	Cerebral cells absorb hypo-osmolar fluid more quickly than other cells.
Progressive Central nervous system (CNS)	Behavioral changes: progressive apprehension, irritability, disorientation, confusion Drowsiness, incoordination Blurred vision Elevated intracranial pressure (ICP)	Hypo-osmolar body fluids usually pass into cerebral cells first. Swollen cerebral cells can cause behavioral changes and elevate ICP.
Vital signs (VS)	Blood pressure ↑ Bradycardia (slow pulse rate) Respiration ↑	VS are the opposite of shock. VS are similar to those in increased ICP.
Later (CNS)	Neuroexcitability (muscle twitching) Projectile vomiting Papilledema Delirium Convulsions, then coma	Severe CNS changes occur when water intoxication is not corrected.
Skin	Warm, moist, and flushed	

17. most; Hypo-osmolar body fluids pass into cerebral cells; swollen cerebral cells cause behavioral changes.

18. apprehension, irritability, disorientation, and confusion

19. increased

17.

Central nervous system symptoms are (least/most) _____ prominent with water intoxication. Explain why? *_____

_____

18.

Name four behavioral changes that occur with progressive symptoms of water intoxication. *_____

_____

19.

The intracranial pressure is (increased/decreased) _____ with water intoxication.

20. a. increased; b. decreased, or bradycardia; c. increased

21. muscle twitching, projectile vomiting, papilledema, delirium, and convulsions

22. warm, moist, and flushed

23. water retention or water intoxication

24. water intoxication or ICFVE (due to intake of copious amounts of hypo-tonic fluids)

20.
With progressive ICFVE, the vital sign measurements reflect:
   a. Blood pressure _____
   b. Pulse rate *_____
   c. Respiration _____

21.
Name five later symptoms of water intoxication. *_____
_____
_____

22.
The skin in the later stages of water intoxication is *_____
_____.

● CLINICAL APPLICATIONS

23.
It is difficult for a person to drink himself into water intoxication unless the renal mechanisms for elimination fail or psychogenic polydipsia occurs.

   If excessive water has been given and the kidneys are not functioning properly, what is most likely to occur? *_____
_____

24.
The most common occurrence of water intoxication is seen in postoperative patients when oral and intravenous fluids have been forced without compensatory amounts of salt. In these situations, the amount of water taken in exceeds that which the kidneys can excrete.

   A postoperative patient receiving several liters of 5% dextrose in water (D_5W) with ice and sips of water PO (by mouth) can develop a fluid imbalance called *_____
_____.

25.
Also, after surgery, an overproduction of the antidiuretic hormone (ADH), known as the syndrome of inappropriate ADH

secretions (SIADH), can occur due to trauma, anesthesia, pain, and narcotics. Because of the overproduction of ADH, water excretion (increases/decreases) _____, causing the urine volume to (rise/drop) _____ and the vascular (intravascular) fluid volume to (rise/drop) _____.

25. decreases; drop; rise

● CLINICAL MANAGEMENT

The overall objective of clinical management for ICFVE is to reduce excess water in the body. Two ways to reduce water intoxication in the body are to reduce the water intake and promote water excretion.

26.

In *less* severe cases of water intoxication, water restriction may be sufficient, or an extracellular replacement solution such as lactated Ringer's or normal saline solution may be given to increase the osmolality of the extracellular fluid.

    The overall objective in the clinical management of water intoxication is *_____

_____.

    Name two ways in which this objective is accomplished.

*_____

26. to reduce excess water in the body; reduce water intake and promote water excretion

27.

Concentrated saline (3% NaCl) may be given in severe cases of water intoxication to raise extracellular electrolyte concentration in hope of drawing water out of the (intracellular space/interstitial space) *_____ and (increasing/decreasing) _____ urinary output.

27. intracellular space; increasing

28.

However, administration of additional salt to a person who already has too much water can result in expansion of the interstitial fluid and blood volume and the development of (water intoxication/edema) _____.

    An osmotic diuretic, e.g., mannitol, includes diuresis and a loss of retained fluid, especially from the cerebral cells.

28. edema

29. water restriction; extracellular replacement solution, such as lactated Ringer's or normal saline solution (0.9% NaCl); concentrated saline solution; and osmotic diuretics, such as mannitol or other diuretics

30. water restriction; extracellular replacement solution; intravenous concentrated saline solution; osmotic diuretics

31. diuresis and a loss of retained fluid, especially from cerebral cells

29.

Identify at least three methods for promoting water excretion.

*_____

_____

_____

_____

_____

30.

For less severe cases of water intoxication, the clinical management includes *_____ and/or *_____

_____

   For more severe cases of water intoxication, identify two possible clinical management interventions. *_____

_____

and/or *_____

31.

An osmotic diuretic induces *_____

_____.

● CLINICAL CONSIDERATIONS

1. ICFVE is also known as water intoxication, excess water in the cells. It usually results from an excess of hypo-osmolar vascular fluid. Water intoxication is not the same as edema. Edema usually results from sodium retention whereas water intoxication results from excess water.

2. In ICFVE, cerebral cells are usually the first cells involved in the fluid shift from the vascular to the cellular (cell) space. Large amounts of fluid shifting into the cerebral cells can result in cerebral edema, or increased intracranial pressure (ICP).

3. Continuous administration of intravenous solutions that are hypotonic or the continuous use of 5% dextrose in water can result in ICFVE. In the latter case, dextrose is metabolized rapidly in the body; thus water remains. At least 1 or 2 liters of the dextrose solution should contain a percentage of a saline solution or be administered in combination with solutes such as lactated Ringer's.

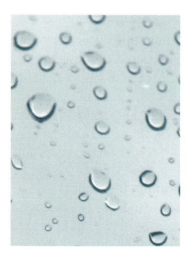

4. Headache and nausea and vomiting are early signs and symptoms of ICFVE. As ICFVE progresses, behavioral changes such as irritability, disorientation, and confusion may occur. Drowsiness and blurred vision may result.

5. Changes in vital signs are similar to those of cerebral edema: increased blood pressure, decreased pulse rate, increased respiration.

6. A concentrated saline solution (3% NaCl) can be administered for severe ICFVE. It is given if the serum sodium is <115 mEq/L. Also it draws the water out of the swollen cells.

7. Water restriction is suggested for mild ICFVE.

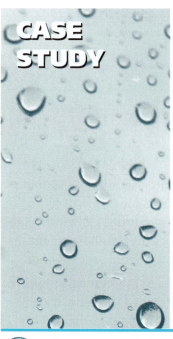

CASE STUDY

REVIEW

A 19-year-old female, returned from having an appendectomy performed. She received 1 liter of 5% dextrose in water during the procedure and another liter postoperatively. She was allowed to have crushed ice and sips of water. That evening she became nauseated, and the third liter of 5% dextrose in water was added. The following day she received 2 more liters of 5% dextrose in water. She took several glasses of crushed ice. Her first day postoperatively she complained of a headache. Later she was drowsy, disoriented, and confused. Her blood pressure evidenced a slight increase, and a drop in her pulse rate was noted.

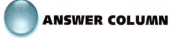 **ANSWER COLUMN**

1. water intoxication or intracellular fluid volume excess

1. The nurse assessed the patient's fluid state. From the history and her symptoms, the nurse assessed a fluid imbalance was present indicative of *_____

_____.

2. water intoxication; With 5% dextrose in water, the dextrose is metabolized by the body, leaving water. The intravenous solution and crushed ice cause the plasma to become hypo-osmolar.

3. Headache. If your answer was nausea—possibly; however, early nausea is most likely the result of the surgery and anesthesia.

4. drowsiness, disorientation, and confusion

5. increased intracranial pressure, ICP, or cerebral edema

6. yes; After surgery, there can be an increased secretion of ADH, due to trauma, anesthesia, pain, and narcotics. This increases water retention and, with the hypo-tonic fluids she received, could increase the state of water intoxication.

7. concentrated saline solution, such as 3% saline, hypertonic solution to "pull" water out of the cells

8. She should have received intravenous fluids containing saline (solute) together with dextrose.

2. Excessive amounts of 5% dextrose in water along with glasses of crushed ice without any other solute intake can cause *_____

   Explain why. *_____

   _____

   _____

   _____

3. Name the patient's early symptoms of ICFVE.

   *_____

4. As the fluid imbalance progressed, name three symptoms that indicated water intoxication or ICFVE. _____

   _____

5. Her vital signs were similar to those of *_____

   _____.

6. Can an overproduction of ADH increase her water intoxication? _____ Explain how. *_____

   _____

   _____

   _____

7. Name the type of intravenous solution to be administered to correct severe cases of water intoxication. *_____

   _____

   _____

   _____

8. Identify how this fluid imbalance could have been prevented.

   *_____

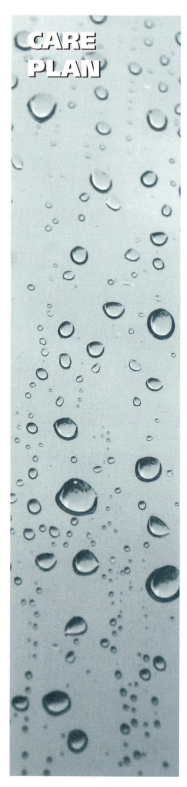

PATIENT MANAGEMENT: INTRACELLULAR FLUID VOLUME EXCESS (ICFVE)

Assessment Factors

● Complete a history to identify possible causes of ICFVE such as excessive administration of hypo-tonic solutions [continuous use of D_5W without solutes (saline)], oral fluid without solutes, major surgical procedure that might cause SIADH, and kidney dysfunction in which urine output is decreased.

● Assess vital signs. Obtain baseline data that can be compared with past and future vital signs. Note if the systolic blood pressure increases even slightly, pulse rate decreases, and respirations increase. These signs are indicative of an accumulation of cerebral fluid (cerebral edema).

● Assess for behavioral changes, such as confusion, irritability, and disorientation. Headache is an early symptom of ICFVE. These symptoms can result when hypo-osmolar fluid in the vascular space shifts to the cells, increasing cellular fluid. Cerebral cells are usually the first cells affected.

● Assess for weight changes. With ICFVE or water intoxication, there is normally an acute weight gain. With peripheral edema, the weight gain occurs more slowly.

Nursing Diagnosis 1

Excess fluid volume: water intoxication related to excessive ingestion and infusion of hypo-osmolar fluids and solutions, major surgical procedure causing SIADH.

Interventions and Rationale

1. Monitor fluid replacement. Assess osmolality of fluid replacement and consult with the health care provider for appropriate replacement balance. Report if the patient is receiving only 5% dextrose in water continuously. Dextrose

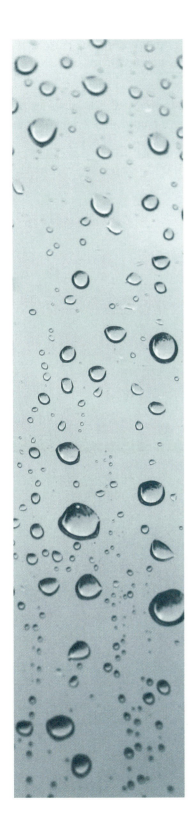

is metabolized rapidly by the body, leaving water, a hypo-osmolar solution.

2. Offer fluids that contain solutes, such as broth and juices, to the postoperative patient. Giving plain water and ice chips increases the hypo-osmolar state. Immediately post-operatively and for 24–48 hours, there may be an over-production of ADH [SIADH, or secretion (syndrome) of inappropriate antidiuretic hormone], causing an increase in water reabsorption.

3. Monitor fluid balance. The urine output after surgery and trauma can be compromised. The SIADH is frequently seen following surgery and trauma, which causes more water to be reabsorbed from the kidney tubules and dilution of the vascular fluid. Urine output is decreased due to water reabsorption.

Nursing Diagnosis 2

Risk for injury: related to cerebral edema secondary to ICFVE.

Interventions and Rationale

1. Monitor vital signs and observe for behavioral changes. Assess the patient for progressive signs and symptoms of water intoxication such as headache, behavioral changes (irritability, drowsiness, confusion, disorientation, delirium), changes in the vital signs (increased blood pressure, decreased pulse, increased respiration), and warm, moist, flushed skin.

2. Protect the patient from injury during periods of confusion and disorientation. Keep bed rails up, assist the patient with ambulation, assist the patient with meals, and frequently reorient to place and time.

3. Observe for signs of seizure activity. Convulsions usually occur with severe ICFVE.

Evaluation/Outcome

1. Confirm that the cause of ICFVE has been corrected or controlled.

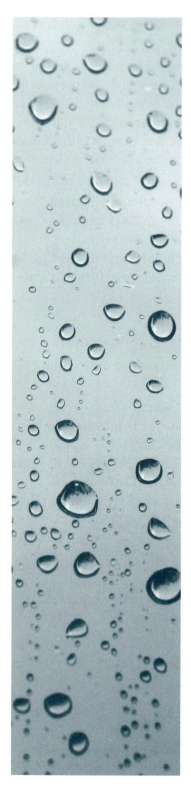

2. Evaluate the effects of clinical management for ICFVE: hypotonic/hypo-osmolar solutions discontinued, solutes offered with fluids.

3. Remain free of signs and symptoms of ICFVE or water intoxication. Vital signs return to normal ranges. Headaches have been lessened or absent.

4. Responds clearly without confusion.

5. Maintain a support system for patient.

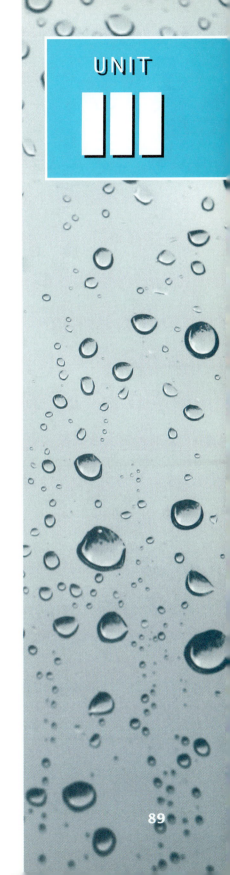

ELECTROLYTES AND THEIR INFLUENCE ON THE BODY

● LEARNING OUTCOMES

Upon completion of this unit, the reader will be able to:

- Describe the relationship of nonelectrolytes, electrolytes, and ions in body fluids.
- Name the principal cation and anion of the extracellular and intracellular fluids.
- Describe the physiologic functions of potassium, sodium, calcium, magnesium, phosphorus, and chloride.
- List the normal ranges of serum and urine potassium, sodium, calcium, magnesium, phosphorus, and chloride.
- Identify the various clinical causes (etiology) of potassium, sodium, calcium, magnesium, phosphorus, and chloride deficits or excesses.
- List the signs and symptoms of hypo-hyperkalemia, hypo-hypernatremia, hypo-hypercalcemia, hypo-hypermagnesemia, hypo-hyperphosphatemia, and hypo-hyperchloremia.
- Relate the electrolyte imbalances to drug action and interaction.
- Describe methods commonly utilized in electrolyte replacement therapy.
- Explain the assessment factors, diagnoses, and interventions to selected clinical situations (clinical applications).
- List foods that are rich in potassium, sodium, calcium, magnesium, phosphorus, and chloride.

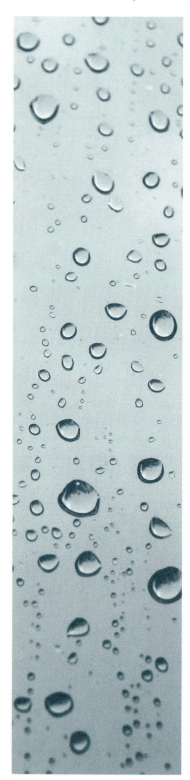

● INTRODUCTION

Chemical compounds may react in one of two ways when placed in solution. In one way, their molecules may remain intact as in urea, dextrose, and creatinine in the body fluid. These molecules do not produce an electrical charge and are considered nonelectrolytes.

In the other reaction, the compound develops a tiny electrical charge when dissolved in water. The compound breaks up into separate particles known as ions; this process is referred to as ionization, and the compounds are known as electrolytes. Some electrolytes develop a positive charge (cations) when placed in water; others develop a negative charge (anions).

The chemical composition of seawater and human body fluid is very similar. The principal cations of seawater are sodium, potassium, magnesium, and calcium, and so it is with the body fluid. The seawater contains as principal anions chloride, phosphate, and sulfate, the same as body fluid.

In Unit III, six electrolytes [potassium, sodium, calcium, magnesium, phosphorus (phosphate), and chloride] are discussed in relation to human body needs (functions), pathophysiology, etiology, clinical manifestations, and clinical management. Normal serum and urine levels, drug-laboratory test interactions, and foods rich in these electrolytes are presented. Clinical applications, clinical considerations, and case studies are discussed using the nursing process format—assessment, diagnoses, interventions, and evaluation/outcome.

An asterisk (*) on an answer line indicates a multiple-word answer. The meanings for the following symbols are: ↑ increased, ↓ decreased, > greater than, < less than.

ELECTROLYTES: CATION AND ANION

ANSWER COLUMN

1.

Electrolytes are compounds that when placed in solution, conduct an electric current.

Pure water does not conduct electricity, but if a pinch of salt, which contains sodium and chloride, is dropped into it, what do you think happens to the water? *_____
_____.

1. Salt (sodium and chloride) would produce an electrical charge. The water would conduct electricity

2.

Ions are dissociated particles of electrolytes that carry either a positive charge called a *cation* or a negative charge called an *anion.*

Dissociated particles of electrolytes are called _____.
The particles that carry a positive charge are called _____, and those that carry a negative charge are called _____.

2. ions; cations; anions

3. A cation carries a positive charge and an anion a negative charge.

3.

What is the difference between a cation and an anion? *_____
_____

Table U3-1 gives the principal cations and anions in human body fluid. Since we will be referring to these elements and their symbols throughout the program, take a

Table U3-1	Cations and Anions		
Cations		**Anions**	
Na^+	(Sodium)	Cl^-	(Chloride)
K^+	(Potassium)	HCO_3^-	(Bicarbonate)
Ca^{2+}	(Calcium)	HPO_4^{2-}	(Phosphate)
Mg^{2+}	(Magnesium)		

few minutes now to memorize them. Be sure to note the + and − symbols.

4.

Place a C in front of the cations and an A in front of anions.

_____ a. K   _____ e. Na

_____ b. Mg   _____ f. Ca

_____ c. Cl   _____ g. HPO_4

_____ d. HCO_3

4. a. C; b. C; c. A; d. A; e. C; f. C; g. A

5.

For electrical balance, the quantities of cations and anions in a solution, expressed in milliequivalents (mEq), always equal each other.

    Electrolytes differ in their chemical activity, for sodium has one positive charge and calcium has *_____.

5. two positive charges

6.

In studying serum chemistry alterations and concentrations, one is concerned with how much the ions or chemical particles weigh. The weight of ions and chemical particles is measured in milligrams percent (mg%), which is the same as mg/100 ml or mg/dl. The number of electrically charged ions is measured in milliequivalents per liter (1000 ml), or mEq/L.

    The term *milliequivalent* involves the chemical activity of elements, whereas milliosmol involves the _____ activity of the solution.

    How do milligrams and milliequivalents differ? *_____

6. osmotic; *Milligrams*, the weight of ions; *Milliequivalents*, the chemical activity of the ions.

7.

Milliequivalents provide a better method of measuring the concentration of ions in the serum than milligrams.

    Milligrams measure the _____ of ions and give no information concerning the number of ions or the electrical charges of the ions.

7. weight

8.

The following is a simple analogy to compare milligrams and milliequivalents.

    If you were having a party and wanted to invite equal numbers of males and females, which would be more

8. 15 females and 15 males; Otherwise you would have an unequal number of males and females for not every child weighs exactly 100 pounds.

accurate—inviting 1500 pounds of females and 1500 pounds of males or inviting 15 females and 15 males? *_____ Why? *_____

_____

9.

From the example in question 8, which would be more accurate in determining the serum chemistry of chemical particles or ions in the body—milliequivalents or milligrams? _____

9. milliequivalents

You will find both measurements used in this book and in your clinical settings for determining changes in our serum chemistry. However, when referring to ions, milliequivalents will be used in this book.

10.

The term *milliequivalents* is used to express the number of ionic charges of each electrolyte on an equal basis. It measures the _____ activity of ions or elements.

10. chemical; anions

The total cations in milliequivalents must equal the total _____ in milliequivalents.

11.

Milliequivalents consider electrolytes in terms of their

11. chemical activity

*_____ rather than their weight.

12.

Electrolytes have different weights but are considered during therapy in terms of their chemical activity, which is expressed as (milliequivalents/milligrams) _____.

12. milliequivalents

Table U3-2 gives the weights and equivalences of five ions. Note how the weights of the named ions differ but the equivalences remain the same according to their ionic charge.

13.

Name a cation and an anion with the same equivalence but different weights. *_____

13. sodium and chloride or potassium and chloride

_____

Table U3-2	**Electrolyte Equivalents**	
Ion	**Weight (mg)**	**Equivalence (mEq)**
Na^+	23	1
K^+	39	1
Cl^-	35	1
Ca^{++}	40	2
Mg^{++}	24	2

14.

The electrolyte composition of fluid differs within the two main classes of body fluid.

The two main classes of body water are *_____ fluid. What are the two main compartments of extracellular fluid?

*_____

14. intracellular and extracellular; intravascular and interstitial

Table U3-3 gives the ion concentrations of the intravascular fluid (which is frequently referred to as plasma), interstitial fluid, and intracellular fluid. Refer back to Table U3-3 when necessary.

15.

According to Table U3-3, the cation that is most plentiful in the extracellular body fluid is _____ and the cation that is most plentiful in the intracellular body fluid is _____.

15. sodium; potassium

Table U3-3	**Electrolyte Composition of Body Fluid (mEq/L)**		
	Extracellular		
Ions	**Intravascular or Plasma**	**Interstitial**	**Intracellular**
Na^+	142	145	10
K^+	5	4	141–150
Ca^{++}	5	3	2
Mg^{++}	2	1	27
Cl^-	104	116	1
HPO_3^-	27	30	10
HPO_4^{--}	2	2	100

16. sodium or Na, chloride
or Cl, and bicarbonate or
HCO$_3$; same as in
intravascular fluid;
potassium or K,
magnesium or Mg, and
phosphate or HPO$_4$

16.
What are the three principal ions in intravascular fluid? *_____

_____

What are the three principal ions in interstitial fluid? *_____

_____

What are the three principal ions in intracellular fluid? *_____

_____

Figure U3-1 shows the various cations and anions in extracellular and intracellular fluids. Refer to Figure U3-1 when necessary.

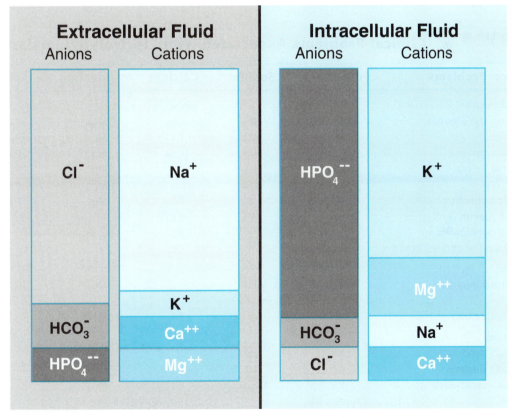

FIGURE U3-1 Anions and cations in body fluid.

17. sodium or Na; potassium
   or K

17.

The principal cation in extracellular fluid is _____.

The principal cation in intracellular fluid is _____.

18. chloride or Cl; phosphate
   or HPO₄

18.

The principal anion in extracellular fluid is _____.

The principal anion in intracellular fluid is _____.

Table U3-4 is a summary of the five electrolytes that either increase or decrease their specific electrolyte level 3, arranged according to clinical problems and drugs.

Table U3-4 **Clinical Problems Associated with Electrolyte Imbalances**

Clinical Problems	Potassium	Sodium	Calcium	Magnesium	Phosphorus
Gastrointestinal					
Vomiting and diarrhea	K↓	Na↓	Ca↓	Mg↓	P↓
Malnutrition	K↓	Na↓	Ca↓	Mg↓	P↓
Anorexia nervosa	K↓	Na↓	Ca↓	Mg↓	P↓
Intestinal fistula	K↓	Na↓		Mg↓	P↓
GI surgery	K↓	Na↓		Mg↓	P↓
Chronic alcoholism	K↓	Na↓	Ca↓	Mg↓	P↓
Lack of vitamin D			Ca↓		
Hyperphosphatemia			Ca↓		
Transfusion of citrated blood			Ca↓		
Cardiac					
Myocardial infarction	K↓	Na↓		Mg↓	
		Hypervolemia			
Heart failure (HF)	K↓/N	Na↑		Mg↓/N	
Endocrine					
Cushing's syndrome	K↓	Na↑		Mg↓	
Addison's disease	K↑	Na↓		Mg↑	
Diabetic ketoacidosis	K↑	Na↑/↓	Ca↓	Mg↑	P↓/N
	Diuresis K↓		(ionized)	Diuresis Mg↓	
Parathyroidism					
Hypo:			Ca↓		P↑
Hyper:			Ca↑		P↓
Renal					
Acute renal failure	Oliguria K↑	Na↑		Mg↑	P↑
	Diuresis K↓				
Chronic renal failure	K↑	Na↑	Ca↑/↓	Mg↑	P↑
					(continues)

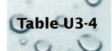

Table U3-4 **Clinical Problems Associated with Electrolyte Imbalances—***continued*

Clinical Problems	Potassium	Sodium	Calcium	Magnesium	Phosphorus
Miscellaneous					
Cancer	K↓/↑	Na↓	Ca↑	Mg↓	P↓
Bone destruction			Ca↑		
Burns	K↓/↑	Na↓	Ca↓	Mg↓	P↓
Acute pancreatitis			Ca↓		
SIADH (syndrome of inappropriate antidiuretic hormone)		Na↓			
Metabolic acidosis	K↑		Ca↓		
Metabolic alkalosis	K↓				
Drugs					
Diuretics					
Potassium wasting	K↓	Na↓	Ca↑/↓	Mg↓	
Potassium sparing	K↑/N	Na↓		Mg↓	
ACE inhibitors	K↑	Na↓/N			

Potassium Imbalances

 INTRODUCTION

Potassium (K) is the most abundant cation in the body cells. Ninety-seven percent of the body's potassium is found in the intracellular fluid, and 2–3% is found in the extracellular fluid (intravascular and interstitial fluids).

ANSWER COLUMN

1. intracellular; cation

1.

Although potassium is present in all body fluids, it is found predominantly in _____ fluid.

What kind of ion is potassium? _____

Figure 6-1 tells the effect of too much potassium or not enough in our body cells. Memorize the normal range of serum potassium. You may wonder why the range of serum potassium and not cell potassium is used to measure the potassium level, since the cells have the highest concentration of potassium. Serum potassium can be aspirated from the intravascular fluid but cannot be aspirated from potassium cells. When you are ready, go ahead to the frames following the figure and refer to Figure 6-1 when necessary.

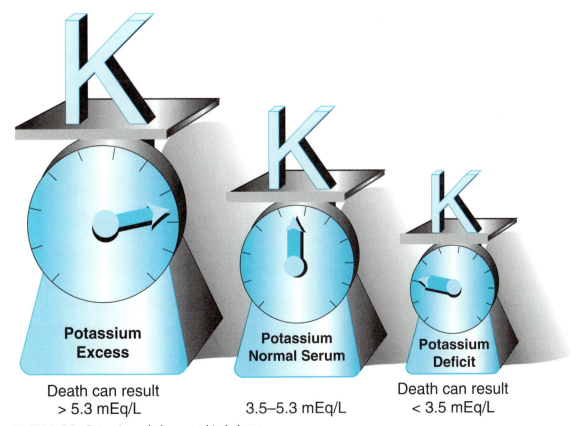

Potassium
Excess

Potassium
Normal Serum

Potassium
Deficit

Death can result
> 5.3 mEq/L

3.5–5.3 mEq/L

Death can result
< 3.5 mEq/L

FIGURE 6-1 Potassium—balance and imbalance.

2.

2. 3.5–5.3; Excess potassium buildup, leading to death.

The normal serum potassium range is _____ mEq/L. The intracellular potassium level is 150 mEq/L, but the concentration cannot be determined.

The kidneys excrete 80–90% of the potassium lost from the body. If the kidneys fail to function, what might result? * _____

_____

3.

3. Too much potassium causes irritability of the heart muscle, increasing and then decreasing the rate.; Too little potassium changes the conduction rate of nerve impulses and weakens the heart muscle, causing the heart to beat irregularly.

Either too much or too little potassium can cause a cardiac arrest. The heart needs potassium for conducting nerve impulses and contracting the heart muscle.

Why do you think too much potassium can cause a cardiac arrest? * _____

_____

Why do you think too little potassium can cause a cardiac arrest? * _____

_____

Note: If the answers are unknown, refer to the section on Functions and Pathophysiology and, particularly, question 11.

● FUNCTIONS

Table 6-1 gives the various functions of potassium according to body systems. Study Table 6-1 and refer to it as needed.

Table 6-1	Potassium and Its Functions
Body Involvement	**Function**
Neuromuscular	Transmission and conduction of nerve impulses
	Contraction of skeletal and smooth muscles
Cardiac	Nerve conduction and contraction of the myocardium
Cellular	Enzyme action for cellular energy production
	Deposits glycogen in liver cells
	Regulates osmolality of intracellular (cellular) fluids

4. nerve impulses; skeletal and smooth muscle and the myocardium

5. enzyme action and glycogen deposits in liver, also regulates intracellular osmolality

6. Potassium shifts into the cells after 1 hour of K ingestion. Renal excretion of potassium decreases the serum potassium level. (Renal excretion is a slower process.)

7. 50–100; 40–60

8. Consume bananas and other fruits as well as vegetables.

4.

Potassium is needed for transmission and conduction of
*_____. Also potassium is needed for the
contraction of *_____ muscles.

5.

Name two cellular activities of potassium. *_____

6.

The average daily oral intake of potassium is 50–100 mEq/day. Within the first hour, potassium from oral absorption shifts into the cells. Renal excretion is slower in response to increased potassium level. It takes 4–6 hours for the kidneys to excrete potassium.

    Identify two ways the body avoids excessive serum potassium levels after large oral potassium consumptions.
*_____
_____
_____

7.

Because potassium is not well stored in body cells, a daily potassium intake of 40–60 mEq is needed. Dietary potassium restriction does not necessarily cause a low serum potassium level unless the decreased potassium intake is prolonged or severely deficient.

    The average daily oral potassium intake is _____ mEq. The daily potassium intake needed for body function is _____ mEq.

8.

Foods rich in potassium include fruits (fresh, dry, and juices), vegetables, meats, and nuts. Particularly rich sources include bananas, dry fruits, and orange juice. If a person's serum potassium level is slightly decreased (3.4 mEq/L), what would you suggest? *_____
_____

9.

Potassium is continually moving between the intracellular fluid and the extracellular fluid, which is controlled by the sodium-potassium pump. Hormones increase the sodium-potassium pump activity. Insulin promotes cellular potassium uptake by shifting glucose and potassium into the cells. Aldosterone promotes potassium excretion and cellular potassium uptake.

The two hormones that can decrease the serum potassium level and increase the cellular potassium level are *_____

_____

9. insulin and aldosterone

10.

Insulin (increases/decreases) _____ the sodium-potassium pump activity.

10. increases

● PATHOPHYSIOLOGY

11.

A serum potassium level below 3.5 mEq/L is known as (hypokalemia/hyperkalemia) _____, and a serum potassium level above 5.3 mEq/L is called _____.

Cardiac arrest may occur if the serum potassium level is less than 2.5 mEq/L or greater than 7.0 mEq/L. Too little potassium (<3.5 mEq/L) changes the conduction rate of nerve impulses to the heart, causing dysrhythmia. Also too much potassium (>5.3 mEq/L) can cause irritability of the heart muscle, increasing and then decreasing the heart rate.

Match the serum potassium levels on the left with the type of potassium imbalance or balance.

_____ 1. 3.7 mEq/L   a. Hypokalemia
_____ 2. 4.8 mEq/L   b. Hyperkalemia
_____ 3. 5.9 mEq/L   c. Normal
_____ 4. 2.7 mEq/L
_____ 5. 3.1 mEq/L
_____ 6. 6.8 mEq/L

11. hypokalemia; hyperkalemia; 1. c; 2. c; 3. b; 4. a; 5. a; 6. b

12.

If the patient's serum potassium level is less than 2.5 mEq/L, what might occur? *_____

12. cardiac arrest

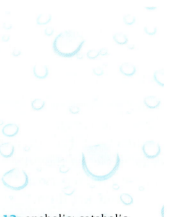

13.

The assimilative processes involved in the formation of new tissue (the synthesis of complex molecules from simple molecules) are referred to as *anabolism*, and the reactions concerned with tissue breakdown (the breakdown of complex molecules to simple molecules with a release of chemical energy) are referred to as *catabolism*.

When cellular activity is *anabolic* (state of building up), potassium enters the cells. When cellular activity is *catabolic* (state of breaking down), potassium leaves the cells.

Potassium enters the cells in _____ states and leaves the cells in _____ states.

13. anabolic; catabolic

14.

Potassium may leave the cells under various conditions. When tissues are destroyed as a result of trauma, starvation, or wasting diseases, large amounts of potassium *_____.

Potassium leaves the cells in _____ states.

14. leave the cells; catabolic

15.

During exercise, when muscles contract, the cells lose potassium and absorb a nearly equal quantity of sodium from the extracellular fluid. After exercise, when the muscles are recovering from fatigue, potassium reenters the cells and most of the sodium goes back into the extracellular fluid.

During exercise which ion may be increased over usual levels in the extracellular fluid—the potassium ion or the sodium ion? *_____

_____

15. The potassium ion. Of course it depends on how much exercise.

16.

During exercise, potassium leaves the cells, causing muscular fatigue.

After exercise, potassium *_____.

Potassium enters the cells in _____ states.

16. reenters the cells; anabolic

17.

After releasing potassium from the cells, the muscles are soft.

The soft muscles are a result of (hyperkalemia/hypokalemia) _____.

17. hypokalemia

18. trauma, exercise, starvation, wasting disease

18.

Name as many conditions as you can in which potassium might leave the cells. *_____

_____

19.

In stress caused by a harmful condition or severe emotional strain, an excessive amount of potassium is lost through the kidneys. The potassium leaves the cells, depleting the cells' supply. From the adrenal gland one of the adreno-cortical hormones, aldosterone, is produced in abundance during stress. This hormone influences the kidneys to excrete potassium and to retain sodium, chloride, and water.

Frequently the cations K and Na have an opposing effect on each other in the extracellular fluid. When one is retained, the other is excreted.

Therefore, with an excessive production of aldosterone, what happens to the cations K and Na in the extracellular fluid?

19. Potassium will be excreted and Na will be retained.

*_____

20.

When kidney function is normal, the excess potassium is slowly excreted by the kidneys. The range of potassium excreted daily by the kidneys is 20–120 mEq/L.

If potassium intake is decreased or if no potassium is taken orally or given intravenously, potassium is still excreted by the kidneys. Potassium is lost from the cells and the extracellular fluid (ECF) when potassium intake is diminished or absent. What type of potassium imbalance occurs?

20. hypokalemia

_____

21.

If the kidneys are injured or diseased and the urine output is markedly decreased, which of the following happen?

( ) a. The potassium concentration increases in the extracellular fluid.

( ) b. The potassium concentration increases in the intracellular fluid.

( ) c. The potassium is excreted through the skin.

21. a

● ETIOLOGY

The causes of hypokalemia and hyperkalemia are divided into two separate tables. Table 6-2 lists the etiology and rationale for hypokalemia and Table 6-3 gives the etiology and rationale for hyperkalemia. Study both tables carefully, noting the causes and reasons for these changes. Then proceed to the questions that follow. Refer to Tables 6-2 and 6-3 as needed.

22.
malnutrition and alcoholism (also reducing diets, anorexia nervosa)

22.
Name two causes of hypokalemia related to dietary changes.

*_____

23.
What is the daily potassium need for body function?

_____

23. 40–60 mEq

24. The diuretics promote loss of water, sodium, and potassium

24.
A major cause of potassium deficit is potassium-wasting diuretics. Why? *_____

25.
Gastrointestinal (GI) losses account for the second major cause of potassium deficit. List three GI causes of hypokalemia.

*_____

25. vomiting, diarrhea, and GI suctioning (also laxative abuse, bulimia)

26. deficit; Potassium is lost from the cells due to tissue injury with normal kidney function.

26.
Trauma and injury to tissues as a result of burns and surgery can cause potassium (deficit/excess) _____. Why?

*_____

27. hypokalemia; Licorice has an aldosteronelike effect, thus promoting potassium excretion and sodium retention.

27.
Excessive ingestion of licorice can cause (hypokalemia/hyperkalemia) _____.

Why? *_____

_____

Table 6-2	Causes of Hypokalemia (Serum Potassium Deficit)
Etiology	**Rationale**
Dietary Changes Malnutrition, starvation, alcoholism, unbalanced reducing diets, anorexia nervosa, crash diets	Potassium is poorly conserved in the body. For a potassium deficit to occur, a prolonged, inadequate potassium intake must occur.
Gastrointestinal Losses Vomiting, diarrhea, gastric/intestinal suctioning, intestinal fistula, laxative abuse, bulimia, enemas	Potassium is plentiful in the GI tract. With the loss of GI secretions, large amounts of potassium ions are lost.
Renal Losses Diuretics, diuretic phase of acute renal failure, hemodialysis and peritoneal dialysis	The kidneys excrete 80–90% of the potassium lost. Diuretics are the major cause of hypokalemia, especially potassium-wasting diuretics [thiazides, loop (high-ceiling), osmotic]
Hormonal Influence Steroids, Cushing's syndrome, stress, excessive intake of licorice, Insulin	Steroids, especially cortisone and aldosterone, promote potassium excretion and sodium retention. Stress increases the production of steroids in the body. In Cushing's syndrome, there is an excess production of adrenocortical hormones (corticol and aldosterone). Licorice contains glyceric acid, which has an aldosteronelike effect. Insulin moves glucose and potassium into the cells.
Cellular Damage Trauma, tissue injury, surgery, burns	Cellular and tissue damage cause potassium to be released in the intravascular fluid. More potassium is needed to repair injured tissue.
Acid-Base Imbalance Metabolic alkalosis	Metabolic alkalosis promotes the movement of potassium into cells.
Drugs Promoting Hypokalemia Sympathomimetics (adrenergics) Epinephrine, decongestants, bronchodilators, beta$_2$-adrenergic agonists	These drugs promote potassium excretion.
Amphotericin B, aminoglycosides, large doses of penicillin	These drugs promote renal excretion of potassium.
Electrolyte Loss Magnesium deficit	Hypomagnesemia can cause renal excretion of potassium. Usually potassium deficit is not corrected until magnesium deficit is corrected.

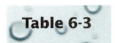

Table 6-3	Causes of Hyperkalemia (Serum Potassium Excess)
Etiology	**Rationale**
Excessive Potassium Intake Oral potassium supplements, salt substitutes, nutritional supplements, and herbal juices	A potassium consumption rate greater than the potassium excretion rate increases the serum potassium level. Many salt substitutes are rich in potassium. Nutritional supplements and herbal juices can be high in potassium.
IV potassium infusions	Adequate urinary output must be determined when giving a potassium supplement.
Decreased Renal Function Acute renal failure Chronic renal failure	Because potassium is generally excreted in the urine, anuria and oliguria cause a potassium buildup in the plasma.
Altered Cellular Function Severe traumatic injury	Cellular injury increases potassium loss due to cell breakdown. Potassium excretion may be greater than cellular K reabsorption. Potassium can accumulate in the plasma.
Acid-Base Imbalance Metabolic acidosis	In acidosis, the hydrogen ion moves into the cells and potassium moves out of the cells, increasing the serum potassium level.
Old Blood Blood for transfusion that is 1–3 weeks old	As stored blood for transfusion ages, hemolysis (breakdown of red blood cells) occurs; potassium from the cells are released into the ECF.
Hormonal Deficiency Addison's disease	Reduced secretion of the adrenocortical hormones causes a retention of potassium and a loss of sodium.
Drugs-Potassium-Sparing Diuretics, ACE inhibitors, beta blockers	Potassium-sparing diuretics can cause an aldosterone deficiency, promoting potassium retention; see Table 6-8.
Pseudohyperkalemia Hemolysis	With hemolysis, ruptured red blood cells release potassium into the ECF.
Tourniquet application Phlebotomy, clenching of the fist	A tourniquet that has been applied too tightly or rapidly drawing blood with a small needle lumen (<18 gauge) can cause a falsely elevated potassium level in the blood specimen.

28. Insulin moves potassium into the cells along with glucose, and alkalosis (metabolic) promotes the exchange of potassium ions for hydrogen ions in the cells. Either can cause a low serum potassium level (hypokalemia).

28.

How do insulin and alkalotic states affect potassium balance?

*_____

_____

29. a. diarrhea, vomiting, gastric suction; b. starvation, anorexia nervosa, bulimia; c. diuretics—potassium wasting; d. burns; e. trauma or injury; f. surgery; Also: stress; increase of adreno-cortical hormones (steroids); metabolic alkalosis

30. The kidneys excrete 80–90% of excess potassium. With increased potassium ingestion and poor urine output, hyperkalemia can result.

31. hyperkalemia

32. metabolic acidosis
33. hyperkalemia (potassium excess); Most salt substitutes contain potassium instead of sodium. If the potassium cannot be excreted because of renal insufficiency, potassium excess occurs.

34. hemolysis or a tightly applied tourniquet to obtain blood sample; also, rapidly drawing blood through a small needle lumen and clenching of the fist

29.

List six clinical conditions causing a potassium deficit:

a. _____

b. _____

c. _____

d. _____

e. _____

f. _____

30.

The serum potassium level should be monitored for patients taking large doses of a potassium supplement. This is especially true when the daily urine output is diminished.

Why? *_____

_____

31.

A patient should not receive more than 10 mEq of IV potassium per hour that has been diluted in intravenous solution.

Usually 20–40 mEq of potassium chloride is diluted in 1 liter of IV fluids.

Potassium in IV fluids administered at a rate faster than 20 mEq/L per hour for 24–72 hours can result in (hypokalemia/hyperkalemia) _____.

32.

Hyperkalemia may occur during (metabolic alkalosis/metabolic acidosis) *_____

33.

A patient having renal impairment is taking salt substitutes to decrease sodium intake. What type of electrolyte imbalance is likely to occur when using salt substitutes? _____

Why? *_____

_____

34.

Pseudohyperkalemia may occur due to _____ or

_____

*_____.

35.

Which of the following are causes of potassium excess (hyperkalemia)?

( ) a. Potassium-wasting diuretics
( ) b. Potassium-sparing diuretics
( ) c. Adrenal gland insufficiency
( ) d. Vomiting, diarrhea
( ) e. Multiple transfusions of old blood
( ) f. Metabolic acidosis with poor kidney function
( ) g. Renal shutdown

35. b, c, e, f, g

● CLINICAL MANIFESTATIONS

36.

Although 98% of potassium is found in cells, focus is placed on the extracellular fluid, for it is more readily available for study. Intracellular levels are not clinically available.

The normal serum potassium level (in extracellular fluid) is _____ mEq/L.

36. 3.5–5.3

Table 6-4 lists the signs and symptoms associated with hypokalemia and hyperkalemia. Clinical manifestations can be determined by the serum potassium level, electrocardiography (ECG/EKG), and signs and symptoms related to gastrointestinal, cardiac, renal, and neurologic abnormalities. The serum potassium level and the ECG play the most important role in determining the severity of the potassium imbalance.

Patients with hypokalemia and hyperkalemia can be found in many clinical settings. You may save a patient's life by recognizing and reporting symptoms of potassium imbalance.

37.

Hypokalemia causes the muscle to become soft, like "half-filled water bottles," and weak. The abdomen becomes bloated due to smooth-muscle weakness and not due to flatus. The blood pressure goes down (hypotension) and dizziness occurs. Malaise or uneasiness occurs.

37. dysrhythmia (arrhythmia)

The heart beat is irregular, known as _____. Eventually, if the irregularity of the heart beat is not corrected, bradycardia occurs and finally cardiac arrest.

Table 6-4	Clinical Manifestations of Potassium Imbalances	
Body Involvement	**Hypokalemia**	**Hyperkalemia**
Gastrointestinal Abnormalities	*Anorexia Nausea *Vomiting Diarrhea †Abdominal distention †Decreased peristalsis or silent ileus	*Nausea *Diarrhea †Abdominal cramps
Cardiac Abnormalities	†Cardiac dysrhythmias †Vertigo Cardiac arrest when severe	Tachycardia, later †bradycardia, and finally cardiac arrest (severe)
ECG/EKG	†Flat or inverted T wave Depressed ST segment	†Peaked, narrow T wave Shortened QT interval Prolonged PR interval followed by disappearance of P wave Prolonged QRS interval if level continues to rise
Renal Abnormalities	Polyuria	†Oliguria or anuria
Neuromuscular Abnormalities	†Malaise Drowsiness †Muscular weakness Confusion Mental depression Diminished deep tendon reflexes Respiratory paralysis	Weakness, numbness, or tingling sensation Muscle cramps
Laboratory Values Serum potassium	<3.5 mEq/L	>5.3 mEq/L

†Most commonly seen symptoms of hypo-hyperkalemia.
*Commonly seen symptoms of hypo-hyperkalemia.

38. hypokalemia

38.
A weak grip, an irregular pulse, and dizziness upon standing may be signs of _____.

39.
The T wave on the ECG/EKG differs with the potassium imbalance. With a low serum potassium level, the T wave will become flat or invert, and with an elevated serum potassium level, the T wave will peak. See Figures 6-2 and 6-3.

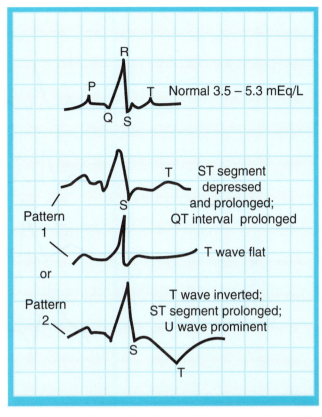

FIGURE 6-2 Electrocardiographic changes in serum potassium deficit.

Match the T wave changes on the left with the type of potassium imbalance.

_____ 1. Peaked T wave   a. Hypokalemia

_____ 2. Flat T wave   b. Hyperkalemia

_____ 3. Inverted T wave

40.

Name the six most commonly seen symptoms of hypokalemia.
*
_____

_____

41.

With hyperkalemia, the heart beats very fast, which is known as _tachycardia._ The heart goes into a block, with few or no impulses being transmitted, and finally cardiac arrest occurs.

You recall that the kidneys are responsible for excreting excessive amounts of potassium not needed by the body.

39. 1. b; 2. a; 3. a

40. abdominal distention, decreased peristalsis or silent ileus, dizziness, dysrhythmia/ arrhythmia, malaise, and muscular weakness

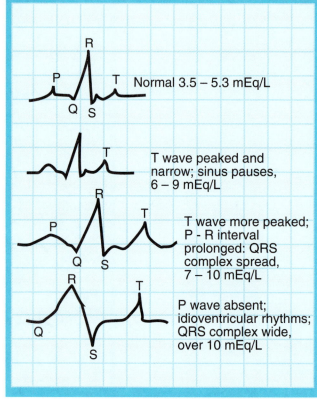

FIGURE 6-3 Electrocardiographic changes in serum potassium concentration. Changes are most marked in the precordial leads over the right side (V1–V4 position) of the heart.

41. Increase in potassium (hyperkalemia); Increase (tachycardia) and later decrease (bradycardia)

If the kidneys excrete a small amount of urine, known as *oliguria,* or no urine, known as *anuria,* what can occur to the potassium level? *_____.

What would you think happens to the heart rate? *_____
_____.

42. abdominal cramps, tachycardia and later bradycardia, and oliguria or anuria

42.

Name the three most commonly seen symptoms of hyperkalemia. *_____
_____

43.

With prolonged hypokalemia, circulatory failure and eventual heart failure can result. The electrocardiogram frequently shows a flat or inverted T wave. With potassium excess, the electrocardiogram shows a peaked T wave.

Serum potassium levels below 2.5 mEq/L and above 7.0 mEq/L are extremely dangerous and need immediate attention. Without correction, what type of heart condition can occur?

*_____

43. cardiac arrest

Figures 6-2 and 6-3 note electrocardiographic changes found with hypo-hyperkalemia.

A brief review of the electrocardiogram. The ECG measures the electrical activity from various areas of the heart and records this as P, QRS, and T waves.

The *P wave* measures the electrical activity initiating contraction of the atrium or the atrial muscle.

The *QRS wave complex* measures the electrical activity initiating contraction of the ventricle, which is the thickest part of the heart muscle responsible for forcing blood from the heart into the circulation. A "heart attack," also known as myocardial infarction, frequently affects this part of the heart muscle.

The *T wave* is the electrical recovery of the ventricles.

Abnormal potassium levels affect the T wave of the electrocardiogram. Note the normal T wave structure in Figure 6-2 and compare the normal with the abnormal, with patterns 1 and 2. Study Figure 6-2 and then proceed to the questions.

44.

The two abnormal changes in the T wave that occur with hypokalemia are *_____.

44. flat T wave and inverted T wave

45.

The ST segment is prolonged in both patterns in Figure 6-2. This change relates to a *_____.

45. potassium deficit

46.

With a serum potassium *deficit* which of the following electrocardiographic changes may occur?

( ) a. Flat T wave
( ) b. Inverted T wave
( ) c. High-peaked T wave
( ) d. Depressed and prolonged ST segment

46. a, b, d

High-peaked T waves are an early electrocardiographic sign of hyperkalemia. Heart block can result from severe hyperkalemia, e.g., 8–10 mEq/L of serum potassium. Study Figure 6-3 carefully, noting especially the T waves, QRS complex, and P wave.

47.

47. high-peaked T wave

Name the abnormal change in the T wave occurring with hyperkalemia. *_____

48.

48. hypokalemic; hyperkalemic

A flat or inverted T wave on an electrocardiogram frequently indicates a _____ state, whereas a high-peaked T wave can indicate a _____ state.

49.

Which of the following electrocardiographic changes can occur with a high serum potassium?

   (   ) a. Flat T wave
   (   ) b. Inverted T wave
   (   ) c. High-peaked T wave
   (   ) d. Depressed and prolonged ST segment
   (   ) e. QRS complex spread
   (   ) f. Prolonged P-R interval

49. c, e, f

50.

Match the following ECG changes on the left with the electrolyte abnormalities on the right. Refer to Figures 6-2 and 6-3 as needed.

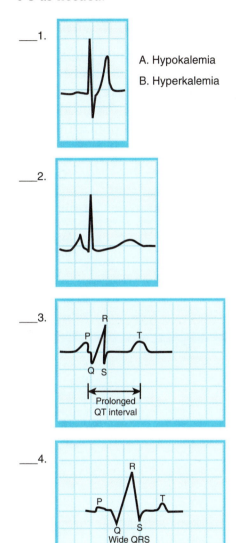

___1.

A. Hypokalemia

B. Hyperkalemia

___2.

___3.

___4.

50. 1. b; 2. a; 3. a; 4. b

● CLINICAL MANAGEMENT

Clinical management of hypokalemia consists of oral supplements (tablets, capsules, liquid) and/or IV potassium diluted in an IV solution. To correct hyperkalemia, potassium intake is restricted and various drugs can be used to lower the serum potassium level. First, potassium replacement for hypokalemia is discussed and, then, drug modalities are presented for correcting hyperkalemia.

Potassium Replacement

Oral potassium supplements help to replace potassium losses due to potassium-wasting diuretics, inadequate nutritional intake, and disease entities that increase potassium losses. Table 6-5 contains examples of frequently ordered oral potassium supplements.

Table 6-5	Oral Potassium Supplements
Preparation	**Drug**
Liquid	Potassium chloride 10% = 20 mEq/15 ml; 20% = 40 mEq/15 ml
	Kay Ciel (potassium chloride)
	Kaochlor 10% (potassium chloride)
	Kaon Cl 20% (potassium chloride)
	Potassium triplex (potassium acetate, bicarbonate, citrate)
Tablet/capsule	Potassium chloride (enteric-coated tablet)
	Kaon—plain (potassium gluconate)
	Kaon Cl (potassium chloride)
	Slow K (potassium chloride—8 mEq)
	Kaochlor (potassium chloride)
	K-Lyte—plain (potassium bicarbonate-effervescent tablet)
	K-Lyte/Cl (potassium chloride)

51.

51. potassium chloride (liquid or tablet)

Name a drug that corrects serum potassium and serum chloride deficits. *_____

52.

52. Potassium triplex and K-Lyte-plain (also Kaon—plain). The gluconate in Kaon is converted to bicarbonate. Kaon comes with or without Cl.

Oral potassium may be extremely irritating to the gastric mucosa and should be diluted in at least 6–8 ounces of water or juice.

Name two oral potassium supplements that contain bicarbonate. *_____

_____

53. no; Because 80–90% of potassium is excreted from the body by the kidneys; hyperkalemia might result.

53.

There have been reports of deaths related to hyperkalemia caused by oral potassium supplements.

 Would oral potassium supplements be recommended for a person with poor kidney function? _____

 Why? * _____

_____

54. hyperkalemia; potassium accumulation in the ECF; also ECG changes, even death.

54.

Severe serum hyperkalemia may occur from administering an intravenous potassium solution too rapidly, thus not allowing enough time for the potassium to pass into the cells.

 The normal dose of intravenous potassium is 20–40 mEq in 1 liter of solution to run over 8 hours or no more than 10 mEq of KCl per hour. What might result from administering 40 mEq of potassium per hour? _____

 Why? * _____

55. Cardiac arrest. Potassium concentration is extremely irritating to the myocardium (heart muscle); phlebitis (inflammation of the vein) and infiltration (tissue sloughing or necrosis)

55.

Intravenous potassium is irritating to blood vessels (can cause phlebitis) and tissues (can cause sloughing and necrosis).

 Potassium should NEVER be given as a bolus (injected directly into the vein).

 What might happen if a bolus injection of potassium chloride (KCl) is given?

 * _____

 The nurse should assess the infusion site when the patient is receiving intravenous KCl for _____ and

_____.

56. 20–40 mEq/L

56.

For severe hypokalemia (<3.0 mEq/L) 40–60 mEq of KCl can be diluted in 1 liter of IV fluids, and no more than 20 mEq per hour should be given.

 For a life-threatening hypokalemic situation (<2.6 mEq/L), 30–40 mEq of KCl can be diluted in 100–150 ml of D_5W and administered through a central venous line in 1 hour.

 What is the recommended KCl dosage to be diluted in 1 liter of IV fluids? * _____

57.

In hypokalemia, if the serum potassium level is 3.0–3.5 mEq/L, 100–200 mEq of KCl is needed to raise the serum level 1 mEq/L. Remember, do not administer the KCl all at once; a high concentration is toxic to the heart muscle and irritating to the blood vessels.

If the serum potassium level is below 3.0 mEq/L, 200–400 mEq of KCl is needed to raise the serum level 1 mEq/L.

If an individual has a serum potassium level of 2.7 mEq/L, how much KCl, administered, is needed to raise the serum level to 3.7 mEq/L? *_____

57. 200–400 mEq

58.

The daily potassium requirement is 40–60 mEq. A patient with a serum potassium of 3.3 mEq/L must (increase/decrease) _____ daily potassium intake.

58. increase

Hyperkalemia Correction

In mild hyperkalemic conditions (5.4–5.6 mEq/L), correcting the cause of the potassium excess and restricting the potassium intake may correct the hyperkalemic state. Interventions to temporarily correct a moderate hyperkalemic state (6.0 mEq/L) include IV sodium bicarbonate infusion, insulin and glucose infusion, and IV calcium salt. Correcting the cause of the potassium excess is often successful in lowering the serum potassium level. In severe hyperkalemic conditions (>6.7 mEq/L), Kayexalate and sorbitol are usually prescribed.

Table 6-6 describes various methods used to correct a potassium excess (hyperkalemia). Study Table 6-6 carefully and refer to it as needed.

59.

To correct mild hyperkalemia, restriction of potassium intake is suggested.

Would you correct a hyperkalemia of 7.0 mEq/L by restricting potassium intake? _____

Why? *_____

59. no; It is severe hyperkalemia, and this method is too slow.

Table 6-6	Correction of Potassium Excess (Hyperkalemia)
Treatment Methods	**Rationale**
Potassium restriction	Restriction of potassium intake slowly lowers the serum level. For mild hyperkalemia (slightly elevated K levels), i.e., 5.4–5.6 mEq/L, potassium restriction is normally effective.
IV sodium bicarbonate ($NaHCO_3$)	By elevating the pH level, potassium moves back into the cells, thus lowering the serum level. This is a temporary treatment.
10% Calcium gluconate	Calcium decreases the irritability of the myocardium resulting from hyperkalemia. It is a temporary treatment and does not promote K loss. *Caution:* Administering calcium to a patient on digitalis can cause digitalis toxicity.
Insulin and glucose (10–50%)	The combination of insulin and glucose moves potassium back into the cells. It is a temporary treatment, effective for approximately 6 hrs, and is not always as effective when repeated.
Kayexalate (sodium polystyrene) and sorbitol 70%	Kayexalate is used as a cation exchange for severe hyperkalemia and can be administered orally or rectally. Approximate dosages are as follows: *Orally:* Kayexalate—10–20 g 3 to 4 times daily Sorbitol 70%—20 ml with each dose *Rectally:* Kayexalate—30–50 g Sorbitol 70%—50 ml; mix with 100–150 ml water (Retention enema—20–30 mins)

60.

For temporary correction of a moderate potassium excess, indicate which methods are most effective:

( ) a. Potassium restriction diet
( ) b. IV sodium bicarbonate
( ) c. 10% Calcium gluconate
( ) d. Insulin and glucose
( ) e. Kayexalate and sorbitol

60. b, c, d

61.

If a patient is taking digoxin and has a serum potassium of 7.4 mEq/L, is 10% calcium gluconate indicated for temporary correction of hyperkalemia? _____

Explain. * _____

61. no; Calcium administration enhances the action of digitalis, causing digitalis toxicity.

62.

Drugs such as Kayexalate (sodium polystyrene sulfonate), a cation exchange resin, and sorbitol 70% are given for severe hyperkalemia. They cause a sodium-potassium ion exchange, and the potassium is excreted.

What treatment is suggested for mild hyperkalemia?
*_____

What treatment is suggested for severe hyperkalemia?
*_____

62. Restrict potassium intake.; Kayexalate and sorbitol—ion exchange.

Drugs and Their Effect on Potassium Balance

63.

Diuretics are divided into two categories: potassium wasting and potassium sparing. Potassium-wasting diuretics excrete potassium and other electrolytes such as sodium and chloride in the urine. Potassium-sparing diuretics retain potassium but excrete sodium and chloride in the urine.

Indicate the electrolytes that are lost when potassium-sparing diuretics are taken:
( ) a. Potassium
( ) b. Sodium
( ) c. Chloride

63. b, c

Table 6-7 lists the trade and generic names of potassium-wasting and potassium-sparing diuretics and a combination of potassium-wasting and potassium-sparing diuretics. Study the types of diuretic in each category and refer to Table 6-7 as needed.

64.

Name the potassium imbalance that is most likely to occur in patients taking a potassium-sparing diuretic, who have poor kidney function. *_____

64. potassium excess (hyperkalemia)

65.

Potassium-wasting diuretics can cause (hypokalemia/hyperkalemia) _____.

65. hypokalemia

Table 6-7	Potassium-Wasting and Potassium-Sparing Diuretics

Potassium-Wasting Diuretics	Potassium-Sparing Diuretics
Thiazides	Aldosterone antagonist
Chlorothiazide/Diuril	Spironolactone/Aldactone
Hydrochlorothiazide/HydroDiuril	Triamterene/Dyrenium
Loop diuretics	Amiloride/Midamor
Furosemide/Lasix	
Ethacrynic acid/Edecrin	*Combination: K-Wasting and*
Carbonic anhydrase inhibitors	*K-Sparing Diuretics*
Acetazolamide/Diamox	Aldactazide
Osmotic diuretic	Spironazide
Mannitol	Dyazide
	Moduretic

66.

Enter W for potassium-wasting, S for potassium-sparing, and C for a combination of potassium-wasting and potassium-sparing diuretics for the following drugs. Refer to Table 6-7 as needed:

( ) a. Chlorothiazide/Diuril
( ) b. Aldactazide
( ) c. Triamterene/Dyrenium
( ) d. Acetazolamide/Diamox
( ) e. Amiloride/Midamor
( ) f. Dyazide
( ) g. Spironolactone/Aldactone
( ) h. Hydrochlorothiazide/HydroDiuril
( ) i. Furosemide/Lasix
( ) j. Ethacrynic acid/Edecrin
( ) k. Mannitol

66. a. W; b. C; c. S; d. W; e. S; f. C; g. S; h. W; i. W; j. W; k. W

Laxatives, corticosteroids, antibiotics, potassium-wasting diuretics, and beta$_2$ agonists are the major drug groups that can cause a potassium deficit, or hypokalemia. The drug groups attributed to potassium excess, or hyperkalemia, are oral and intravenous potassium salts, central nervous system (CNS) agents, potassium-sparing diuretics, ACE inhibitors, beta blockers, heparin, and NSAIDs. Table 6-8 lists the drugs that affect potassium balance. Refer to the table as needed.

Table 6-8	**Drugs Affecting Potassium Balance**	
Potassium Imbalance	**Substances**	**Rationale**
Hypokalemia (serum potassium deficit)	Laxatives	Laxative abuse can cause potassium depletion.
	Enemas (hyperosmolar)	
	Corticosteroids	
	Cortisone	Ion exchange agent.
	Prednisone	Steroids promote potassium loss and sodium retention.
	Kayexalate	Exchange potassium ion for a sodium ion.
	Licorice	Licorice action is similar to aldosterone, promoting K loss and Na retention.
	Levodopa/L-dopa	Increases potassium loss via urine.
	Lithium	
	Antibiotic I	
	Amphotericin B	Toxic effect on renal tubules, thus decreasing potassium reabsorption.
	Polymyxin B	
	Tetracycline (outdated)	
	Gentamicin	
	Neomycin	
	Amikacin	
	Tobramycin	
	Cisplatin	
	Antibiotic II	
	Penicillin	Potassium excretion is enhanced by the presence of nonreabsorbable anions.
	Ampicillin	
	Carbenicillin	
	Ticarcillin	
	Nafcillin	
	Piperacillin	
	Azlocillin	
	Alpha-adrenergic blockers	These agents promote movement of potassium into cells, thus lowering the serum potassium level.
	Insulin and glucose	
	Beta$_2$ agonists	
	Terbutaline	These beta$_2$ agonists promote potassium loss.
	Albuterol	
	Estrogen	
	Potassium-wasting diuretics	See Table 6-7.

(continues)

Table 6-8 **Drugs Affecting Potassium Balance—*continued***

Potassium Imbalance	Substances	Rationale
Hyperkalemia (serum potassium excess)	Potassium chloride (oral or IV) Potassium salt (substitute) K penicillin KPO$_4$ enema Angiotensin-converting enzyme (ACE) inhibitors	Excess ingestion or infusion of these agents can cause a potassium excess.
	Captopril (Capoten) Quinapril HCl (Accupril) Ramipril (Altace) and others Angiotensin II receptor antagonists	Increase the state of hypoaldosteronism (decrease sodium and increase potassium) and impair renal potassium excretion.
	Losartan potassium (Cozaar)	Decrease adrenal synthesis of aldosterone; potassium is retained and sodium excreted.
	Beta-adrenergic blockers Propranolol (Inderal) Nadolol (Corgard) and others	Decrease cellular uptake of potassium and decrease Na-K-ATPase function.
	Digoxin	Therapeutic dose is not affected; however, with overdose, potassium excess may occur.
	Heparin (> 10,000 units/d)	Inhibits adrenal aldosterone production.
	Low-molecular-weight heparin (LMWH)	Decreases potassium homeostasis; renal excretion of potassium is reduced.
	Immunosuppressive drugs Cyclosporine Tacrolimus Cyclophosphamide Nonsteroidal anti-inflammatory drugs (NSAIDs)	Reduce potassium excretion by induction of hypoaldosteronism; loss of potassium from cells.
	Ibuprofens and others Indomethacin	Impair potassium homeostasis and block cellular potassium uptake.
	Succinylcholine: intravenous	Allows for leakage of potassium out of cells.
	CNS agents Barbiturates Sedatives Narcotics Heroin Amphetamines	These CNS agents are usually characterized by muscle necrosis and cellular shift of potassium from cells to serum.
	Potassium-sparing diuretics	See Table 6-7.

67.

Enter KD for potassium deficit/hypokalemia and KE for potassium excess/hyperkalemia beside the drugs that can cause a potassium imbalance. Refer to Table 6-8 as needed:

_____ a. Laxatives

_____ b. Corticosteroids

_____ c. Barbiturates

_____ d. Narcotics

_____ e. ACE inhibitors

_____ f. Licorice

_____ g. Antibiotics

_____ h. Levodopa

_____ i. Heparin

_____ j. Potassium chloride

_____ k. Succinylcholine/Anectine

_____ l. Terbutaline/Brethine

67. a. KD; b. KD; c. KE; d. KE; e. KE; f. KD; g. KD; h. KD; i. KE; j. KE; k. KE; l. KD

68.

Digoxin is a drug that strengthens the heart muscle and slows down the heart beat. A serum potassium deficit, or hypokalemia, enhances the action of digoxin and causes the drug to become more potent. Digitalis toxicity or intoxication (slow and irregular pulse, nausea and vomiting, anorexia) can result from a low serum potassium level.

Thiazides and loop diuretics can cause (hypokalemia/hyperkalemia) _____.

The nurse needs to be alert for what type of drug toxicity when a patient is taking potassium-wasting diuretics and digoxin? _____

68. hypokalemia; digitalis toxicity

69.

Common symptoms of digitalis toxicity are bradycardia (slow heart beat) and/or dysrhythmia (arrhythmia).

Can you name two other symptoms of digitalis toxicity?

a. * _____

b. _____

69. a. nausea and vomiting; b. anorexia

70. more

71. it enhances the action of digitalis; it decreases the action of quinidine

72. hypokalemia or potassium deficit; Hypokalemia precipitates digitalis toxicity by enhancing the action of digoxin.

73. increase; ACE inhibitors impair renal potassium excretion and cause hypoaldosteronism. Beta-adrenergic blockers decrease cellular uptake of potassium.

74. Heparin and low-molecular-weight heparin decrease potassium homeostasis and reduce renal potassium excretion.

75. Nonsteroidal anti-inflammatory drugs (NSAIDs); potassium excess or hyperkalemia

70.

A serum potassium excess (hyperkalemia) inhibits the action of digoxin. If a person has a serum potassium of 5.8 mEq/L, (more/less) _____ digoxin will be needed to obtain the appropriate digoxin dosage.

71.

Quinidine is an antidysrhythmic drug used to correct irregular heart rates. Hypokalemia blocks the effects of quinidine; therefore more quinidine may be needed to produce therapeutic action. Hyperkalemia enhances the action of quinidine and can produce quinidine toxicity and myocardium depression.

   Explain the effect of hypokalemia:
On digitalis * _____
On quinidine * _____

72.

Cortisone causes excretion of potassium and retention of sodium. If a person takes digoxin hydrochlorothiazide/HydroDiuril, and prednisone/cortisone daily, what type of severe electrolyte imbalance can result? * _____

   Explain the effect this imbalance has on digoxin.

* _____

73.

ACE inhibitors and beta blockers (decrease/increase) _____ the serum potassium level.

   Explain. * _____

74.

Heparin and LMWH may increase serum potassium level.
   Explain. * _____

75.

What type of drug are the ibuprofens? * _____

   They may cause what type of potassium imbalance if taken in excess or if the patient has renal insufficiency?

* _____

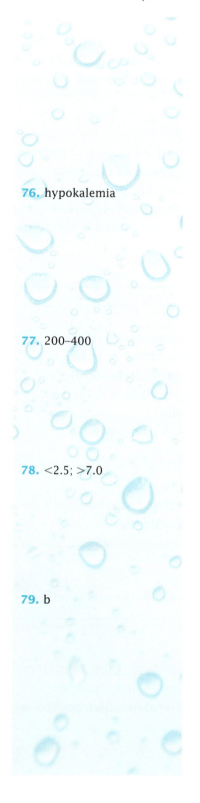

● CLINICAL APPLICATIONS

76.

Approximately 2% of healthy adults develop hypokalemia. Twenty to 80% of persons taking potassium-wasting diuretics develop hypokalemia. Hypokalemia is present in about 20% of hospitalized patients, and hyperkalemia occurs in approximately 10% of hospitalized patients.

   The most common potassium imbalance in hospitalized patients is (hypokalemia/hyperkalemia) _____.

76. hypokalemia

77.

Five percent of hospitalized patients with hypokalemia have a serum potassium level lower than 3.0 mEq/L. One to 2% of hospitalized clients having hyperkalemia have a serum potassium level greater than 6.0 mEq/L.

   A patient with a serum potassium level below 3.0 mEq/L requires approximately _____ mEq of potassium to raise the serum potassium level 1 mEq/L.

77. 200–400

78.

An example of a severe serum potassium deficit that is life threatening is a serum potassium level of _____ mEq/L. An example of a severe serum potassium excess that is life threatening is _____ mEq/L.

78. <2.5; >7.0

79.

Eighty to 90% of potassium excretion is lost in the urine, and only a very small percentage is lost in the feces.

   Which of the following promotes a greater loss of potassium?
   ( ) a. An individual taking a laxative
   ( ) b. An individual taking a diuretic

79. b

80.

Hyperglycemia, an increased blood sugar, is a symptom of diabetes mellitus. Cells cannot utilize glucose; thus, catabolism (cellular breakdown) occurs, and potassium leaves the cells and is excreted by the kidneys. If the kidneys are not functioning adequately (<600 ml/day), potassium can accumulate and serum potassium excess can occur.

When cells do not receive their proper nutrition, what happens to the cells? *_____

_____

In hyperglycemia (hypokalemia/hyperkalemia) _____ occurs due to cellular breakdown and polyuria. If there is kidney shutdown, (hypokalemia/ hyperkalemia) _____ occurs.

80. catabolism—cellular breakdown with loss of potassium; hypokalemia; hyperkalemia

81.

Administering glucose and insulin to correct abnormal cellular metabolism in a diabetic patient may lead to rapid transfer of potassium from the extracellular fluid to the cell. In this situation, the serum potassium rapidly (increases/decreases) _____.

81. decreases

82.

When oliguria develops because of poor renal function, potassium is no longer excreted, which results in a high serum potassium level.

If there is poor renal function, do you think potassium should be administered? *_____

Why? *_____

82. no, NEVER with poor renal function; Hyperkalemia can be brought to a dangerous level.

83.

Potassium therapy should not be administered to patients with untreated adrenal insufficiency and *_____.

83. renal failure or poor renal function

84.

In the cirrhotic patient with degenerated liver cells, hypokalemia can precipitate hepatic coma or liver failure.

As a nurse caring for a patient with cirrhosis you would alert the healthcare provider of any low serum K levels, and you should watch for symptoms of *_____.

84. hypokalemia and hepatic coma

85.

Increasing potassium intake can lower blood pressure and reduce strokes and cardiovascular diseases. Hypertensive African Americans have a three times greater systolic blood pressure reduction after taking potassium supplements than Caucasians.

85. a

86. African American

87. b

88. cardiac dysrhythmias

89. yes; ACE inhibitor would not be sufficient to raise the serum potassium level, especially because of a low-average serum potassium level and the patient taking a loop diuretic (potassium-wasting diuretic).

Hypertensive patients may decrease their blood pressure by
( ) a. Increasing potassium intake
( ) b. Restricting potassium intake
( ) c. Making no changes in dietary or potassium supplement intake

86.
The cultural/racial group with hypertension who benefits most by increasing potassium intake is (Caucasian/African American/Asians) _____.

87.
Patients with cardiac ischemia, heart failure, or left ventricular hypertrophy who have mild to moderate potassium loss have an increased chance of cardiac dysrhythmias.
   To decrease cardiac dysrhythmias in these patients with cardiac conditions, what would you think their serum potassium level should be?
( ) a. > 3.0 mEq
( ) b. > 4.0 mEq
( ) c. > 5.0 mEq

88.
A potassium-sparing diuretic is sometimes prescribed for cardiac patients to increase their serum potassium level to approximately 4.0 mEq plus. Cardiac patients with a low or low-average serum potassium level are more prone to develop
*_____
_____.

89.
Angiotensin-converting enzyme (ACE) inhibitors can increase potassium but not to the extent needed by patients with low potassium levels.
   Would a patient with a 3.7 mEq/L potassium level who is taking a loop diuretic (Lasix), digoxin, and an ACE inhibitor take a potassium supplement? _____ Explain.
*_____

90. no; Magnesium deficit usually needs to be corrected first, which may automatically correct potassium deficit by making potassium that is given usable by the body.

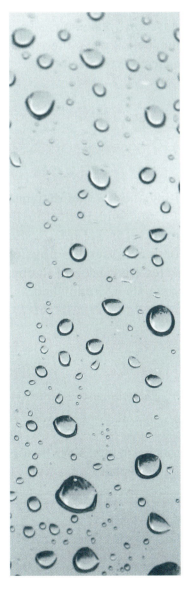

90.

The serum levels of magnesium, chloride, and protein should be checked when correcting hypokalemia. Low serum levels of Mg, Cl, and protein inhibit potassium utilization by the body.

If hypokalemia and hypomagnesemia (Mg deficit) are present, should a potassium deficit be corrected by giving potassium chloride? _____ Why? *_____
_____

● CLINICAL CONSIDERATIONS

1. Oral potassium should be taken with food and/or 8 ounces of fluid. Potassium is irritating to the gastric mucosa and can cause a gastric ulcer.

2. Mild hypokalemia, 3.4 mEq/L, can be avoided by eating foods rich in potassium, i.e., fresh/dry fruits, fruit juices, vegetables, meats, nuts.

3. IV potassium should be well diluted in IV solution. NEVER administer IV potassium as a bolus (IV push). It can cause cardiac arrest.

4. Normal dose for IV potassium is 20–40 mEq in 1 liter of IV fluids to run for 8 hours.

5. Infiltration of IV potassium salt in solution causes sloughing of the subcutaneous tissues. IV potassium is irritating to blood vessels, and with prolonged use, phlebitis might occur.

6. Potassium should NOT be administered if the urine output is, <600ml/day. Eighty to 90% of potassium is excreted in the urine.

7. Potassium deficit can enhance the action of digoxin; digitalis toxicity could result.

8. Potassium-wasting diuretics, i.e., thiazides [hydrochlorothiazide (HydroDiuril)], and loop/ high-ceiling [furosemide (Lasix)] cause potassium loss via kidneys. Steroids promote potassium loss and sodium retention.

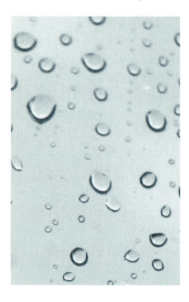

9. ACE inhibitors, beta blockers, NSAIDs, and potassium-sparing diuretics increase the serum potassium level. The serum potassium levels should be monitored when taking these drug groups, especially in older adults and those with renal insufficiency.

10. Increasing serum potassium level to > 4.0 mEq/L can aid in lowering blood pressure and reduce the risk of stroke and cardiovascular diseases.

11. High sodium diet can cause an increase in urinary potassium loss.

12. Magnesium is a cofactor for potassium uptake. It is also impossible to correct a potassium deficit when there is a magnesium deficit. Both serum electrolytes need to be checked.

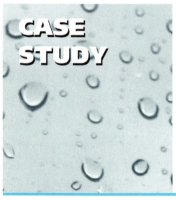

CASE STUDY

REVIEW

A 68-year-old male, has been vomiting and has had diarrhea for 2 days. He takes digoxin, 0.25 mg, and HydroDiuril, 50 mg, daily. His serum potassium level is 3.2 mEq/L. He complains of being dizzy. The nurse assesses his physiologic status and notes that his muscles are weak and flabby, his abdomen is distended, and peristalsis is diminished.

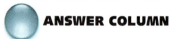

ANSWER COLUMN

1. hypokalemia

2. 3.5–5.3 mEq/L

3. yes; Hypokalemia enhances the action of digoxin, causing digitalis toxicity.

4. loss

1. What was his potassium imbalance? _____

2. The "normal" range of potassium balance is * _____.

3. Should the nurse have checked his pulse rate, since he was receiving digoxin? _____ Explain. * _____
_____

4. Vomiting can cause a potassium (gain/loss) _____.

5. dizziness; muscles weak and flabby; distended abdomen; diminished peristalsis

6. hypokalemia

7. 40–60 mEq/L

8. hyperkalemia, which is toxic to heart muscle and can cause phlebitis (irritated blood vessel)

9. abdominal cramps, tachycardia and later bradycardia, and oliguria

10. Potassium chloride. Also potassium triplex, Kaon, or K-Lyte since the chloride level is normal.

11. causes loss of potassium

12. Aldactone or Dyrenium

5. Name the signs and symptoms of his potassium deficit. _____, * _____, * _____, and * _____

   His heart activity was monitored with an ECG. He received 1 liter of 5% dextrose in water with 40 mEq/L of KCl.

6. A flat T wave would be indicative of _____.

7. The daily potassium requirement is * _____.

8. A concentration of KCl in IV fluids higher than 40 mEq/L can cause * _____ _____

9. List at least three common symptoms found with hyperkalemia. * _____ _____

   A week after his acute illness, his serum potassium was 3.7 mEq/L and his serum chloride was in the "normal" range. The health care provider ordered an oral potassium supplement with his daily digoxin and HydroDiuril (hydrochlorothiazide) and prednisone 4 times a week was ordered for his arthritis.

10. Name an oral potassium supplement that can be prescribed. * _____ _____

11. Explain the effect of cortisone on potassium in the body. * _____

12. If a potassium supplement was not prescribed, name a potassium-sparing diuretic that can be taken in conjunction with hydrochlorothiazide _____.

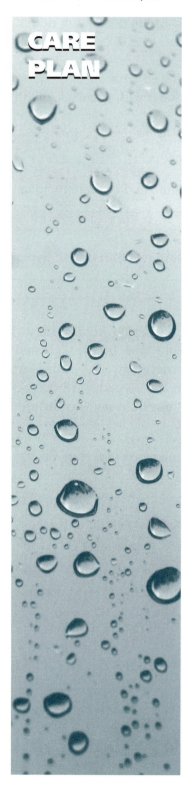

CARE PLAN

PATIENT MANAGEMENT: HYPOKALEMIA

Assessment Factors

● Obtain a history observing for a clinical health problem that may cause hypokalemia, i.e., vomiting, diarrhea, fad-reducing diet, potassium-wasting diuretics.

● Assess for signs and symptoms of hypokalemia, i.e., dizziness, dysrhythmia, soft muscles, abdominal distention, and decreased peristalsis or paralytic ileus.

● Check the serum potassium level that can be used as a baseline for comparison of future serum potassium levels. A serum potassium level below 3.5 mEq/L indicates hypokalemia. A serum potassium level below 2.5 mEq/L may cause cardiac arrest.

● Check the ECG/EKG strips for changes in the T wave (flat or inverted) that may indicate hypokalemia.

● Assess the urine output for 24 hours. Excess urine excretion increases the amount of potassium being excreted.

● Assess for signs and symptoms of digitalis toxicity (i.e., nausea, vomiting, anorexia, bradycardia, dysrhythmias) when a patient is receiving a potassium-wasting diuretic and/or steroids with a digoxin. Hypokalemia enhances the action of digoxin.

Nursing Diagnosis 1

Risk for injury: vessels, tissues, or gastric mucosa related to phlebitis from concentrated potassium solution, infiltration of potassium solution into subcutaneous tissues, or ingestion of concentrated oral potassium, irritating and damaging to the gastric mucosa.

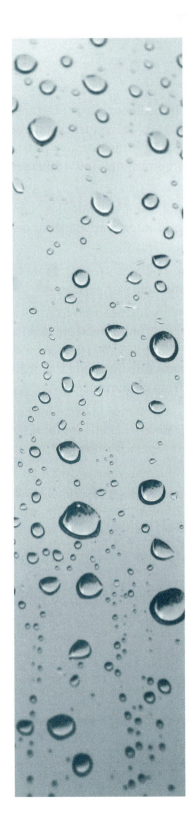

Interventions and Rationale

1. Dilute oral potassium supplements in at least 8 ounces of water or juice. Concentrated potassium is irritating to the gastric mucosa.

2. Check infusion site for phlebitis or infiltration when KCl is given intravenously. Potassium is irritating to blood vessels and subcutaneous tissue. NEVER administer potassium intravenously as a bolus or IV push.

3. Monitor serum potassium levels. A serum potassium level less than 3.5 mEq/L can cause neuromuscular dysfunction and injury to tissues.

4. Monitor the ECG for changes that indicate hypokalemia such as a flat or inverted T wave. Report changes immediately.

Nursing Diagnosis 2

Imbalanced nutrition: less than body requirements, related to insufficient intake of foods rich in potassium or potassium losses (gastric suctioning etc.).

Interventions and Rationale

1. Instruct patients to eat foods rich in potassium when hypokalemia is present or when they are taking potassium-wasting diuretics and steroids. Examples of such foods are fresh fruits, fruit juices, dry fruits, vegetables (especially leafy green vegetables), meats, nuts, potato skins, cocoa, and cola.

2. Monitor the serum potassium level of clients receiving potassium-wasting diuretics and steroids (cortisone preparations).

3. Irrigate GI tube with normal saline solution to prevent electrolyte loss. Gastrointestinal fluid loss from GI suctioning, vomiting, and diarrhea should be measured.

4. Recognize other drugs and substances (i.e., glucose, insulin, laxatives, lithium carbonate, salicylates, tetracycline, and licorice) that decrease serum potassium levels.

5. Monitor serum magnesium, chloride, and protein when hypokalemia is present. Attempts to correct the potassium deficit may not be effective when hypomagnesemia, hypochloremia, and hypoproteinemia are also present.

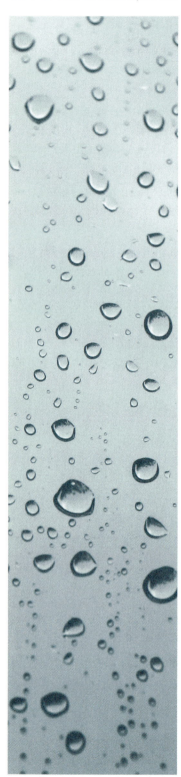

HYPERKALEMIA

Assessment Factors

● Obtain a history of clinical health problems or procedures that may cause hyperkalemia (i.e., renal insufficiency or failure, administration of large doses of intravenous potassium or rapid administration of potassium, and Addison's disease).

● Assess for signs and symptoms of hyperkalemia [i.e., cardiac dysrhythmia (tachycardia and later bradycardia), decreased urine output, abdominal cramps].

● Check the ECG/EKG strips for changes in the T wave (peaked) that may indicate hyperkalemia.

● Check the serum potassium level, which can be used as a baseline for comparison of future serum potassium levels. A serum potassium level greater than 5.3 mEq/L is indicative of hyperkalemia. A serum potassium level greater than 7.0 mEq/L can be a factor in causing cardiac arrest.

● Assess urine output for 24 hours. A decrease in urine output of less than 600 ml/day can indicate an inadequate fluid intake, decreased cardiac output, or renal insufficiency.

● Check the age of whole blood before administering it to a patient with hyperkalemia. Blood, for transfusion, that is 10 or more days old has an elevated serum potassium level due to the hemolysis of aging blood cells.

Nursing Diagnosis 1

Risk for decreased cardiac output: related to dysrhythmia secondary to hyperkalemia.

Interventions and Rationale

1. Monitor vital signs. Report presence of tachycardia or bradycardia.

2. Monitor ECG strips. Report presence of peaked T wave, wide QRS complex, and prolonged P-R interval.

3. Monitor serum potassium levels. Report precipitous decrease or increase in serum potassium level.

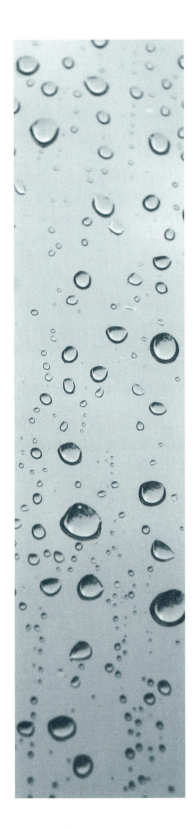

Nursing Diagnosis 2

Impaired urinary elimination: related to renal dysfunction, cardiac insufficiency.

Interventions and Rationale

1. Monitor daily urine output. Urine output that is less than 600 ml per day should be reported.

2. Monitor urine output for patients receiving potassium supplements (orally or intravenously). If urine output is poor while the patient is receiving potassium supplements, the serum potassium level will be increased.

3. Regulate the flow rate of intravenous fluid with potassium so that no more than 10 mEq/L of KCl is administered per hour. Rapidly administered KCl can cause hyperkalemia.

4. Monitor medical treatments for hyperkalemia. Know which corrective treatments are used for mild, moderate, and severe hyperkalemia.

5. Note if the patient is on digoxin when calcium gluconate is ordered for temporary correction of hyperkalemia. Hypercalcemia enhances the action of digitalis, causing digitalis toxicity.

6. Recognize that ACE inhibitors, beta blockers, and potassium-sparing diuretics increase serum potassium levels and should be monitored in older adults and those with renal insufficiency.

7. Administer Kayexalate and sorbitol orally or rectally, according to the amount prescribed by the healthcare provider. The serum potassium should be checked frequently during treatment to prevent hypokalemia resulting from overcorrection of hyperkalemia.

8. Administer fresh blood (blood transfusion) to patients with hyperkalemia. The serum potassium level of fresh blood is 3.5–5.5 mEq/L. With blood that is 3 weeks old, the serum potassium level can be as high as 25 mEq/L.

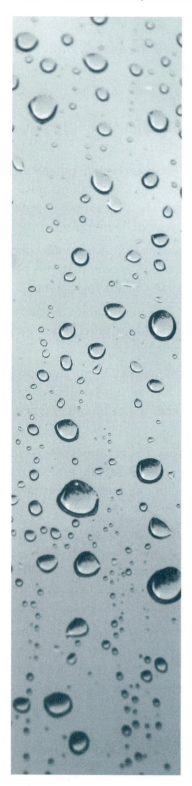

Evaluation/Outcomes

1. Confirm that the cause of potassium imbalance has been corrected.

2. Confirm that the therapeutic regimen corrected the potassium imbalance. The serum potassium levels are within normal range.

3. Remain free of clinical signs and symptoms of hypokalemia or hyperkalemia. Patient's ECG, vital signs, and muscular tone are or return to a normal pattern.

4. Diet includes foods rich in potassium while taking drugs that promote potassium loss.

5. Urine output is adequate (> 600 ml/day).

6. Document compliance with the prescribed drug therapy and medical and dietary regimens.

7. Patient and family recognize risk factors related to hypokalemia.

8. Maintain a support system, i.e., health professionals, family members, friends.

9. Schedule follow-up appointments.

Sodium and Chloride Imbalances

INTRODUCTION

Sodium (Na) and chloride (Cl) are the principal cations and anions in the extracellular fluid (ECF). Sodium and chloride levels in the body are regulated by the kidneys and are influenced by the hormone aldosterone. Sodium is mainly responsible for water retention, which influences the serum osmolality level.

ANSWER COLUMN

1.

Sodium is the main cation found in ＿＿＿＿＿＿＿＿＿＿ fluid.

2.

Chloride is a(n) (anion/cation) ＿＿＿＿＿＿＿＿＿＿.
   The chloride ion frequently appears in combination with the sodium ion. Which fluid has the greatest concentration of chloride—intracellular or extracellular? *＿＿＿＿＿＿＿＿＿＿.

3.

Sodium loss from the skin is negligible under normal conditions. Environmental conditions related to temperature and humidity, fever, and/or muscular exercise can influence the loss of sodium.
   If an individual runs a race and the atmospheric temperature is 100, what do you think happens to the sodium in his or her body? *＿＿＿＿＿＿＿＿＿＿.

4.

The normal concentration of sodium in the extracellular fluid is 135–146 mEq/L.
   The normal concentration of sodium in perspiration is 50–100 mEq, which is less than the concentration found in the *＿＿＿＿＿＿＿＿＿＿.

5.

Perspiration is regarded as a by-product of temperature regulation. Therefore, when the body's sodium level is elevated, perspiration is not a means of regulating sodium excretion.
   Bones contain as much as 800–1000 mEq of sodium, but only a portion of the sodium is available for exchange with sodium in other parts of the body.
   The normal concentration of sodium in the extracellular fluid is ＿＿＿＿＿＿＿＿＿＿ mEq/L.

6. more

6.

Bones contain (more/less) _____ sodium than extracellular fluid.

7.

Thirst often leads to the replacement of water, but not of sodium.

    One (can/cannot) _____ replace sodium by drinking lots of water.

7. cannot

8.

Ocean water is about three times as salty as our body fluid—far too salty for our body organs, i.e., stomach and intestines.

    Ocean water is a (hypo-osmolar/hyperosmolar) _____ fluid. Therefore, in cases of ocean water ingestion, the water is drawn from the body fluid into the stomach and intestines by the process of (osmosis/diffusion) _____.

8. hyperosmolar; osmosis

9.

An elevated serum sodium is known as sodium excess or *hypernatremia* and a decreased serum sodium is known as sodium deficit or *hyponatremia.*

    Hypernatremia is also known as *_____.
Hyponatremia is also known as *_____.

9. sodium excess; sodium deficit

10.

One of the main functions of sodium is to influence the distribution of water in the body. Water accompanies sodium.

    A name for a sodium excess is _____.
    A name for a sodium deficit is _____.
    A function of sodium is to influence the distribution of
*_____.

10. hypernatremia; hyponatremia; body water (water accompanies sodium)

11.

The normal serum chloride (Cl) range is 95–108 mEq/L. The chloride concentration in the intracellular fluid is 1 mEq/L.

    A serum chloride level less than 95 mEq/L is called (hypochloremia/hyperchloremia) _____.
    A serum chloride level greater than 108 mEq/L is called (hypochloremia/hyperchloremia) _____.

11. hypochloremia; hyperchloremia

● FUNCTIONS

Sodium action is influenced by the kidneys, the posterior pituitary gland, and the adrenal glands. The kidneys have an important role in maintaining homeostasis of body sodium. The hypothalamus produces ADH (antidiuretic hormone) and the posterior hypophysis (posterior pituitary gland) stores and secretes ADH. This hormone facilitates the absorption of large quantities of water from the kidneys. The adrenal glands are composed of two sections, the cortex and the medulla, each secreting its own hormones. The hormones from the adrenal cortex are frequently referred to as steroids. Table 7-1 explains how one organ and two glands influence serum sodium. Study Table 7-1 carefully.

12.

The chief regulation of sodium occurs within the _____.

13.

Explain the effect of cortisone and aldosterone on the regulation of sodium and potassium. *_____

_____

12. kidneys

13. They stimulate the kidneys, to absorb sodium and excrete potassium.

Table 7-1	**Influences Affecting Serum Sodium**
Organ Kidneys	Kidneys are regulators that maintain homeostasis through excretion or absorption of water and sodium from the renal tubules according to excess or deficit of serum sodium.
Glands 1. Posterior hypophysis or posterior pituitary gland	The antidiuretic hormone (ADH), secreted by the pituitary gland, favors water absorption from the distal tubules of the kidneys and thus limits sodium excretion.
2. Adrenal cortex of the adrenal glands	Adrenal cortical hormones, e.g., cortisone and aldosterone, secreted by the adrenal cortex, favor sodium absorption from the renal tubules. These steroids stimulate the kidneys to absorb sodium and excrete potassium.

Table 7-2	**Sodium and Its Functions**
Body Involvement	**Functions**
Neuromuscular	Transmission and conduction of nerve impulses (sodium pump—see Cellular).
Body fluids	Largely responsible for the osmolality of vascular fluids. Doubling Na level gives the approximate serum osmolality.
	Regulation of body fluid (increased sodium levels cause water retention).
Cellular	Sodium pump action. Sodium shifts into cells as potassium shifts out of the cells, repeatedly, to maintain water balance and neuromuscular activity. When Na shifts into the cell, depolarization occurs (cell activity); and when Na shifts out of the cell, K shifts back into the cell, and repolarization occurs.
	Enzyme activity.
Acid-base levels	Assist with the regulation of acid-base balance. Sodium combines readily with chloride (Cl) or bicarbonate (HCO_3) to regulate the acid-base balance.

Table 7-2 explains the functions of sodium. The two most important functions of sodium are water balance and neuromuscular activity. Study Table 7-2 carefully and refer to the table as needed.

14.

An important function of sodium is neuromuscular activity. Name another electrolyte responsible for neuromuscular activity.

_____

14. potassium, magnesium, or calcium

15.

The concentration or osmolality of vascular fluids is determined by which electrolyte? _____

  A rough estimate of the serum osmolality can be obtained by *_____.

15. sodium; doubling the serum sodium level

16. Sodium shifts in as potassium shifts out of the cells, stimulating depolarization and cell activity. K shifts in and Na shifts out for repolarization (cell rest); water balance and neuromuscular activity

16.

Explain the action of the sodium pump. *_____

_____

Name two purposes for the sodium pump. *_____

_____

17.

What are the two anions that combine with sodium to help regulate acid-base balance? *_____

17. chloride and bicarbonate

18.

Sodium in increased quantities is contained within the following body secretions: saliva, gastric secretions, bile, pancreatic juice, and intestinal secretions.

Indicate which of the following body secretions contain large quantities of sodium:

( ) a. Saliva
( ) b. Thyroid secretions
( ) c. Gastric secretions
( ) d. Bile
( ) e. Parathyroid secretions
( ) f. Pancreatic juice
( ) g. Intestinal secretions

18. a, c, d, f, g

Table 7-3 lists the four functions of the chloride ion. Study Table 7-3 and refer to it as needed.

19.

Chloride, like sodium, influences the serum osmolality.

What two ions are usually increased when the serum osmolality is elevated? *_____

19. sodium and chloride

Table 7-3	Chloride and Its Functions
Body Involvement	**Functions**
Osmolality (tonicity) of ECF	Chloride, like sodium, changes the serum osmolality. When serum osmolality is increased, >295 mOsm/kg, there are more sodium and chloride ions in proportion to the water. A decreased serum osmolality, <280 mOsm/kg, results in less sodium and chloride ions, and a lower serum osmolality.
Body water balance	When sodium is retained, chloride is frequently retained, causing an increase in water retention.
Acid-base balance	The kidneys excrete the anion chloride or bicarbonate, and sodium reabsorbs either chloride or bicarbonate to maintain the acid-base balance.
Acidity of gastric juice	Chloride combines with the hydrogen ion in the stomach to form hydrochloric acid (HCl).

20.

When there is a body water deficit, what occurs to the:

a. Serum sodium and serum chloride levels? _____

b. Serum osmolality? _____

c. Body water? _____

20. a. increases; b. increases; c. is reabsorbed

21.

For every sodium ion absorbed from the renal tubules, a chloride or bicarbonate ion is also absorbed; thus the proportion of sodium and chloride lost can differ.

The organs responsible for electrolyte homeostasis by the excretion and absorption of ions are the _____.

21. kidneys

22.

If metabolic alkalosis is present, the kidneys excrete the bicarbonate ion and sodium is reabsorbed with the (bicarbonate/chloride) _____ ions.

If metabolic acidosis is present, the kidneys excrete (bicarbonate/chloride) _____ ion, and the sodium is reabsorbed with which ion? _____

22. chloride; chloride; bicarbonate

● PATHOPHYSIOLOGY

23.

The pathophysiologic effects of hyponatremia are evidenced in the membranes of the central nervous system (CNS), the neuromuscular tissues, and the smooth muscles of the gastrointestinal (GI) tract.

The cells of the CNS are more sensitive to a decreased serum sodium level than other cells. The cardiac muscle is usually not affected by changes in the serum sodium level.

Hyponatremia has an effect on the membranes of:

a. * _____

b. * _____

c. * _____

23. a. central nervous system; b. neuromuscular tissues; c. smooth muscles of the GI tract

24. hyponatremia

24.

Hyponatremia can occur when the kidneys are unable to excrete enough urine. Reduced urine excretion increases the amount of body water, which in turn dilutes the serum sodium concentration.

The type of electrolyte imbalance that can result when the body fluid volume is increased is known as (hyponatremia/hypernatremia) _____.

25. increased; less

25.

When the serum sodium level is increased, sodium passes more freely across the cell membranes, accelerating the rate of depolarization. This can cause (decreased/increased) _____ cellular activity (irritability). As the hypernatremic state intensifies, less sodium passes across the cell membrane, ultimately resulting in (more/less) _____ cellular activity.

26. increases. The serum osmolality is the concentration of solutes in the plasma.

26.

An increased serum sodium level (hypernatremia) (increases/decreases) _____ the serum osmolality. Explain why _____.

27. a

27.

Three types of hyponatremia are hypo-osmolar hyponatremia (most common), iso-osmolar hyponatremia, and hyperosmolar hyponatremia. The serum osmolality aids in identifying the type of hyponatremia. (Refer to "osmolality" in Chapter 1.)

The most common type of hyponatremia is

( ) a. hypo-osmolar

( ) b. iso-osmolar

( ) c. hyperosmolar

28. 280–295 mOsm/kg (some references use 275–295 mOsm/kg)

28.

Normal range for serum osmolality is *_____.

29. iso-osmolar hyponatremia

29.

A serum sodium of 130 mEq/L and a serum osmolality of 285 mOsm/kg can indicate *_____.

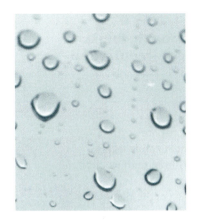

The body fluid volume status with hyponatremia should also be considered in order to correct the underlying cause of hyponatremia.

There are three types of body fluid volume imbalances associated with hyponatremia: hypovolemic (decrease volume), euvolemic (normal volume), and hypervolemic (increased volume). If the urine sodium spot testing is <30 mEq/L, hypovolemic and hypervolemic hyponatremia are likely; if the urine sodium spot testing is >30 mEq/L, euvolemic hyponatremia is likely. Table 7-4 lists some of the causes of body fluid volume imbalances that occur with hyponatremia.

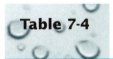 **Table 7-4**	**Causes of Hyponatremia and Hypochloremia (Serum Sodium and Chloride Deficit)**
Etiology	**Rationale**
Dietary Changes Low-sodium diet Excessive plain water intake "Fad" diets/fasting Anorexia nervosa Prolonged use of IV D_5W	A low-sodium intake over several months can lead to hyponatremia. Drinking large quantities of plain water dilutes the ECF. Administration of continuous IV D_5W dilutes the ECF and can cause water intoxication. Gastric juice is composed of the acid hydrogen chloride (HCl).
Gastrointestinal Losses Vomiting, diarrhea GI suctioning Tap-water enemas GI surgery Bulimia	Sodium and chloride are in high concentration in the gastric and intestinal mucosas. Sodium and chloride losses occur with vomiting, diarrhea, GI suctioning, and GI surgery.
Loss of potassium	Loss of potassium is accompanied by loss of chloride.
Renal Losses Salt-wasting kidney disease Diuretics	In advanced renal disorders, the tubules do not respond to ADH; therefore, there is a loss of sodium, chloride, and water. The extensive use of diuretics or excessively potent diuretics can decrease the serum sodium and chloride levels.
Hormonal Influences Antidiuretic hormone (ADH), syndrome of inappropriate ADH (SIADH)	ADH promotes water reabsorption from the distal renal tubules. Surgical pain, increased use of narcotics, and head trauma, cause more water to be reabsorbed, thus diluting the ECF.
Decreased adrenocortical hormone: Addison's disease	Decreased adrenocortical hormone production related to decreased adrenal gland activity (Addison's disease) causes sodium loss and potassium retention.

(continues)

Table 7-4	Causes of Hyponatremia and Hypochloremia (Serum Sodium and Chloride Deficit)—*continued*
Etiology	**Rationale**
Altered Cellular Function	
Hypervolemic state: HF, cirrhosis	In hypervolemic states due to HF, cirrhosis, and nephrosis, the ECF is increased, thus diluting the serum sodium and chloride levels.
Burns	Great quantities of sodium and chloride are lost from burn wounds and from oozing burn surface areas.
Skin	Large amounts of sodium and chloride are lost from the skin due to increased environmental temperature, fever, and large skin wounds.
Acid-Base Imbalance	
Metabolic alkalosis	An increase in the concentration of bicarbonate ions is associated with a decrease in the concentration of chloride ions.

30.
A urine sodium spot testing showing >30 mEq/L usually occurs with what type of volemic hyponatemia?
( ) a. hypovolemic
( ) b. euvolemic
( ) c. hypervolemic

30. b

31.
Patients with heart failure or cirrhosis of the liver may have what type of volemic hyponatremia? _____

31. hypervolemic

32.
To determine the type of volemic hyponatremia, the three test values need to include serum sodium, serum osmolality, and _____.

32. urine sodium

33.
Hypernatremia is mostly associated with hyperosmolar state. Hypernatremia results from water (loss/retention) _____ and sodium (loss/retention) _____.

33. loss; retention

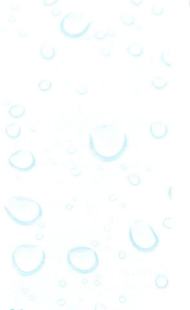

⬤ ETIOLOGY

The general causes of hyponatremia and hypochloremia are GI losses, altered cellular function, renal losses, electrolyte-free fluids, and hormonal influences. Table 7-4 lists the various causes and gives the rationale concerning the sodium and chloride loss.

34.

The hemodilution of body fluids that can cause hyponatremia and hypochloremia includes which of the following symptoms:

( ) a. Drinking excessive amounts of plain water
( ) b. Increased adrenocortical hormone
( ) c. SIADH
( ) d. Gastric suction
( ) e. Hypervolemic state due to HF
( ) f. Increased environmental temperature

34. a, c, e

35.

Vomiting and diarrhea can (increase/decrease) _____ the serum sodium and chloride levels. Explain. *_____

_____

35. decrease; The high concentrations of sodium and chloride in the GI tract are reduced.

36. sweating, increased environmental temperature and humidity, fever, and muscular exercise

36.

Name four conditions that cause an increased sodium and chloride loss through the skin. *_____

_____

37.

Wound drainage, bleeding, and vomiting postoperatively can cause a sodium and chloride (deficit/retention) _____.

SIADH may occur following surgery. Explain how it causes a sodium and chloride deficit. *_____

_____

37. deficit; Excess or continuous ADH secretion (SIADH) causes water to be reabsorbed from the kidney, thus diluting ECF.

38. decreased; metabolic alkalosis

38.

Increased bicarbonate ion concentration (HCO_3) is associated with a(n) (increased/decreased) _____ chloride ion concentration.

What type of acid-base imbalance results? * _____

39. hyponatremia; Gastric and intestinal secretions are lost through the gastric tube/suction.

39.

The use of gastric suction for the purpose of drainage can cause (hypernatremia/hyponatremia) _____. Why?

* _____

_____

40. insufficiency; loss

40.

Addison's disease occurs when there is an adrenocortical hormone (insufficiency/overproduction) _____.

In Addison's disease, there is a sodium (loss/gain) _____.

41. water, sodium, and chloride loss; due to oozing at the burn surface

41.

Patients recovering from burn injuries experience numerous fluid shifts as the body attempts to compensate for the trauma to its tissues. Burns promote increased * _____. Why? * _____

Table 7-5 lists the various causes and gives the rationale concerning sodium excess.

42. hypernatremia; hyperchloremia; Water loss is greater than sodium and chloride loss (hypovolemic with hypernatremic/ hyperchloremic effect).

42.

Severe vomiting and diarrhea can cause (hyponatremia/ hypernatremia) and (hypochloremia/hyperchloremia) _____. Why? * _____

_____

43.

Which of the following situations can cause an increased serum sodium and chloride level:

( ) a. Excessive use of table salt

( ) b. Continuous use of canned vegetables and soups

( ) c. Increased water intake

( ) d. Use of intravenous 3% saline solutions

( ) e. Use of diuretics

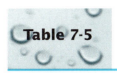

Table 7-5	**Causes of Hypernatremia and Hyperchloremia (Serum Sodium and Chloride Excess)**
Etiology	**Rationale**
Dietary Changes Increased sodium intake Decreased water intake Administration of 3% saline solutions	Inadequate fluid intake and increased use of table salt, canned vegetables, and soups can increase the serum sodium and chloride levels. Administration of concentrated 3% saline solutions can cause hypernatremia and hyperchloremia.
GI Disorders Vomiting (severe) Diarrhea	With severe vomiting, water loss can be greater than sodium loss, causing a dangerously high serum sodium level. This is particularly true in babies who have diarrhea. Their loss of water can be greater than their loss of sodium.
Decreased renal function	Reduced glomerular filtration causes an excess of sodium in the body.
Environmental Changes Increased temperature and humidity	Increased environmental and body temperatures may cause profuse perspiration.
Water loss	Water loss can be greater than sodium and chloride losses.
Hormonal Influence Increased adrenocortical hormone production: oral or IV cortisone	Excess adrenocortical hormone can cause a sodium and chloride excess in the body whether it is due to cortisone ingestion or hyperfunction of the adrenal gland (Cushing's syndrome).
Altered Cellular Function HF, renal diseases	Usually with HF and renal disease, the body's sodium and chloride are greatly increased. If water retention is greatly enhanced, pseudohyponatremia may result.
Trauma: head injury	Chloride ions are frequently retained with the sodium.
Acid-base imbalance: metabolic acidosis	Increased chloride (Cl) ion concentration is associated with a decreased bicarbonate ion concentration.

( ) f. Large doses or prolonged uses of oral cortisone therapy

( ) g. Severe vomiting

43. a, b, d, f, g

44. retention; Reduced glomerular filtration. Sodium retention usually causes an increase in body fluid and may give a false indication that the serum sodium level is normal or low.

44.

Heart failure (HF) or obstruction of the arterial blood supply to the kidney can cause sodium and chloride (excretion/retention) _____. Why? *_____

_____

45.

Cushing's syndrome occurs when there is an adrenocortical hormone (insufficiency/overproduction) _____.

In Cushing's syndrome, there is a sodium and chloride _____.

45. overproduction; retention

46.

An increased chloride level is associated with a(n) (increased/decreased) _____ bicarbonate (HCO$_3$) level. What type of acid-base imbalance occurs? *_____

46. decreased; metabolic acidosis

● CLINICAL MANIFESTATIONS

The severity of the clinical manifestations of hypo-hypernatremia varies with the onset and extent of sodium deficit or excess. Mild hypernatremia is normally asymptomatic, and early nonspecific symptoms such as nausea and vomiting may be overlooked. Table 7-6 gives the signs and symptoms associated with hypo-hypernatremia. Study

Table 7-6   **Clinical Manifestations of Sodium Imbalances**

Body Involvement	Hyponatremia	Hypernatremia
Gastrointestinal Abnormalities	*Nausea, vomiting, diarrhea, abdominal cramps	*Nausea, vomiting, anorexia *Rough, dry tongue
Cardiac Abnormalities	Tachycardia, hypotension	*Tachycardia, possible hypertension
Central Nervous System (CNS)	*Headaches, apprehension, lethargy, confusion, depression, seizures	*Restlessness, agitation, stupor, elevated body temperature
Neuromuscular Abnormalities	*Muscular weakness	Muscular twitching, tremor, hyperreflexia
Integumentary Changes	Dry skin, pale, dry mucous membrane	*Flushed, dry skin, dry, sticky membrane
Laboratory Values		
Serum sodium	<135 mEq/L	>146 mEq/L
Urine sodium		<40 mEq/L
Specific gravity	<1.008	>1.025
Serum osmolality	<280 mOsm/kg	>295 mOsm/kg

Note: *Most common clinical manifestations of hyponatremia and hypernatremia.

Table 7-6 carefully. Refer back to Table 7-6 as needed to complete the questions on hypo-hypernatremia.

47.

In hyponatremia, the serum sodium level is below
_____ mEq/L. What is the serum value in hypernatremia?
*_____ mEq/L

47. 135; above 146

48.

Headaches, lethargy, depression, and muscular weakness are clinical manifestations of (hyponatremia/hypernatremia)
_____.

48. hyponatremia

49.

Which of the following signs and symptoms indicate hypernatremia?

( ) a. Rough, dry tongue
( ) b. Tachycardia
( ) c. Apprehension, confusion
( ) d. Flushed, dry skin
( ) e. Restlessness, agitation
( ) f. Elevated body temperature

49. a, b, d, e, f

50.

A serum osmolality below 280 mOsm/L can indicate (hyponatremia/hypernatremia) _____, while a serum osmolality above 295 mOsm/L can indicate
_____.

50. hyponatremia (also indicates ECF dilution caused by a sodium deficit or excess water retention); hypernatremia

51.

Hypochloremia neuromuscular abnormalities are similar to the symptoms of tetany. Tetany symptoms are evidenced as (hypo/hyper) _____ excitability of the nerves and muscles. Examples of these symptoms are _____ and _____.

51. hyper; tremors; twitching

52.

With hyperchloremic neuromuscular abnormalities, there is a decrease in nerve and muscle activity. Two examples of these symptoms are *_____.

52. weakness and lethargy

53.

In hypochloremia, the respiratory symptom is similar to metabolic alkalosis.

Indicate which type of breathing occurs with a chloride deficit.

(　) a. Slow, shallow breathing
(　) b. Deep, rapid, vigorous breathing
Explain why. *_____

_____

53. a; The lungs conserve carbon dioxide ($CO_2 + H_2O = H_2CO_3$) or carbonic acid to increase acid and restore the pH.

54.

In hyperchloremia, the respiratory symptom is similar to metabolic acidosis.

Indicate which type of breathing occurs with a chloride excess.

(　) a. Slow, shallow breathing
(　) b. Deep, rapid, vigorous breathing
Do you know why? *_____

_____

54. b; The lungs below off carbon dioxide to prevent the formation of H_2CO_3—carbonic acid.

Table 7-7 lists the clinical manifestations of hypochloremia and hyperchloremia according to the body areas affected. Hypochloremic symptoms are similar to metabolic alkalosis, and hyperchloremic symptoms are similar to metabolic acidosis. Study Table 7-7 carefully and refer to it as needed.

Table 7-7   **Clinical Manifestations of Chloride Imbalances**

Body Involvement	Hypochloremia	Hyperchloremia
Neuromuscular Abnormalities	Hyperexcitability of the nerves and muscles (tremors, twitching)	Weakness Lethargy Unconsciousness (later)
Respiratory Abnormalities	Slow and shallow breathing	Deep, rapid, vigorous breathing
Cardiac Abnormalities	↓ Blood pressure with severe Cl and ECF losses	
Laboratory Values Milliequivalent per liter	<95 mEq/L	>108 mEq/L

● CLINICAL MANAGEMENT

Sodium Correction

55.

The majority of Americans consume 3–5 g of sodium per day (some consume 8–15 g daily). Daily sodium requirements are 2–4 g. A teaspoon of salt has 2.3 g of sodium.

When sodium intake increases, what happens to the water intake and to the body fluids? * _____

56.

To restore the sodium balance due to a sodium deficit, either normal saline solution (0.9% NaCl) or a 3% salt solution is recommended. Several health professionals suggest that the serum sodium fall below 130 mEq/L before giving saline and ≤115 mEq/L before giving a concentrated salt solution, i.e., 3% saline.

Remember, a rapid infusion of concentrated salt solutions can result in pulmonary edema. Explain why. * _____

_____

57.

Excessive intravenous administration of dextrose and water can cause sodium dilution. Dextrose is metabolized, leaving free water. Copious amounts of plain water can cause sodium

_____.

Explain how sodium can be diluted. * _____

_____

Drugs and Their Effect on Sodium Balance

Diuretics, certain antipsychotics, antineoplastics, and barbiturates can cause a sodium deficit. Corticosteroids and the ingestion and infusion of sodium are the major causes of a sodium excess. Table 7-8 lists the drugs that affect sodium balance.

---

55. Sodium holds water. Extracellular fluid (ECF) is increased.

56. Sodium retains fluid. A high concentration of sodium pulls intracellular fluid from cells, thus overexpanding the vascular compartment. Fluid collects in the lungs.

57. dilution; Following the utilization of dextrose, the remaining water dilutes the sodium and other electrolytes.

Table 7-8   **Drugs Affecting Sodium Balance**

Sodium Imbalance	Drugs	Rationale
Hyponatremia (serum sodium deficit)	Diuretics	Diuretics, either K wasting or K sparing, cause sodium excretion.
	Lithium	Lithium promotes urinary sodium loss.

	Antineoplastics/Anticancer
	    Vincristine
	    Cyclophosphamide
	    Cisplatin
		Anticancer drugs, antipsychotics, and antidiabetics stimulate ADH release and cause hemodilution and decrease sodium level.

	Antipsychotics
	    Amitriptyline (Elavil)
	    Thioridazine (Mellaril)
	    Thiothixene (Navane)
	    Tranylcypromine (Parnate)	

	Antidiabetics
	    Chlorpropamide (Diablenease)
	    Tolbutamide (Orinase)	

	CNS depressants
	    Morphine
	    Barbiturates
	    Ibuprofens (Motrin)
	    Nicotine
	    Clonidine (Catapres)	

Hypernatremia (serum sodium excess)	Corticosteroids
	    Cortisone
	    Prednisone
		Steroids promote sodium retention and potassium excretion.

	Hypertonic saline
	    Sodium salicylate
	    Sodium phosphate
	    Sodium bicarbonate
	    Cough medicines
		Administration of sodium salts in excess.

	Antibiotics
	    Azlocillin Na
	    Penicillin Na
		Many of the antibiotics contain the sodium salt, which increases drug absorption.

	Mezlocillin Na
	    Carbenicillin
	    Ticarcillin disodium
		Ion exchange.

	Cholestyramine	These miscellaneous drugs promote urinary water loss without sodium.

	Amphotericin B
	    Demeclocycline
	    Propoxyphene (Darvon)	

	Lactulose	Water loss in excess of sodium via GI tract.

58.

Enter SD for sodium deficit/hyponatremia and SE for sodium excess/hypernatremia beside drugs that affect sodium balance. Refer to Table 7-8 as needed.

_____ a. Lithium

_____ b. Cortisone

_____ c. Diuretics

_____ d. Sodium penicillin

_____ e. Antipsychotic agents

_____ f. Ibuprofen/Motrin

_____ g. Amphotericin B

_____ h. Lactulose

_____ i. Barbiturates

_____ j. Cyclophosphamide/Cytoxan

_____ k. Tolbutamide/Orinase

58. a. SD; b. SE; c. SD; d. SE; e. SD; f. SD; g. SE; h. SE; i. SD; j. SD; k. SD

59.

Patients who are receiving steroids, such as cortisone and prednisone, should be cautioned in the use of excess salt. Explain. *_____

59. Steroids promote sodium retention (sodium retaining effect).

60.

Hyponatremia enhances the action of quinidine and hypernatremia reduces or decreases the action of quinidine.

   With a serum sodium of 156 mEq/L would the action of quinidine be (increased/decreased)? _____

60. decreased

61.

Cough medicines, most antibiotics, and sulfonamides can (increase/decrease) _____ the serum sodium level.

61. increase

● CLINICAL APPLICATIONS

62.

You have a cardiac patient who has edema and his serum sodium concentration is reduced. Why do you think this occurs?

*_____

_____

62. Hyponatremia thus results from hemodilution. May be receiving a low-sodium diet and taking a diuretic.

63. yes; A low urine sodium indicates sodium retention in the body, especially with symptoms of overhydration. A low serum sodium level can be misleading. Hyponatremia can also occur with a fluid volume excess (hypervolemia), by causing the sodium to be diluted.

63.

A 24-hour urine sodium test is helpful for determining sodium retention or loss within the body. A normal range for a 24-hour urine sodium is 40–220 mEq/L.

A patient's 24-hour urine sodium is 32 mEq/L, the serum sodium level is 133 mEq/L, and the patient has symptoms of heart failure. Do you think the patient is retaining sodium? _____ Explain. *_____
_____

64.

A normal urine chloride level in 24 hours is 150–250 mEq/L. The amount of chloride excreted depends on the amount of salt intake, body fluid imbalance, and acid-base imbalance.

With a body fluid deficit, the serum chloride and sodium levels are increased due to hemoconcentration. In this situation do you expect the urine chloride level to be (increased/decreased)? _____

64. decreased

65.

With hospital patients, hyponatremia is one of the leading causes of electrolyte disorders. It may be due to numerous conditions, such as heart failure, cancer, surgery, or drugs. Conventional treatment has been fluid restriction and/or administration of hypertonic saline (3% saline).

New treatment for hyponatremia is AVP (arginine vasopressin) antagonist, for example, conivaptan. AVP promotes water reabsorption from the renal collecting tubules. Reabsorption of water promotes water (retention/excretion). _____. The serum sodium would most likely be (increased/decreased) _____.

65. retention; decreased

66.

A leading cause of electrolyte disorder in hospital patients is _____. A new suggested treatment for this electrolyte disorder may be (AVP agent/AVP antagonist) _____

66. hyponatremia; AVP antagonist

67. hyponatremia; The release of AVP causes water reabsorption; also possible hypotonic fluid (IV or oral).

67.

Following surgery, postoperative period, the patient may develop (hypernatremia/hyponatremia) _____. Why?
_____

68.

If your patient is vomiting following a surgical intervention and is receiving dextrose and water intravenously, one may expect a sodium and chloride (excess/deficit) _____ if the vomiting persists.

A patient experiencing severe vomiting without water replacement is at high risk for a sodium (excess/deficit) _____. Why? *_____ _____

68. deficit; excess; The loss of water is greater than the loss of sodium in severe vomiting.

69. retention; Poor circulation reduces the glomerular filtration; therefore, Na and Cl are retained.

69.

In heart failure, there is sodium and chloride (retention/ excretion) _____ Why? *_____ _____

70.

If a feeble or debilitated patient receives numerous tap-water enemas for the purpose of cleaning the bowel, the enemas can cause a sodium and chloride _____.

70. loss (deficit)

71.

Frequently some marathon runners experience hyponatremia, which is more common in women than men.

Excessive amount of fluid consumption is the primary cause of a low serum sodium level and not the composition of fluid consumed. The cause of most athletes having hyponatremia is because of fluid (deficit/overload) _____.

71. overload

72.

Diarrhea can cause either a sodium deficit or a sodium excess. Babies having diarrhea can lose more _____ than the sodium; therefore, a sodium _____ can result.

72. water; excess

73.

Hypochloremia usually indicates alkalosis (hypochloremic alkalosis) due to increased levels of bicarbonate.

Persistent vomiting and gastric suction cause a loss of hydrogen and chloride ions. A loss in hydrogen and chloride results in *_____.

73. hypochloremic alkalosis

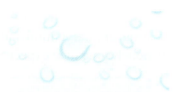

74.

A potassium deficit cannot be fully corrected until a chloride deficit is corrected.

   With vomiting, what potassium supplement is needed to replace the potassium and chloride deficits (K-Lyte/potassium chloride/Kaon)? *_____.

   Explain. *_____

74. potassium chloride; Both chloride and potassium are lost due to vomiting.

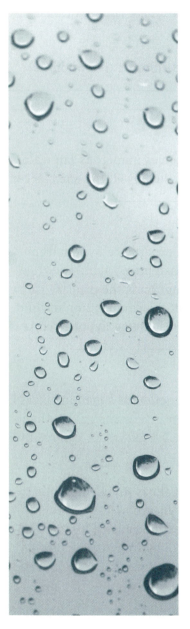

● CLINICAL CONSIDERATIONS

1. Serum osmolality of body fluids (ECF) can be estimated by *doubling the serum sodium level.* For a more accurate serum osmolality level, use the formula

$$2 \times \text{serum Na} + \frac{\text{BUN}}{3} + \frac{\text{glucose}}{18} = \text{serum osmolality (mOsm/kg)}$$

   The normal serum osmolality range is 280–295 mOsm/kg.

2. Sodium causes water retention.

3. One teaspoon of salt is equivalent to 2.3 g of sodium. The daily sodium requirement is 2–4 g. Most Americans consume 3–5 g of sodium per day, and some consume 8–15 g daily.

4. Vomiting causes sodium and chloride losses, and diarrhea causes sodium, chloride, and bicarbonate losses.

5. A 3% saline solution should be given when there is a severe serum sodium deficit, e.g., <115 mEq/L. When administering a 3% saline solution, check for signs and symptoms of pulmonary edema.

6. A serum potassium deficit cannot be fully corrected until the chloride deficit is corrected.

7. Sodium and potassium have opposite effects on cellular activity. The sodium pump effect causes sodium to shift into the cells resulting in depolarization. When sodium shifts out of the cells, potassium shifts into cells and repolarization occurs. The sodium pump action is continuously repeated.

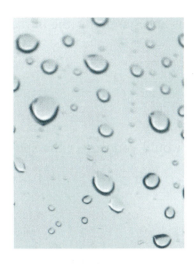

8. Continuous use of a saline solution causes a calcium loss.

9. Steroids promote sodium retention and, thus, water retention. Cough medicine, sulfonamides, and some antibiotics containing sodium can increase the serum sodium level.

10. If hypovolemic hyponatremia is present, normal saline solution is usually given. If hypervolemic hyponatremia occurs, salt and water restriction is ordered and loop diuretics may also be prescribed. If euvolemic hyponatremia occurs, water restriction is necessary.

11. Patients with heart failure or cirrhosis of the liver usually have hypervolemic hyponatremia.

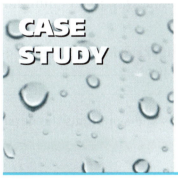

CASE STUDY

REVIEW

A middle-aged female is suffering from a high temperature and diaphoresis. She has been nauseated and has taken only ginger ale for the last several days. Her serum sodium is 129 mEq/L.

 ANSWER COLUMN

1. sodium deficit or hyponatremia

2. 135–146 mEq/L

3. fever; diaphoresis; ginger ale intake for several days (lack of food)

1. Identify the type of sodium imbalance she has.
   * _____
   _____

2. Give the "normal" serum sodium range. * _____

3. Give some of the reasons for her imbalance.
   a. * _____
   b. * _____

4. abdominal cramps; muscular weakness; headaches; nausea and vomiting

5. a. 1.010 or below

6. yes; She could have a loss of potassium from lack of food and due to illness. Arrhythmia may be a sign of hypokalemia.

7. flushed skin; elevated body temperature; rough, dry tongue; tachycardia

8. It reduces or decreases quinidine's action.

9. They increase the hypernatremic state. Cortisone causes sodium, chloride, and water retention, and certain antibiotics increase sodium levels.

10. During cell catabolism, potassium leaves the cells and sodium enters the cells.

4. Name some of the clinical signs and symptoms the nurse might observe.

a. *_____

b. *_____

c. *_____

d. *_____

5. When testing her urine, what would you expect the specific gravity level to be?

( ) a. 1.010 or below

( ) b. 1.015

( ) c. 1.020 or above

She was given 3% sodium chloride solution. Her serum sodium level rose to 152 mEq/L. She was given quinidine for her irregular pulse rate.

6. Do you think her serum potassium should have been evaluated? _____ Why not? *_____
_____

7. Name some of the clinical signs and symptoms the nurse observes with hypernatremia.

a. *_____

b. *_____

c. *_____

8. Explain the effect of hypernatremia on quinidine. _____
_____

9. If she received cortisone and antibiotic, penicillin G Na, what would this do to her hypernatremic state?

*_____
_____

10. Sodium is most plentiful in the extracellular compartment. Explain why sodium might enter the cells. *_____
*_____

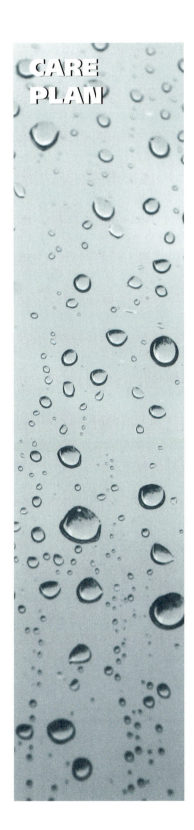

CARE PLAN

PATIENT MANAGEMENT: SODIUM AND CHLORIDE IMBALANCES:

Hyponatremia and Hypochloremia

Assessment Factors

● Obtain a history of high-risk factors for decreased serum sodium and chloride levels, i.e., GI loss from vomiting, diarrhea, or GI suctioning; eating disorders such as anorexia nervosa and bulimia; SIADH as a result of surgery; hypervolemic state resulting in hemodilution; use of potent diuretics with a low-sodium diet; or continuous use of D_5W.

● Assess for signs and symptoms of hyponatremia, i.e., headache, nausea, vomiting, lethargy, confusion, tachycardia, and/or muscular weakness.

● Obtain serum sodium and chloride levels that can be used as baseline values for comparison. A serum sodium level less than 135 mEq/L would indicate hyponatremia. A sodium level less than 125 mEq/L should be reported immediately to the health care provider. A serum chloride level below 95 mEq/L is indicative of hypochloremia.

● Check other electrolytes, such as potassium and chloride, when serum sodium levels are not within normal range.

● Check the serum osmolality level and urine specific gravity. A serum osmolality level of less than 280 mOsm/kg indicates hyponatremia. A specific gravity below 1.010 can indicate hyponatremia.

Nursing Diagnosis 1

Ineffective health maintenance: related to vomiting, diarrhea, gastric suction, SIADH resulting from surgery, potent diuretics.

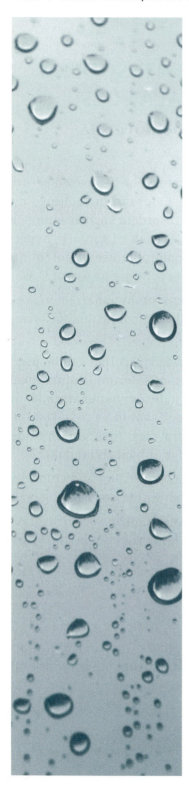

Interventions and Rationale

1. Monitor the serum sodium and chloride levels. Sodium replacement with chloride may be needed if the serum sodium deficit is due to GI losses. Hypervolemic conditions such as HF can indicate a pseudohyponatremia.

2. Keep an accurate intake and output record. Excess water intake can cause hyponatremia and hypochloremia due to hemodilution.

3. Observe changes in vital signs, especially the pulse rate. If hyponatremia is due to hypovolemia (loss of fluid and sodium), shocklike symptoms such as tachycardia can occur. Frequently, hyponatremia is due to hemodilution from an excess fluid volume.

4. Check for signs and symptoms of water intoxication, i.e., headaches and behavioral changes, when hyponatremia is due to SIADH.

5. Restrict water when hyponatremia is due to hypervolemia (excess fluid volume).

6. Monitor serum CO_2 or arterial HCO_3. An increased serum CO_2, >32 mEq/L, and/or increased arterial HCO_3, >28 mEq/L, can indicate metabolic alkalosis and hypochloremia (hypochloremic alkalosis).

7. Observe for respiratory difficulties, i.e., slow, shallow breathing due to hypochloremic alkalosis.

Hypernatremia and Hyperchloremia
Assessment Factors

● Obtain a history of high-risk factors for increased serum sodium and chloride levels, i.e., increased sodium intake, decreased water intake, administration of concentrated saline solutions, renal diseases, and increased adrenocortical hormone production.

● Assess for signs and symptoms of hypernatremia, i.e., nausea, vomiting, tachycardia, elevated blood pressure, flushed, dry skin, dry sticky membrane, restlessness, and elevated body temperature. Obtain serum sodium and chloride

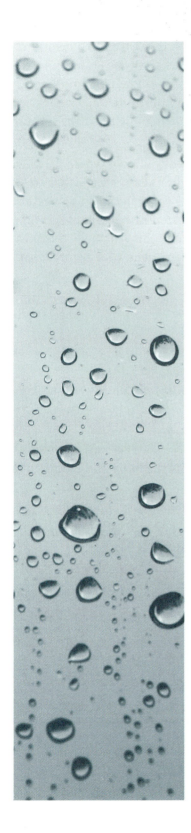

values. Serum sodium levels greater than 146 mEq/L indicate hypernatremia. A serum chloride level greater than 108 mEq/L is indicative of hyperchloremia.

● Check the serum osmolality level and urine specific gravity. A serum osmolality level greater than 295 mOsm/kg can indicate hypernatremia. A specific gravity above 1.025 can indicate hypernatremia.

Nursing Diagnosis 1

Imbalanced nutrition: more than body requirements, related to excess intake of foods rich in sodium.

Interventions and Rationale

1. Instruct the patient with hypernatremia to avoid foods rich in salt, i.e., canned foods, lunch meats, ham, pork, pickles, potato chips, and pretzels.

2. Identify drugs that have a sodium-retaining effect on the body, i.e., cortisone preparations, cough medicines, and certain laxatives containing sodium.

3. Monitor the serum sodium level. Check for chest crackles and for edema in the lower extremities.

4. Monitor the serum sodium levels daily or as ordered. A serum sodium level above 146 mEq/L can indicate hypernatremia. A serum sodium level above 160 mEq/L should be reported immediately to the health care provider. Report serum chloride level greater than 108 mEq/L.

5. Monitor serum CO_2 or arterial HCO_3. A decreased serum CO_2 level, <22 mEq/L, and/or decreased arterial HCO_3, <24 mEq/L, can indicate metabolic acidosis and hyperchloremia.

6. Observe for respiratory difficulties, i.e., deep, rapid, vigorous breathing due to hyperchloremia and an acidotic state (metabolic acidosis).

7. Check the serum osmolality level and the urine specific gravity. A serum osmolality level exceeding 295 mOsm/kg can indicate hypernatremia. Sodium is primarily responsible for the serum osmolality value.

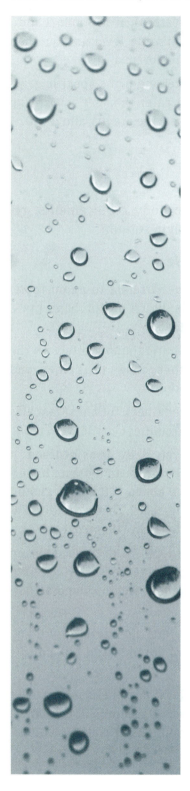

8. Check the urine sodium level. A decreased urine sodium, <40 mEq/L, frequently indicates sodium retention in the body, even though the serum sodium level may be within normal range (caused by hemodilution). Also check for crackles in the lung and for pitting edema from sodium and fluid retention.

9. Check for signs and symptoms of pulmonary edema when the patient is receiving several liters of normal saline (0.9% NaCl) or 3% saline. Sodium holds water in the blood vessels, and when administering a concentrated saline solution, overhydration can occur. Symptoms include dyspnea, cough, chest crackles, and neck and hand vein engorgement.

10. Keep an accurate intake and output record. A decrease in urine output could indicate hypervolemia due to sodium excess.

Nursing Diagnosis 2

Impaired tissue integrity: related to peripheral edema secondary to sodium and water excess.

Interventions and Rationale

1. Provide skin care to the body, especially the edematous areas.

2. Change the patient's positions frequently to maintain skin integrity.

3. Promote increased mobility.

4. Use lotions as needed to keep skin moist.

Evaluation/Outcomes

1. Confirm that the cause of sodium and chloride imbalances has been corrected or controlled.

2. Evaluate the effect of the therapeutic regimen in correcting sodium and chloride imbalances. Serum sodium and chloride levels should be periodically checked.

3. Remain free of signs and symptoms of hyponatremia and hypernatremia.

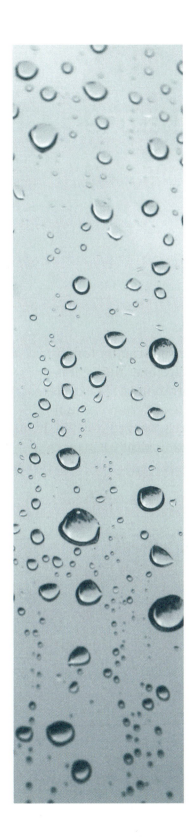

4. Check that fluid imbalances are not contributing to sodium and chloride imbalances. The patient is not dehydrated or overhydrated.

5. Urine output is adequate (>600 ml/day).

6. Maintain a support system, i.e., health professionals, family members, friends.

CHAPTER
8

Calcium Imbalances

 ## INTRODUCTION

Calcium (Ca) is an electrolyte that can be found in both the extracellular and intracellular fluids; it is in somewhat of a greater concentration in the extracellular fluid. Approximately 55% of serum calcium is bound to protein and 45% is free, ionized calcium. It is the free calcium that is physiologically active.

ANSWER COLUMN

1. cation; both;
extracellular fluid

2. calcium

3. teeth and bone;
phosphorous

4. No. For calcium to cause
a physiologic response,
it must be free, ionized
calcium; 4.5–5.5; 9–11

1.
Calcium is a(n) (anion/cation) _____ found in the
(extracellular/intracellular/both) _____ body
fluids.
  Which body fluid has the greater calcium concentration?
*
_____

2.
Calcium is a durable chemical substance of the body that is
the last element to find its place in the adult body
composition and the last element to leave after death.
  The element that preserves the bony remains of dead
creatures and is responsible for the x-ray photograph of bones
is _____.

3.
The normal range of the serum (plasma) calcium concentration
level in the blood is 4.5–5.5 mEq/L, or 9–11 mg/dl.
  Thirty percent is absorbed from food and 99% is combined
with phosphorus in the skeletal system.
  Approximately 99% of the body's calcium is in teeth and bone.
The remaining 1% is in the extracellular and intracellular fluids.
  Most of the body's calcium is in the _____ and
_____. Calcium is combined with _____
in the skeletal system.

4.
About one-half of the body's serum calcium is bound to
plasma proteins and the other half is free, ionized calcium
that serves as a catalyst to stimulate a physiologic cellular
response. Do you think the calcium that is bound to protein
can cause a cellular response? _____ Why?
_____.
  The serum calcium level is _____ mEq/l, or
_____ mg/dl.

5.

When calcium becomes unbound from the plasma protein, the calcium is free, active calcium. This free calcium (can/cannot) _____ cause a physiologic cellular response.

5. can

6.

Today's blood analyzers allow the ionized calcium (iCa) level to be measured. The normal serum ionized calcium level is 2.2–2.5 mEq/L, or 4.25–5.25 mg/dl.

   Certain changes in the blood composition can either increase or decrease the serum iCa level. During acidosis, decreased pH, calcium is released from the serum proteins, which (increases/decreases) _____ the serum iCa level.

   With alkalosis, there is an increased pH level that (increases/decreases) _____ the calcium bound to protein. This results in a(n) (increase/decrease) _____ in the amount of free serum calcium, and thus, the serum iCa level is (increased/decreased) _____.

6. increases; increases; decrease; decreased

7.

The normal serum calcium (Ca) range is _____ mEq/L, or _____ mg/dl.

   The normal ionized calcium (iCa) range is _____ mEq/L, or _____ mg/dl.

7. 4.5–5.5; 9–11; 2.2–2.5; 4.25–5.25

● FUNCTIONS

8.

Vitamin D is an element that is needed for calcium absorption from the gastrointestinal tract. The anion phosphorus (P) inhibits calcium absorption. Thus, the actions of these two ions on the body have an opposite physiologic effect. When the serum calcium level is increased, the serum phosphorus level (increases/decreases) _____. However, both calcium and phosphorus are stored in the bone and are excreted by the kidneys.

8. decreases

9.

The parathyroid glands, which are four small oval-shaped glands located on the posterior thyroid gland, regulate the serum level of calcium. These glands secrete the parathyroid hormone (PTH), which is responsible for the homeostatic regulation of the calcium ion in the body fluids.

When the serum calcium level is low, the parathyroid gland secretes more parathyroid hormone. Explain what happens when the serum calcium level is high. * _____

_____

9. It inhibits or limits the secretion of the parathyroid hormone (PTH).

10.

Calcitonin from the thyroid gland increases calcium return to the bone, thus decreasing the serum calcium level. Figure 8-1 diagrams the sequence of PTH and calcitonin which are secreted from the thyroid and parathyroid glands, and their effects on bone and serum Ca levels.

The parathyroid hormone (PTH) can (increase/decrease) _____ the serum calcium level by promoting calcium release from the bone as needed.

Indicate which of the hormones listed on the left increase or decrease the serum calcium levels.

_____ 1. Calcitonin   a. Increase

_____ 2. PTH   b. Decrease

10. increase; 1. b; 2. a

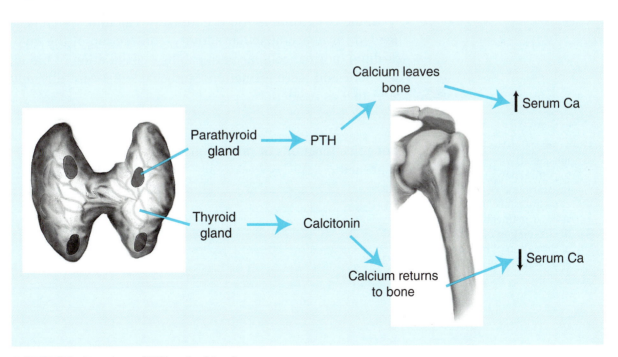

FIGURE 8-1   Functions of PTH and calcitonin.

11. secrete parathyroid hormone (PTH); It inhibits the secretion of parathyroid hormone (PTH) from the parathyroid gland.

11.

The regulation of serum calcium is maintained by the negative-feedback system. A low serum calcium stimulates the parathyroid gland to *_____. What do you think happens when there is a high serum calcium? *_____
_____

12.

A low serum calcium level tells the parathyroid gland to secrete more parathyroid hormone (PTH). The parathyroid hormone increases serum calcium by mobilizing calcium from the bone, increasing renal absorption of calcium and promoting calcium absorption from the intestine in the presence of vitamin D.

PTH increases serum calcium by which of the following mechanisms:

( ) a. Mobilizing calcium from the bone
( ) b. Decreasing renal absorption of calcium
( ) c. Increasing renal absorption of calcium
( ) d. Promoting calcium absorption from the intestine with vitamin D

12. a, c, d

Table 8-1 explains the functions of calcium. Calcium is needed for neuromuscular activity, contraction of the myocardium, normal cellular permeability, coagulation of blood, and bone and teeth formation. Study Table 8-1 carefully, and refer to it as needed.

13.

Name five functions of calcium in the body. Refer to Table 8-1 as needed.

13. a. normal nerve and muscle activity;
b. contraction of myocardium;
c. maintenance of normal cellular permeability;
d. coagulation of blood;
e. formation of bones and teeth

a. *_____
b. *_____
c. *_____
d. *_____
e. *_____

Table 8-1	Calcium and Its Functions
Body Involvement	**Functions**
Neuromuscular	Normal nerve and muscle activity. Calcium causes transmission of nerve impulses and contraction of skeletal muscles. When there is a low serum calcium level, sodium goes into the cells, causing the neuromuscular system to become excited. If calcium deficit is severe, tetany symptoms could result.
Cardiac	Contraction of heart muscle (myocardium).
Cellular and Blood	Maintenance of normal cellular permeability. ↑ calcium decreases cellular permeability and ↓ calcium increases cellular permeability. Coagulation of blood. Calcium promotes blood clotting by converting prothrombin into thrombin.
Bones and Teeth	Formation of bones and teeth. Calcium and phosphorus make bones and teeth strong and durable.

14. decreases; increases

14.

A high serum concentration of calcium (increases/decreases) _____ the permeability of membranes, whereas a low serum concentration of calcium (increases/decreases) _____ the permeability of membranes.

15. Calcium converts prothrombin into thrombin; A calcium deficit causes neuromuscular excitability.

15.

A calcium deficit causes neuromuscular excitability (tetany symptoms). How does calcium promote blood clotting?
*_____.

Explain how tetany occurs. *_____

⬤ PATHOPHYSIOLOGY

16. hypercalcemia; 4.5–5.5 mEq/L, or 9–11 mg/dl

16.

A decrease in the serum calcium level is known as *hypocalcemia.* What do you think an increase in the serum calcium level is called? _____

The normal serum calcium level is *_____.

17. hypocalcemia; hypercalcemia

17.

A serum calcium level less than 4.5 mEq/L is (hypocalcemia/hypercalcemia/normal) _____.

A serum calcium level greater than 5.5 mEq/L is known as (hypocalcemia/hypercalcemia/normal) _____.

18.

Match the serum calcium levels on the left with the type of calcium imbalance or balance.

———————— 1. 5.0 m Eq/L   a. Hypocalcemia

———————— 2. 6.5 mEq/L   b. Hypercalcemia

———————— 3. 5.8 mEq/L   c. Normal

———————— 4. 4.2 mEq/l

———————— 5. 8.2 mg/dl

———————— 6. 9.6 mg/dl

———————— 7. 11.8 mg/dl

18. 1. c; 2. b; 3. b; 4. a; 5. a; 6. c; 7. b

19.

When the parathyroid hormone (PTH) level is low, calcium release from the bones is (increased/inhibited) ————————.

What type of calcium imbalance can occur? ————————

19. inhibited; hypocalcemia

20.

Tissues most affected by hypocalcemia include peripheral nerves, skeletal and smooth muscles, and the cardiac muscle.

A prolonged serum calcium deficit leads to osteoporosis, and a marked serum calcium deficit impairs the clotting time (clot formation).

Neuromuscular excitability of the skeletal, smooth, and cardiac muscles can result from (hypocalcemia/hypercalcemia) ————————.

A decrease in blood coagulation resulting in bleeding may be due to a serum calcium (deficit/excess) ————————.

20. hypocalcemia; deficit

21.

There is a correlation between calcium and magnesium levels. Usually, when there is a magnesium deficit, there is an accompanying calcium deficit.

Hypomagnesemia (serum magnesium deficit) causes a decrease in PTH secretion. A PTH deficiency causes (hypocalcemia/hypercalcemia) ————————.

21. hypocalcemia

22.

With a magnesium deficit, PTH secretions (increase/decrease) ————————.

As a result of the PTH secretion, what happens to the serum calcium level? ————————

22. decrease; It decreases.

23.

Hypercalcemia is frequently the result of calcium loss from the bones. Hypophosphatemia (serum phosphorus deficit) promotes calcium retention.

As a result of hypercalcemia, cellular permeability is _____. (Refer to Table 8-1 as needed.)

23. decreased

24.

Increased calcium enhances hydrochloric acid, gastrin, and pancreatic enzyme release. Hypercalcemia decreases GI peristalsis; thus gastrointestinal motility is (increased/decreased) _____.

24. decreased

25.

Hypercalcemia can decrease the activity of the smooth muscles in the GI system as well as the cardiac muscle activity. Cardiac dysrhythmias, heart block, and ECG/EKG changes are likely to occur from hypercalcemia.

Indicate the effects of a calcium deficit (CD) or calcium excess (CE) for the following physiologic changes:

_____ a. Impaired clotting time
_____ b. Decreased GI peristalsis
_____ c. Increased capillary permeability
_____ d. Neuromuscular excitability of skeletal, smooth, and cardiac muscles
_____ e. Decreased cardiac muscle activity
_____ f. Decreased capillary permeability

25. a. CD; b. CE; c. CD; d. CD; e. CE; f. CE

● ETIOLOGY

The causes of hypocalcemia and hypercalemia are presented in two separate tables. Table 8-2 lists the etiology and rationale for hypocalcemia and Table 8-3 gives the etiology and rationale for hypercalcemia. Proceed to the questions and refer to Tables 8-2 and 8-3 as needed.

26.

Name three causes of hypocalcemia related to dietary changes.

*_____

_____

26. lack of calcium intake, inadequate vitamin D intake, and lack of protein in the diet

27. Vitamin D must be present for calcium absorption.

27.

What effect does vitamin D insufficiency have on calcium?

*

_____

_____

28.

What effect does an inadequate protein diet have on calcium?

*

_____

_____

28. It inhibits the body's utilization of calcium.

Table 8-2	Causes of Hypocalcemia (Serum Calcium Deficit)
Etiology	**Rationale**
Dietary Changes	
Lack of calcium intake, inadequate vitamin D, and/or lack of protein in diet	A calcium (Ca) deficit resulting from lack of Ca intake is rare. Vitamin D must be present for calcium absorption from GI tract. Inadequate protein intake inhibits the body's utilization of calcium.
Hypoalbuminemia (low albumin level)	The most common cause of low total serum calcium level.
Chronic diarrhea	Chronic diarrhea interferes with adequate calcium absorption.
Renal Dysfunction	
Renal failure	Renal failure causes phosphorus and calcium retention. Lack of PTH decreases renal calcium absorption.
Hormonal and Electrolyte Influence	
Decreased parathyroid hormone (PTH)	With hypoparathyroidism, there is less PTH secreted. PTH deficiency decreases renal production of calcitriol, which causes a decrease in calcium absorption from the intestines.
Increased serum phosphorus (phosphate)	Secondary hypoparathyroidism may be caused by sepsis, burns, surgery, or pancreatitis.
Increased serum magnesium	Overuse of phosphate laxatives can decrease calcium retention.
Severe decreased magnesium	Magnesium imbalances inhibit PTH secretion.
Increased calcitonin	
Calcium Binders or Chelators	
Citrated blood transfusions	Rapid administration of citrated blood binds with calcium, inhibiting ionized (free) Ca.
Alkalosis	Alkalosis increases calcium protein binding.
Increased serum albumin level	With an increase in serum albumin, more calcium is bound and less calcium is free and active.

29. hypoalbuminemia; normal; Calcium binds with proteins such as albumin and with a decrease in albumin levels, there is more free ionized calcium.

30. deficit; Less parathyroid hormone (PTH) is secreted.

31. decrease

29.

Total serum calcium level may be low; however, the ionized calcium level can be normal. The total serum calcium level may be low because of (hyperalbuminemia/hypoalbuminemia) _____.

However, the ionized calcium level could be _____.
Explain. *_____
_____

30.

Hypoparathyroidism can cause a calcium (deficit/excess) _____. How? *_____

31.

Calcitriol has a synergistic effect with PTH on bone absorption; it increases calcium absorption from the intestines.
With a calcitriol deficiency, there would be a(an) (increase/decrease) _____ in calcium absorption from the intestine.

Table 8-3	Causes of Hypercalcemia (Serum Calcium Excess)
Etiology	**Rationale**
Dietary Changes: Increased Calcium Salts (supplements)	Excessive use of calcium supplements, calcium salts, and antacids can increase the serum calcium level.
Renal Impairment, Diuretics: Thiazides	Kidney dysfunction and use of thiazide diuretics decrease the excretion of calcium.
Cellular Destruction Bone Immobility	A malignant bone tumor, a fracture, and/or a prolonged immobilization can cause loss of calcium from the bone. Some malignancies cause an ectopic PTH production. Increased immobility promotes calcium loss from the bone.
Hormonal and Drug Influence Increased PTH Decreased serum phosphorus	Hyperparathyroidism increases the production of PTH and increased PTH then promotes the release of calcium from the bone. A decreased phosphorus level can increase the serum calcium level to the extent that the kidneys are unable to excrete excess calcium.
Thiazide diuretics	Thiazides increase the action of PTH on kidneys, promoting calcium reabsorption.
Steroid therapy	Steroids such as cortisone mobilize calcium absorption from the bone.

32.

Which of the following are the effects of an insufficient PTH level?

( ) a. Calcium release from the bone is inhibited.

( ) b. Less calcium is absorbed from the kidney tubules.

( ) c. Calcium release from the bone is promoted.

( ) d. Calcium absorption from the kidneys is promoted.

32. b, c

33.

Calcium and phosphorus, which are found in many foods, are regulated by the parathyroid gland and absorbed together. The serum values of calcium and phosphate (ionized phosphorus) are opposites. With hyperphosphatemia, (hypocalcemia/hypercalcemia) _____ is more likely to occur.

33. hypocalcemia

34.

What effect does prolonged immobilization have on calcium?

_____

_____

34. It increases the serum calcium level by releasing Ca from the bones.

35.

Hypercalcemia occurs because of increased amounts of calcium being released from the bone due to which of the following conditions: (Refer to Table 8-3 as needed.)

( ) a. Fractures

( ) b. Immobilization

( ) c. Decreased parathyroid hormone (PTH) secretion

( ) d. Bone cancer

( ) e. Malignancies promoting PTH production

35. a, b, d, e

36.

Multiple fractures cause the release of calcium into the intravascular fluid, thus (increasing/decreasing) _____ the serum calcium level.

36. increasing

37.

Loop or high-ceiling diuretics (furosemide) decrease the serum calcium level. Thiazide diuretics such as HydroDiuril (increase/decrease) _____ the serum calcium level.

Hypercalcemia (increases/decreases) _____ cellular permeability.

37. increase; decreases

38.

Hypercalcemia occurs in 25–50% of malignancies occurring in the lung, breast, ovaries, prostate, and bladder. These cancers can cause bone destruction due to metastasis or (increased/decreased) _____ ectopic PTH secretion.

38. increased

39.

Prolonged steroid therapy can cause increased serum calcium levels. Explain. *_____

_____

39. Prolonged use of steroids mobilizes calcium release from the bone.

● CLINICAL MANIFESTATIONS

40.

Clinical manifestations of hypocalcemia and hypercalcemia are determined by the signs and symptoms of calcium imbalance, ECG/EKG changes, and the serum calcium level.

The normal serum calcium range is _____ mEq/L, or _____ mg/dl. Levels less than _____ mEq/L indicate hypocalcemia and those greater than _____ mEq/L indicate hypercalcemia.

40. 4.5–5.5; 9–11; 4.5; 5.5

41.

A commonly seen clinical manifestation of hypocalcemia is tetany. A calcium deficit causes sodium to move into the neuromuscular cells, causing excitability. With hypocalcemia, the amount of circulating free, ionized calcium is (increased/decreased) _____.

41. decreased

Table 8-4 lists the clinical manifestations of hypocalcemia and hypercalcemia according to the body areas that are affected. The serum calcium level and the specific ECG changes determine the severity of the calcium imbalance. Study Table 8-4 and refer to it as needed.

42.

Tetany symptoms are due to a decrease in free, (ionized/nonionized) _____ circulating calcium. Symptoms of tetany include which of the following:

_____ a. Twitching around the mouth

Table 8-4

Clinical Manifestations of Calcium Imbalances

Body Involvement	Hypocalcemia	Hypercalcemia
CNS and Muscular Abnormalities	Anxiety, irritability Tetany 　Twitching around mouth 　Tingling and numbness of fingers 　Carpopedal spasm 　Spasmodic contractions 　Laryngeal spasm 　Convulsions Abdominal cramps Muscle cramps	Depression/apathy Muscles are flabby
Chvostek's Sign	Positive	
Trousseau's Sign	Positive	
Cardiac Abnormalities	Weak cardiac contractions	Signs of heart block Cardiac arrest in systole
ECG/EKG	Lengthened ST segment Prolonged QT interval	Decreased or diminished ST 　segment Shortened QT interval
Blood Abnormalities	Blood does not clot normally, 　reduction of prothrombin.	
Skeletal Abnormalities	Fractures occur if deficit persists.	Pathologic fractures Deep pain over bony areas Thinning of bones apparent
Renal Abnormalities		Flank pain Calcium stones formed in the kidney
Laboratory Values		
Serum Ca	<4.5 mEq/L	>5.5 mEq/L
Ionized serum Ca	<2.2 mEq/L	>2.5 mEq/l
Serum Ca	<9.0 mg/dl	>11.0 mg/dl
Ionized serum Ca	<4.25 mg/dl	>5.25 mg/dl

＿＿＿＿＿＿＿＿＿ b. Tingling and numbness of the
　　　　　　　　　　extremities

＿＿＿＿＿＿＿＿＿ c. Carpopedal spasms

＿＿＿＿＿＿＿＿＿ d. Laryngeal spasm

＿＿＿＿＿＿＿＿＿ e. Spasmodic contractions

42. ionized; a, b, c, d, e　＿＿＿＿＿＿＿＿＿ f. Muscular hypertrophy

43. absent; With metabolic acidosis, more calcium is freed from protein-binding sites. When the acidotic state is corrected, calcium will bind again with albumin/protein and the tetany symptoms can occur.

44. deficit

45. 1. b; 2. a

43.

Tetany symptoms are (present/absent) _____ when the patient with hypocalcemia is in an acidotic state (metabolic acidosis). Explain your response. *_____

_____

44.

Two tests, Chvostek and Trousseau, may be used to test for severe hypocalcemia and presence of tetany. Figure 8-2 describes the technique for checking for positive Chvostek and Trousseau signs.

   A positive test for Chvostek and/or Trousseau indicates a calcium (deficit/excess) _____.

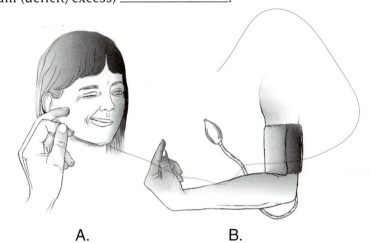

A.   B.

FIGURE 8-2 Testing for Chvostek and Trousseau's signs. A. Chvostek's sign: The face is tapped over the facial nerve (2 cm anterior to the earlobe). A positive Chvostek is evidenced as spasms of the cheek and mouth. B. Trousseau's sign: Inflate a blood pressure cuff (20–30 mm Hg) on the upper arm to constrict circulation. A positive Trousseau is evidenced as the occurrence of a carpopedal spasm of the fingers and hand within 1–5 minutes.

45.

Match the symptoms of hypocalcemia on the left with the appropriate test for tetany.

_____ 1. Carpopedal spasm   a. Chvostek's sign
_____ 2. Facial muscle twitching   b. Trousseau's sign

46.

With hypercalcemia, kidney stones (calcium) may occur. This may result when calcium leaves the bones due to immobilization, bone tumors, or increased PTH associated with a secondary malignancy. Increased PTH promotes

_____.
*

46. calcium release from the bone

47.

For the following clinical manifestations, indicate which is the result of a calcium deficit (CD) or a calcium excess (CE).

_____ a. Muscles are flabby

_____ b. Tetany symptoms

_____ c. Muscle cramps

_____ d. Positive Chvostek's sign

_____ e. Deep pain over bony areas

_____ f. Kidney stones

_____ g. Blood does NOT clot normally

47. a. CE; b. CD; c. CD; d. CD; e. CE; f. CE; g. CD

Figures 8-3A and B note the electrocardiographic changes found with hypocalcemia and hypercalcemia. The normal ECG/EKG tracing is found on page 100. The ECG changes that may occur with hypocalcemia are shown in Figure 8-3A.

The ECG changes that may occur with hypercalcemia are shown in Figure 8-3B.

48.

The hypocalcemia effect on the ECG causes the ST segment to be _____ and the QT interval to be _____. It may progress to heart block.

48. lengthened; prolonged

49.

The hypercalcemia effect on the ECG causes the ST segment to be _____ and the QT interval to be

_____.

Severe hypercalcemia can lead to complete heart block and cardiac arrest.

49. decreased; shortened

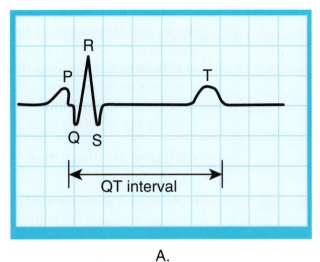

A.

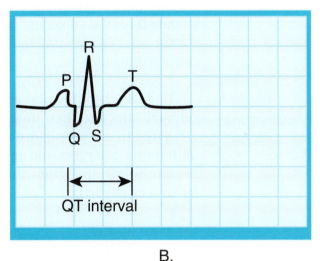

B.

FIGURE 8-3 A. Lengthened ST segment; prolonged QT interval.
B. Decreased ST segment; shortened QT interval.

● CLINICAL MANAGEMENT

Clinical management of hypocalcemia consists of oral supplements and intravenous calcium diluted in 5% dextrose in water (D_5W). Calcium should not be diluted in normal saline solution (0.9% NaCl) since the sodium encourages calcium loss.

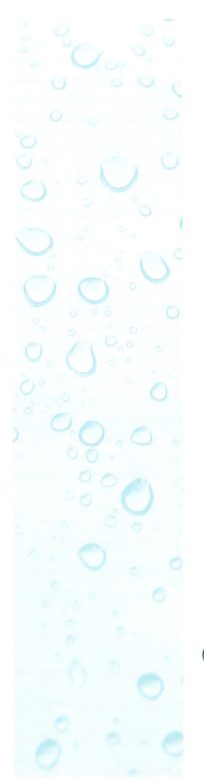

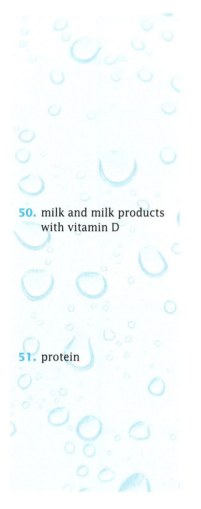

The goal of management for hypercalcemia is to correct the underlying cause of the serum calcium excess. Drugs such as calcitonin or IV saline solution administered rapidly and followed by a loop diuretic can be used to promote urinary excretion of calcium. Plicamycin (Mithracin), an anticancer antibiotic, lowers the serum calcium level by prohibiting calcium loss from the bone.

Calcium Replacement

50.

Identify food products high in calcium that can be used to prevent or correct the body's calcium deficit. * _____

50. milk and milk products with vitamin D

51.

Normally, calcium is not required for IV therapy since there is a tremendous reservoir in the bone. However, the body needs vitamin D for the utilization of dietary calcium.

What other essential composition of the diet is needed for calcium utilization? _____

51. protein

Table 8-5 lists the oral and intravenous preparations of calcium salts and their dosages and drug form. The drugs are listed in alphabetic order. The drug dosage is given in milligrams per gram and indicates the elemental calcium amount within that gram. Study Table 8-5 carefully and refer to it as needed.

Table 8-5	Calcium Preparations	
Calcium Name	**Drug Form**	**Drug Dose**
Orals		
Calcium carbonate	650–1500-mg tablets	400 mg/g*
Calcium citrate	950-mg tablet	211 mg/g*
Calcium lactate	325–650-mg tablets	130 mg/g*
Calcium gluconate	500–1000-mg tablets	90 mg/g*
Intravenous		
Calcium chloride	10 ml size	272 mg/g*; 13.5 mEq
Calcium gluceptate	5 ml size	90 mg/g*; 4.5 mEq
Calcium gluconate	10 ml size	90 mg/g*; 4.5 mEq

*Elemental calcium is 1 gram (1 g).

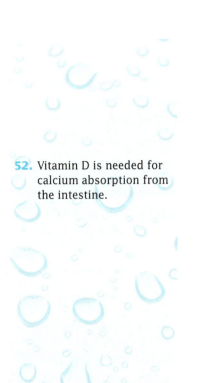

52.

Asymptomatic hypocalcemia is normally corrected with oral calcium gluconate, calcium lactate, and calcium carbonate. Calcium carbonate can cause GI upset due to carbon dioxide (CO_2) formation. For better calcium absorption, a calcium supplement containing vitamin D should be given 30 minutes before meals.

Why should the calcium supplement contain vitamin D?

*_____

52. Vitamin D is needed for calcium absorption from the intestine.

53.

Acute hypocalcemia with tetany symptoms needs immediate correction. Intravenous 10% calcium chloride or 10% calcium gluconate is given slowly, 1–3 ml/min, to avoid hypotension, bradycardia, and other dysrhythmias.

Calcium chloride provides more ionized calcium than calcium gluconate; however, it is more irritating to the subcutaneous tissue, and if calcium chloride infiltrates, sloughing of the tissue results.

For intravenous administration calcium salts should be diluted in which of the following solution(s):

( ) a. Normal saline (0.9% NaCl)

( ) b. Five percent dextrose in water

53. b

54.

The suggested rate of IV flow for a calcium solution is *_____. If the rate of IV flow is too rapid, what might occur? *_____

54. 1–3 ml/min; cardiac dysrhythmias (bradycardia), hypotension

Table 8-6 gives the suggested clinical management for hypocalcemia.

Table 8-6	Suggested Clinical Management for Hypocalcemia
Calcium Deficit	**Suggested Clinical Management**
Mild	Oral calcium salts with vitamin D, take twice a day.
	10% IV calcium gluconate (10 ml) in D_5W solution. Administer slowly, 1–3 ml/min.
Moderate	10% IV calcium gluconate (10–20 ml) in D_5W solution. Administer slowly, 1–3 ml/min.
Severe	10% IV calcium gluconate (100 ml) in 1 liter of D_5W. Administer over 4 hrs.

55. dilute 100 ml of 10% IV calcium gluconate in D$_5$W and administer over 4 hours.

56. does not (elevated calcium level enhances the action of digoxin)

57. decreases; a decrease in the T wave

58. volume expansion or sodium to promote calcium loss; prevent fluid overload

55.

For moderate hypocalcemia, 10–20 ml of 10% IV calcium gluconate is diluted in 5% dextrose and water (D$_5$W). The solution is administered at a rate of 1–3 ml/min.

   For severe hypocalcemia, the suggested clinical management is to *_____.

56.

Care should be taken when administering calcium to a patient who is taking digoxin daily (digitalis preparation). An elevated serum calcium level enhances the action of digoxin; thus digitalis toxicity can result.

   A decreased calcium level (does/does not) _____ cause digitalis toxicity.

57.

Intravenous calcium salts may be used to counteract the effect of a potassium excess on the heart muscle (myocardium). IV calcium (increases/decreases) _____ the effect of hyperkalemia.

   What type of ECG improvement should the nurse observe when using calcium supplements to correct hyperkalemia?

*_____

Hypercalcemia Correction

To treat hypercalcemia, expanding the fluid volume is important to increase renal calcium excretion. The use of normal saline solution (NSS) to increase volume expansion decreases calcium reabsorption in the renal proximal tubules. Sodium in NSS promotes calcium loss. Also a loop diuretic such as furosemide (Lasix) is prescribed to prevent fluid overload. Table 8-7 lists suggested treatments for correcting mild to moderate and severe hypercalcemia.

58.

An intravenous NSS is given for *_____ and furosemide (Lasix) is given intravenously to *_____.

Table 8-7	Suggested Corrections for Hypercalcemia

Mild to Moderate Hypercalcemia 11–14 mg/dl	Severe Hypercalcemia > 14 mg/dl
Normal saline solution (NSS, 0.9% NaCl)	Normal saline solution (NSS, 0.9% NaCl)
Loop diuretics, e.g., furosemide (Lasix)	Loop diuretics, e.g., furosemide (Lasix)
	Calcitonin, 4 units/kg, SC
	Others:
	Corticosteroids
	Antitumor antibiotics, e.g., plicamycin (Mithracin, Mithramycin)

59. b

60. The thiazide HydroDiuril causes increased serum calcium level by promoting calcium reabsorption.

61. furosemide, calcitonin, cortisone, and IV phosphate; also plicamycin

59.

Which diuretic promotes urinary calcium excretion?

_____ a. Hydrochlorothiazide (HydroDiuril)

_____ b. Furosemide (Lasix)

60.

Why would the potassium-wasting (thiazide) diuretic, hydrochlorothiazide (HydroDiuril) not be prescribed for treating hypercalcemia? *_____

61.

Other drugs that can decrease the serum calcium level are:

a. Calcitonin, a thyroid hormone that inhibits the effects of PTH on the bone and increases urinary calcium excretion

b. Glucocorticoids (Cortisone), which compete with vitamin D, thus decreasing the intestinal absorption of calcium

c. Intravenous phosphates, which promote calcium excretion

d. Plicamycin (Mithracin, Mithramycin), which inhibits the action of PTH

The four drugs that may be used to treat hypercalcemia are

*_____

_____.

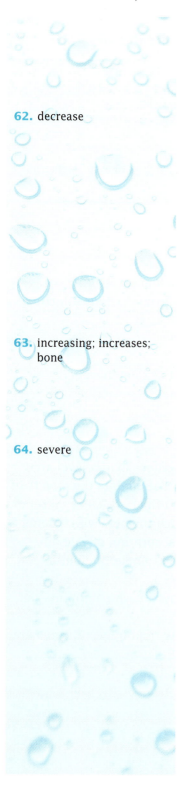

62.

The antitumor antibiotic plicamycin (Mithracin, Mithramycin) inhibits the action of PTH on osteoclasts in bone. Plicamycin is a treatment for malignancy-associated hypercalcemia. The result of this drug action is a(n) (increase/decrease) _____ in the serum calcium level.

62. decrease

63.

Malignancies are a common cause of hypercalcemia. A metastatic bone lesion can destroy the bone, which releases calcium into the circulation, thus (increasing/decreasing) _____ serum calcium level.

   Some cancers promote the secretion of the parathyroid hormone (PTH) and may be referred to as tumor-secreting (ectopic) PTH production. The most common types of cancer that can cause hypercalcemia are lung, breast, ovary, prostate, leukemia, and gastrointestinal cancers.

   Parathyroid hormone (increases/decreases) _____ the release of calcium from the _____.

63. increasing; increases; bone

64.

Corticosteroids (glucocorticoids, Cortisone) are effective in treating calcitriol-induced hypercalcemia. Corticosteroid therapy is a treatment for (mild/moderate/severe) _____ hypercalcemia.

64. severe

Drugs and Their Effect on Calcium Balance

Phosphate preparations, corticosteroids, loop diuretics, aspirin, anticonvulsants, magnesium sulfate, and plicamycin are some of the groups of drugs that can lower the serum calcium level. Excess calcium salt ingestion and infusion and thiazide and chlorthalidone diuretics are drugs that can increase the serum calcium level. Table 8-8 lists drugs that affect calcium balance.

Table 8-8	Drugs Affecting Calcium Balance	
Calcium Imbalance	**Drugs**	**Rationale**
Hypocalcemia (serum calcium deficit)	Magnesium sulfate Propylthiouracil/Propacil Colchicine Plicamycin/Mithracin Neomycin Excessive sodium citrate	These agents inhibit parathyroid hormone/PTH secretion and decrease the serum calcium level.

	Acetazolamide
	Aspirin
	Anticonvulsants
	Glutethimide/Doriden
	Estrogens
	Aminoglycosides
	   Gentamicin
	   Amikacin
	   Tobramycin
		These agents can alter the vitamin D metabolism that is needed for calcium absorption.

	Phosphate preparations:
	Oral, enema, and intravenous
	   Sodium phosphate
	   Potassium phosphate
		Phosphates can increase the serum phosphorus level and decrease the serum calcium level.

	Corticosteroids
	   Cortisone
	   Prednisone
		Steroids decrease calcium mobilization and inhibit the absorption of calcium.

	Loop diuretics Furosemide/Lasix	Loop diuretics reduce calcium absorption from the renal tubules.
Hypercalcemia (serum calcium excess)	Calcium salts Vitamin D	Excess ingestion of calcium and vitamin D and infusion of calcium can increase the serum Ca level.
	IV lipids	Lipids can increase the calcium level.

	Kayexalate, androgens
	Diuretics
	   Thiazides
	   Chlorthalidone/Hygroteon
		These agents can induce hypercalcemia.

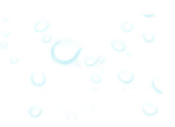

65.

Enter CD for calcium deficit/hypocalcemia and CE for calcium excess/hypercalcemia opposite the following drugs. Refer to Table 8-8 as needed.

_____ a. Magnesium sulfate

_____ b. Aspirin

_____ c. Anticonvulsants

_____ d. Calcium sulfates

_____ e. Thiazide diuretics

_____ f. Corticosteroids

_____ g. Loop diuretics

_____ h. Vitamin D

_____ i. Aminoglycosides

65. a. CD; b. CD; c. CD; d. CE;
e. CE; f. CD; g. CD; h. CE;
i. CD

66.

Plicamycin, an antineoplastic antibiotic, is used to treat hypercalcemia. This agent lowers the serum calcium level.

Steroids and plicamycin (increase/decrease) _____ the serum calcium level.

66. decrease

67.

Hypercalcemia can cause cardiac dysrhythmias. An elevated serum calcium enhances the effect of digitalis and can cause digitalis toxicity.

Give three signs and symptoms of digitalis toxicity.

*_____

_____

67. bradycardia (slow heart rate) with or without dysrhythmias, nausea and vomiting, and anorexia

68.

During a hypercalcemic state the dose of digoxin should be (increased/decreased)? _____

68. decreased

69.

Steroids such as cortisone tend to decrease calcium mobilization and inhibit the absorption of calcium.

Steroids (increase/decrease) _____ the serum calcium level.

69. decrease

70.

A loop (high-ceiling) diuretic affects the renal tubules by reducing the absorption of calcium and increasing calcium excretion. Give the name of a loop diuretic. _____

Name two other electrolytes that are excreted by loop diuretics. *_____

70. furosemide/Lasix; potassium and sodium

⬤ CLINICAL APPLICATIONS

71.

For body utilization, calcium must be in the ionized form. In body fluids, calcium is found in both ionized and nonionized (bound to plasma proteins) forms.

In an alkalotic state (body fluids are more alkaline), large amounts of the calcium become protein bound and cannot be utilized. When the body fluids are more acid (acidotic state), calcium is more likely to be (ionized/nonionized)

_____.

71. ionized (hence calcium can be utilized)

72.

Calcium acts on the central nervous system (CNS).

Let us say you are caring for a debilitated patient who becomes severely agitated. You notice the patient's hands trembling and mouth twitching. These symptoms may indicate a calcium (excess/deficit) _____.

72. deficit

73.

Lack of calcium causes neuromuscular irritability. Explain.

*_____

_____

What does hypocalcemia do to blood clotting? *_____

_____

73. It leads to hyperactivity of the nervous system and painful muscular contractions (symptoms of tetany). It decreases clotting and causes bleeding.

74.

Prolonged vomiting leads to alkalosis due to the loss of hydrogen and chloride ions from the stomach.

When the body fluids are alkaline, what happens to calcium?

*_____

_____

74. Calcium is nonionized; hypocalcemia occurs.

75.

Acidosis (increases/decreases) _____ the ionization of calcium.

75. increases

76. hypercalcemia

77. Eat foods that are high in acid content (meat, fish, poultry, eggs, cheese, peanuts, cereals) and/or drink at least 1 pint (2 glasses) of cranberry juice daily. Orange juice does not make the urine acid.

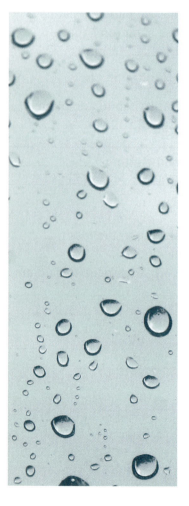

76.

The kidneys excrete approximately 50–250 mg/dl of calcium in the urine daily. If the kidneys excrete less than 50 mg/dl, what type of calcium imbalance is likely to occur? _____

77.

The health intervention for a patient with hypercalcemia is to prevent renal calculi. There are three ways this can be accomplished:
   a. Drink at least 12 glasses of fluid a day.
   b. Keep urine acid.
   c. Prevent urinary tract infections.
How do you think the urine can be kept acid? *_____
_____

● CLINICAL CONSIDERATIONS

   1. Administer an oral calcium supplement containing vitamin D. Vitamin D is necessary for intestinal absorption of calcium.

   2. Oral calcium supplements with vitamin D should be given 30 minutes before meals to improve GI absorption.

   3. Intravenous calcium salts should be diluted in 5% dextrose in water (D_5W). Do NOT dilute calcium salts in a saline solution; sodium promotes calcium loss.

   4. The suggested IV flow rate for a calcium solution is 1–3 ml/min (average: 2 ml/min).

   5. Infiltration of calcium solution, especially calcium chloride, can cause sloughing of the subcutaneous tissues.

   6. An elevated serum calcium level can enhance the action of digoxin, causing digitalis toxicity.

   7. Diuretics such as furosemide (Lasix) can decrease the serum calcium level, and thiazide diuretics tend to increase the serum calcium levels. Steroids decrease serum calcium levels.

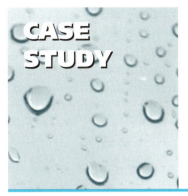

CASE STUDY

REVIEW

A 58-year-old male has had a gastric upset for the past 6 weeks. He has been taking antacids and drinking several glasses of milk each day. His stomach discomfort was not relieved and he was admitted to the hospital to rule out a possible malignant tumor. His serum calcium was 5.9 mEq/L.

ANSWER COLUMN

1. hypercalcemia
2. 4.5–5.5 mEq/l, or 9–11 mg/dl
3. Decrease in ionized calcium for utilization. In alkaline fluids, calcium is nonionized and protein bound. An elevated serum calcium can result from large amounts of milk intake and from a malignant neoplasm. A variety of neoplasms (tumors) can cause hypercalcemia.
4. maintenance of normal cell permeability, formation of bones and teeth, normal clotting mechanism, and normal muscle and nerve activity.
5. elevated; Prolonged immobilization would increase the serum calcium by releasing calcium from the bones.
6. kidney stones
7. Drink at least 12 glasses of fluid a day, eat foods high in acid content to keep urine acid, and prevent urinary tract infections.

1. His serum calcium level indicates what type of calcium imbalance? _____

2. The "normal" range for calcium balance is *_____.

3. Explain what happens to body calcium when there is a decrease in gastric acidity and an increase in body alkaline fluids. *_____
   _____

4. Give four functions of calcium in the body. *_____
   _____
   _____

5. If the patient was bedridden, would you expect his serum calcium to be (elevated/decreased)? _____
   Explain.
   *_____
   _____

6. Identify a health problem that can occur from immobilization. *_____

7. Identify three nursing interventions to prevent renal calculi resulting from hypercalcemia. *_____
   _____

8. Hypercalcemia enhances the action of digoxin, making it more powerful; decreased

8. Previously, he had a "heart condition" and he was started on digoxin. What effect does hypercalcemia have on digoxin? *_____

Should his digoxin dosage be (increased/decreased) _____ until his hypercalcemic state is corrected?

9. hypocalcemia
10. carpopedal spasm, twitching of the mouth, tingling of the fingers, spasm of the larynx, abdominal cramps, and muscle cramps

9. If his serum calcium became 3.9 mEq/L, what type of calcium imbalance would be present? _____

10. Identify five common signs and symptoms of severe hypocalcemia.
* _____
_____

CARE PLAN

PATIENT MANAGEMENT: CALCIUM IMBALANCES

Hypocalcemia Assessment Factors

● Obtain a health history to identify potential causes of hypocalcemia: insufficient diet in protein and calcium, lack of vitamin D intake, chronic diarrhea, hormonal influence [decreased parathyroid hormone (PTH)], drug influence, hypoparathyroidism, metabolic alkalotic state, and rapid administration of a blood transfusion that contains citrate.

● Assess for signs and symptoms of hypocalcemia, i.e., tetany symptoms (twitching around mouth, carpopedal spasms, laryngospasms), abdominal cramps, and muscle cramps.

● Obtain a serum calcium level that can be used as a baseline for comparison of future serum calcium levels. A serum calcium level below 4.5 mEq/L, or 9 mg/dl, or iCa <2.2 mEq/L indicates hypocalcemia.

● Check the ECG/EKG strips for changes in the QT interval. A prolonged QT interval may indicate a serum calcium deficit.

● Identify drugs the patient is taking that may cause a serum calcium deficit, such as furosemide (Lasix), cortisone preparations, phosphate preparations, and massive use of antacids that can interfere with calcium absorption.

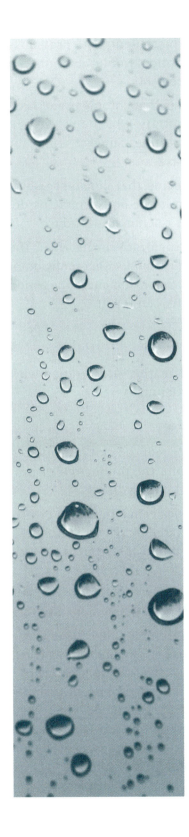

● Determine the acid-base status when hypocalcemia is present. In an acidotic state, calcium is ionized and can be utilized by the body even though there is a calcium deficit. This is not true when alkalosis occurs. Calcium is not ionized in an alkalotic state; and if a severe calcium deficit is present, tetany symptoms occur.

● Assess for positive Trousseau's and Chvostek's signs of hypocalcemia. For Trousseau's sign, inflate the blood pressure cuff for 3 minutes and observe for a carpopedal spasm. For Chvostek's sign, tap the facial nerve in front of the ear for spasms of the cheek and mouth.

Nursing Diagnosis 1

Imbalanced nutrition: less than body requirements, related to insufficient calcium intake, poor calcium absorption due to insufficient vitamin D and protein intake, or drugs (antacids, cortisone preparation) that interfere with calcium ionization.

Interventions and Rationale

1. Monitor serum calcium levels. A serum calcium level under 4.5 mEq/L or iCa <2.2 mEq/L can cause neuromuscular excitability. Tetany symptoms may occur.

2. Monitor ECG and note changes related to hypocalcemia, i.e., prolonged QT interval and lengthened ST segment.

3. Frequently monitor IV solutions containing calcium to prevent infiltration. Calcium is irritating to the subcutaneous tissues and can cause tissue sloughing.

4. Administer oral calcium supplements an hour before meals to enhance intestinal absorption.

5. Regulate IV 10% calcium gluconate or chloride in a liter of 5% dextrose in water (D_5W) to run 1–3 ml/min, or according to the order. Do not administer calcium salts in a normal saline solution (0.9% NaCl). The sodium encourages calcium loss.

6. Instruct patients to eat foods rich in calcium, vitamin D, and protein, especially the older adult. Explain the importance of calcium in the diet to prevent osteoporosis and to aid

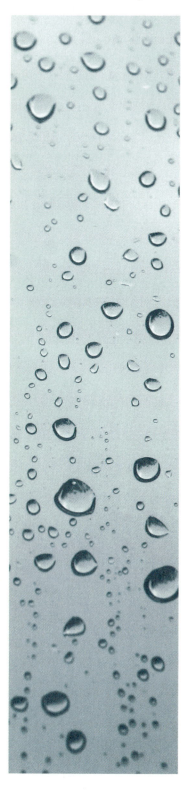

normal clot formation. Tell the patient that protein is needed to aid in calcium absorption. Nonfat dry milk can be used to meet calcium requirements.

7. Teach "bowel-conscious" persons that chronic use of laxatives can increase intestinal motility, which prevents calcium absorption from the intestine. Suggest fruits for bowel elimination, instead of laxatives.

8. Explain to persons using antacids that constant use of antacids can decrease calcium in the body. Antacids decrease acidity, which decreases calcium ionization.

9. Monitor the pulse regularly for bradycardia when the patient is receiving digoxin and calcium, either orally or intravenously. Increased serum calcium enhances the action of digoxin, and digitalis toxicity can result.

Nursing Diagnosis 2

Risk for injury: bleeding related to the interference with blood coagulation secondary to calcium loss.

Interventions and Rationale

1. Check for prolonged bleeding or reduced clot formation. A low serum calcium level inhibits the production of prothrombin, which is needed in clot formation.

2. Observe for symptoms of hypocalcemia in clients receiving massive transfusions of citrated blood. The serum calcium level may not be affected, but the citrates prevent calcium ionization.

Hypercalcemia Assessment Factors

● Obtain a health history to identify probable causes of hypercalcemia, such as excessive use of calcium supplements, bone destruction due to cancer, cancer of the breast, lung, or prostate (ectopic PTH production), prolonged immobilization, multiple fractures, hormone influence (increased PTH, steroid therapy), hyperparathyroidism, and thiazide diuretics. Approximately 20–25% of hypercalcemia is due to continuous use of large doses of thiazide diuretics.

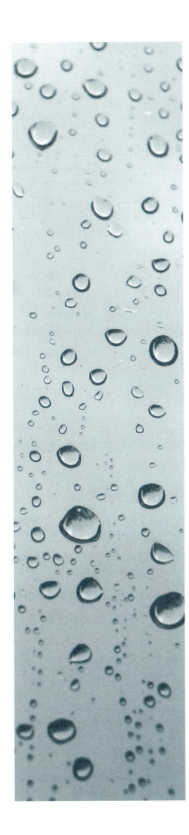

- Assess for signs and symptoms of hypercalcemia, i.e., flabby muscles, pain over bony areas, renal calculi, and pathologic fractures.

- Check ECG/EKG strips for changes in the QT interval. A shortened QT interval may indicate a serum calcium excess.

- Obtain a serum calcium level that can be used as a baseline for comparison of future serum calcium levels. A serum calcium level above 5.5 mEq/L, or 11 mg/dl, or iCa >2.5 mEq/L indicates hypercalcemia.

- Assess for fluid volume depletion and changes in the state of the patient's sensorium. These changes may be indicators of hypercalcemia.

Nursing Diagnosis 1

Risk for injury: related to pathologic fractures due to bone destruction from bone cancer, prolonged immobilization.

Interventions and Rationale

1. Monitor serum calcium levels. Report increased serum calcium levels. Levels exceeding 13.0 mg/dl can be life threatening.

2. Monitor ECG and note changes related to hypercalcemia, i.e., shortened QT interval and decreased ST segment.

3. Monitor patient's state of sensorium. Extreme lethargy, confusion, and a comatose state may be the result of hypercalcemia. Safety precautions may be needed.

4. Promote active and passive exercise for bedridden patients. Immobilization promotes calcium loss from the bone.

5. Handle patients gently who have long-standing hypercalcemia and bone demineralization to prevent fractures.

6. Identify symptoms of digitalis toxicity. When the patient has an elevated serum calcium level and is receiving a digitalis preparation such as digoxin, digitalis toxicity may occur. Elevated serum calcium enhances the action of digitalis. Symptoms of digitalis toxicity include bradycardia, nausea, and/or vomiting.

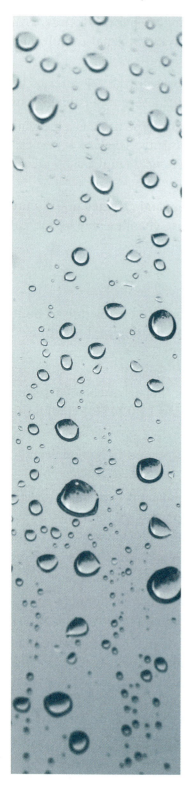

Nursing Diagnosis 2

Imbalanced nutrition: more than body requirements, related to excess calcium intake.

Interventions and Rationale

1. Instruct patients with hypercalcemia to avoid foods rich in calcium and to avoid taking massive amounts of vitamin D supplements.

2. Instruct patients with hypercalcemia to keep hydrated, in order to increase calcium dilution in the serum and urine and to prevent renal calculi formation.

3. Explain to patients with hypercalcemia that the purpose for maintaining an acid urine is to increase solubility of calcium. An acid-ash diet may be ordered that includes meats, fish, poultry, eggs, cheese, cereals, nuts, cranberry juice, and prune juice. Orange juice will not change the urine pH.

Nursing Diagnosis 3

Impaired urinary elimination related to causes of hypercalcemia.

Interventions and Rationale

1. Monitor urinary output and urine pH. Calcium precipitates in alkaline urine and renal calculi may result. Acid-ash foods and juices such as cranberry and prune juices should be encouraged to increase the acidity of the urine.

2. Instruct patients to increase fluid intake to dilute the serum and urine levels of calcium to prevent formation of renal calculi.

3. Administer prescribed loop diuretics to enhance calcium excretion. Thiazide diuretics inhibit calcium excretion and are not indicated in hypercalcemia.

Evaluation/Outcomes

1. Identify the cause of calcium imbalance and document corrective measures taken.

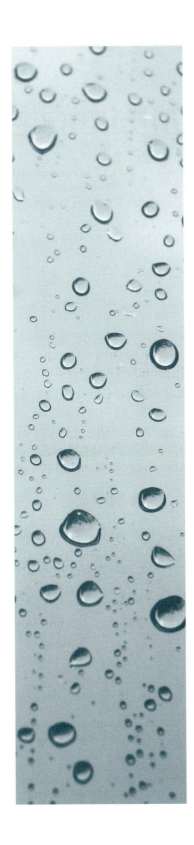

2. Evaluate the effects of prescribed clinical management for hypocalcemia or hypercalcemia. Serum calcium and ionized calcium levels are within normal range.

3. Patient will remain free of signs and symptoms of hypocalcemia. (Tetany signs and symptoms are absent. Vital signs are within normal range.)

4. Recognize risk factors related to hypocalcemia and hypercalcemia.

5. Include foods rich in calcium and take oral calcium supplements, containing vitamin D, as prescribed.

6. Document compliance with the prescribed drug therapy—medical and dietary regimens.

7. Maintain a support system, i.e., health professionals, family, and friends.

8. Schedule follow-up appointment.

Magnesium Imbalances

 INTRODUCTION

Magnesium (Mg), the second most plentiful intra-cellular cation, has similar functions, causes of imbalances, and clinical manifestations as potas-sium. Approximately one-half (50%) of the body's magnesium is contained in the bone, 49% in the body cells (intracellular fluid), and 1% in the extra-cellular fluid. The normal serum magnesium range is 1.5–2.5 mEq/L, or 1.8–3.0 mg/dl.

ANSWER COLUMN

1. cation; intracellular

2. potassium

3. calcium

4. 1.5–2.5 mEq/L, or
1.8–3.0 mg/dl

5. kidneys; feces

1.

Magnesium is a(n) (anion/cation) _____. Its highest concentration is found in what type of body fluid?

_____

2.

What other cation has its highest concentration in the intracellular fluid? _____

3.

Magnesium is widely distributed throughout the body. Half of the body magnesium is in the bone. What other ion is plentiful in the bone? _____

4.

Magnesium has a higher concentration in the cerebrospinal fluid, also known as spinal fluid, than in the blood plasma. The serum concentration of magnesium is *_____.

5.

One-third of magnesium is protein bound and approximately two-thirds is ionized, free magnesium that can be utilized by the body. Magnesium is absorbed from the small intestine. Sixty percent of magnesium is excreted in the feces (magnesium that was not absorbed) and 40% is excreted through the kidneys.

  Forty percent of magnesium is excreted via _____ and 60% is excreted via _____.

6.

The minimum daily magnesium requirement is 200–300 mg for an adult and 150 mg for an infant. Many of the same foods that are rich in potassium are also rich in magnesium. These foods include green vegetables, whole grains, fish and seafood, and nuts.

6. green vegetables, whole grains, and fish and seafood

If your patient has a magnesium deficit, name three foods rich in magnesium that the patient should include in his or her diet.

* _____

_____

7.

A serum magnesium level of less than 1.5 mEq/L is known as (hypomagnesemia/hypermagnesemia) _____. A serum magnesium level of greater than 2.5 mEq/L is called _____.

7. hypomagnesemia; hypermagnesemia

● FUNCTIONS

Table 9-1 describes the various functions of magnesium. Study Table 9-1 and refer to it as needed.

8.

Magnesium plays an important role in enzyme activity. An *enzyme* is a catalyst capable of inducing chemical changes in other substances. Magnesium acts as a coenzyme in the metabolism of carbohydrates and protein.

Magnesium is also involved in maintaining neuromuscular stability. What other ion has this similar function?

_____

8. calcium

Table 9-1	Magnesium and Its Functions
Body Involvement	**Functions**
Neuromuscular	Transmits neuromuscular activity. Important mediator of neural transmissions in the CNS.
Cardiac	Contracts the heart muscle (myocardium).
Cellular	Activates many enzymes for proper carbohydrate and protein metabolism. Responsible for the transportation of sodium and potassium across cell membranes. Influences utilization of potassium, calcium, and protein. Magnesium deficits are frequently accompanied by a potassium and/or calcium deficit.

9.

Indicate which of the following are functions of magnesium:

( ) a. Neuromuscular activity
( ) b. Contraction of the myocardium
( ) c. Exchange of CO_2 and O_2
( ) d. Enzyme activity
( ) e. Responsibility (partial) for Na and K crossing cell membranes.

9. a, b, d, e

10.

When there is a magnesium deficit, what two other cations may also be decreased? _____

All three cations should be closely monitored.

10. potassium and calcium

● PATHOPHYSIOLOGY

11.

Magnesium maintains neuromuscular function. A serum magnesium deficit increases the release of acetylcholine from the presynaptic membrane of the nerve fiber. This increases neuromuscular excitability.

A serum magnesium excess has a sedative effect on the neuromuscular system that may result in a loss of deep tendon reflexes.

Indicate which neuromuscular function may occur from the magnesium imbalances listed below.

_____ 1. Hypomagnesemia   a. Hyperexcitability
_____ 2. Hypermagnesemia   b. Inhibition

11. 1. a (due to increased release of acetylcholine); 2. b (causing a sedative effect)

12.

Cardiac dysrhythmias can result from a serum magnesium deficit. Tachycardia, hypertension, and ventricular fibrillation may result from hypomagnesemia. Hypotension and heart block may result from hypermagnesemia.

What is the most serious cardiac dysfunction that might occur from hypomagnesemia? *_____

From hypermagnesemia? *_____

12. ventricular fibrillation; heart block

13.

Magnesium is regulated by gastrointestinal absorption and renal excretion. In the gastrointestinal (GI) tract, an increase in calcium absorption causes a decrease in magnesium absorption and an increase in magnesium excretion.

What is likely to occur with decreased calcium absorption?

*_____

13. increased magnesium absorption

14.

Magnesium inhibits the release of the parathyroid hormone (PTH). A decrease in the release of PTH (increases/decreases) _____ the amount of calcium released from the bone. This can cause a calcium (excess/deficit) _____.

14. decreases; deficit

15.

Match the serum magnesium levels on the left with the type of magnesium imbalance or balance on the right.

_____	1. 1.2 mEq/L	a. Normal serum
_____	2. 2.0 mEq/L	magnesium level
_____	3. 2.3 mEq/L	b. Hypomagnesemia
_____	4. 2.9 mEq/L	c. Hypermagnesemia
_____	5. 1.0 mEq/L	
_____	6. 3.6 mEq/L	

15. 1. b; 2. a; 3. a; 4. c; 5. b; 6. c

● **ETIOLOGY**

Hypomagnesemia is probably the most undiagnosed electrolyte deficiency. This is most likely due to the fact that hypomagnesemia is asymptomatic until the serum magnesium level approaches 1.0 mEq/L. The total serum magnesium concentration is not representative of the cellular magnesium level. This is why many patients with hypomagnesemia are asymptomatic. Patients with hypokalemia or hypocalcemia who do not respond to potassium and/or calcium replacement may also have hypomagnesemia. Correction of the magnesium deficit is an important consideration when correcting serum potassium and serum calcium imbalances.

The causes of hypomagnesemia and hypermagnesemia are presented in two tables. Table 9-2 lists the etiology and rationale for hypomagnesemia and Table 9-3 lists the

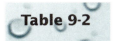

Table 9-2	Causes of Hypomagnesemia (Serum Magnesium Deficit)
Etiology	**Rationale**
Dietary Changes	
Inadequate intake, poor absorption, GI losses	Magnesium is found in various foods, e.g., green, leafy vegetables and whole grains.
Malnutrition, starvation	Inadequate nutrition can result in a magnesium deficit.
Total parenteral nutrition (TPN, hyperalimentation)	Continuous use of TPN without a magnesium supplement can cause a magnesium deficit.
Chronic alcoholism	Alcoholism promotes inadequate food intake and GI loss of magnesium.
Increased calcium intake	Calcium absorption promotes magnesium loss in feces.
Chronic diarrhea, intestinal fistulas, chronic use of laxatives	Chronic diarrhea impairs magnesium absorption. Prolonged use of laxatives can cause a magnesium deficit.
Renal Dysfunction	
Diuresis: diabetic ketoacidosis	Diuresis due to diabetic ketoacidosis causes magnesium loss via the kidneys.
Acute renal failure (ARF)	ARF in the diuretic phase promotes magnesium loss.
Cardiac Dysfunction	
Acute myocardial infarction (AMI)	Hypomagnesemia may occur from the first to the fifth day post-acute MI.
Heart failure (HF)	Prolonged diuretic therapy for HF can cause a magnesium deficit.
Electrolyte and Acid-Base Influences	
Hypokalemia	The cations potassium and calcium are interrelated with
Hypocalcemia	magnesium action.
Metabolic alkalosis	Hypomagnesemia can occur with hypokalemia, hypocalcemia, and metabolic alkalosis.
Drug Influence	
Aminoglycosides, potassium-wasting diuretics, cortisone, amphotericin B, digitalis	These drugs promote the loss of magnesium. Hypomagnesemia enhances the action of digitalis; digitalis toxicity may result.

etiology and rationale for hypermagnesemia. After studying Tables 9-2 and 9-3, proceed to the questions. Refer to the tables as needed.

16.

Magnesium is found in various foods; thus prolonged inadequate nutrient intake can cause (hypomagnesemia/hypermagnesemia) _____.

16. hypomagnesemia

Table 9-3	Causes of Hypermagnesemia (Serum Magnesium Excess)
Etiology	**Rationale**
Dietary Changes Excessive administration of magnesium products IV magnesium sulfate to manage eclampsia and prelabor Antacids with magnesium Laxatives with magnesium	Hypermagnesemia rarely occurs unless there is a prolonged excess use of magnesium-containing antacids (Maalox), laxatives (milk of magnesia), and IV magnesium sulfate.
Renal Dysfunction Renal insufficiency Renal failure	Renal insufficiency or failure inhibits the excretion of magnesium.
Severe Dehydration Diabetic ketoacidosis	Loss of body fluids due to diuresis from diabetic ketoacidosis causes a hemoconcentration of magnesium, which can result in an increased magnesium level.

17.

Chronic alcoholism is a leading cause and problem of hypomagnesemia because of inadequate food intake. This results from GI losses due to diarrhea and poor absorption related to *_____.

Chronic diarrhea is attributed to hypomagnesemia. Why?

*_____

_____

17. inadequate nutritional intake; because of impaired magnesium absorption

18.

The diuretics that promote magnesium loss are the (potassium-wasting diuretics/potassium-sparing diuretics)

*_____

_____.

When does acute renal failure (ARF) cause hypomagnesemia?

*_____.

18. potassium-wasting diuretics; During the diuretic phase of ARF

19.

Two cardiac causes of hypomagnesemia are acute myocardial infarction (AMI) and *_____.

During what period of time during the AMI does a serum magnesium deficit occur? *_____.

19. heart failure (HF); 1–5 days post-AMI

20. no; Large doses of
potassium and calcium
supplements do not fully
correct hypokalemia and
hypocalcemia unless the
magnesium deficit is also
corrected.

20.
Hypokalemia and hypocalcemia may be present along with
hypomagnesemia. Can hypokalemia and hypocalcemia be
corrected without correcting hypomagnesemia?

_____

Explain. *_____

_____

21. inhibit

21.
Magnesium is important for potassium uptake and for
maintaining cellular potassium; therefore, a low magnesium
level will (inhibit/promote) _____ the correction of
a low potassium level.

22.
Indicate which of the following are causes of
hypomagnesemia.
    ( ) a. Chronic alcoholism
    ( ) b. Chronic use of laxatives
    ( ) c. Potassium-sparing diuretics
    ( ) d. Hyperkalemia
    ( ) e. Increased calcium intake
    ( ) f. Malnutrition
    ( ) g. Diuresis due to diabetic ketoacidosis
    ( ) h. Magnesium-containing antacids
    ( ) i. Continuous TPN or salt-free IV fluids

22. a, b, e, f, g, i

23.
Hypermagnesemia occurs primarily because of magnesium
intake, which results from the chronic use of laxatives,
antacids, and many enema preparations. Also those at risk of
hypermagnesemia include older adults and those with
(renal/pulmonary) _____ insufficiency. Explain.

*_____

23. renal; Kidneys excrete
40% of the magnesium.
With lack of kidney
function, Mg increases.

24.
When magnesium-containing antacids and laxatives are taken
continuously for a prolonged period of time, what type of
magnesium imbalance is likely to occur? _____

24. hypermagnesemia, or
magnesium excess;
Maalox and Mylanta; milk
of magnesia (MOM) and
magnesium sulfate
(Epsom salt).

Name an antacid that can cause a magnesium excess when used for a prolonged period of time or in conjunction with renal impairment? *_____

Name a laxative that if used constantly can cause a magnesium excess, especially if there is renal impairment?
* _____

_____

25.

Approximately one-half of magnesium is excreted via the kidneys. With renal insufficiency, the serum magnesium level is (increased/decreased) _____.

What other electrolyte is primarily excreted in the urine?

_____

25. increased; potassium

26.

Place a D for magnesium deficit and an E for magnesium excess in the following situations:

_____ a. Renal insufficiency

_____ b. Prolonged diuresis

_____ c. Constant use of Epsom salt or milk of magnesia

_____ d. Chronic alcoholism

_____ e. Malnutrition

_____ f. Prolonged inadequate nutrient intake

_____ g. Severe diarrhea

_____ h. Constant use of antacids with magnesium hydroxide

26. a. E; b. D; c. E; d. D; e. D;
f. D; g. D; h. E

● CLINICAL MANIFESTATIONS

27.

The normal serum magnesium range is *_____.

A serum magnesium level less than _____ mEq/L is known as hypomagnesemia.

For hypermagnesemia to occur, the serum magnesium level should be greater than _____ mEq/L.

27. 1.5–2.5 mEq/L, or
1.8–3.0 mg/dl; 1.5; 2.5

28.

Severe magnesium imbalance occurs when the serum magnesium level is below 1.0 mEq/L and above 10.0 mEq/L. A cardiac arrest may result with a severe magnesium imbalance.

Severe serum magnesium deficit and excess are life threatening and need immediate action. Would a serum magnesium deficit of 1.3 mEq/L be life threatening?

_____

28. no; greater than 10 mEq/L

For severe hypermagnesemia to be life threatening, the serum magnesium level is *_____.

Table 9-4 lists the clinical manifestations of hypomagnesemia and hypermagnesemia according to the body area affected. The serum magnesium level and the ECG determine the severity of the magnesium imbalance. Study the table carefully and refer to it as needed.

29.

Magnesium influences the nervous system; too much or too little magnesium affects the neuromuscular function.

Table 9-4	Clinical Manifestations of Magnesium Imbalances	
Body Involvement	**Hypomagnesemia**	**Hypermagnesemia**

Neuromuscular abnormalities	Hyperirritability
	Tetany-like symptoms
	  Tremors
	  Twitching of face
	  Spasticity
	Increased tendon reflexes
		CNS depression
		Lethargy, drowsiness, weakness, paralysis
		Loss of deep tendon reflexes

Cardiac abnormalities	Hypertension
	Cardiac dysrhythmias
	  Premature ventricular contractions (PVC)
	  Ventricular tachycardia
	  Ventricular fibrillation
		Hypotension (if severe, profound hypotension)
		Complete heart block
		Bradycardia

ECG/EKG	Flat or inverted T wave Depressed ST segment	Widened QRS complex Prolonged QT interval
Others		Flushing Respiratory depression

Hyperirritability, tremors, and twitching of the face are signs and symptoms of _____.

Lethargy, drowsiness, and loss of deep tendon reflexes are signs and symptoms of _____.

29. hypomagnesemia; hypermagnesemia

30.

Central nervous system depression, inhibited neuromuscular transmission, decreased respiration, and lethargy are signs and symptoms of _____.

30. hypermagnesemia

31.

Match the cardiac signs and symptoms on the left to a magnesium deficit or excess on the right

_____ 1. Hypotension	a. Hypomagnesemia
_____ 2. Ventricular tachycardia	b. Hypermagnesemia
_____ 3. PVC (premature ventricular contraction)	
_____ 4. Heart block	

31. 1. b; 2. a; 3. a; 4. b

32.

Place a D for hypomagnesemia and an E for hypermagnesemia beside the following signs and symptoms:

_____ a. Hyperirritability

_____ b. CNS depression

_____ c. Lethargy

_____ d. Tremors

_____ e. Twitching of the face

_____ f. Convulsion

_____ g. Decreased respiration

_____ h. Loss of deep tendon reflexes

_____ i. Ventricular fibrillation

32. a. D; b. E; c. E; d. D; e. D; f. D; g. E; h. E; i. D

● CLINICAL MANAGEMENT

Clinical management of hypomagnesemia may be corrected by a diet consisting of green vegetables, legumes, whole-grain cereal, nuts (peanut butter), and fruits. Oral or intravenous magnesium salts may be prescribed when there is a marked to severe magnesium deficit.

For hypermagnesemia, correcting the underlying cause and using intravenous saline or calcium salts decreases the magnesium level.

Magnesium Replacement

33.

With asymptomatic hypomagnesemia, oral magnesium replacement is usually prescribed and with symptomatic hypomagnesemia, parenteral (IV, IM) magnesium is usually prescribed.

What would most likely be prescribed for severe magnesium deficit, (oral/parenteral) _____ magnesium agent?

33. parenteral

34.

Oral magnesium comes as sulfate, gluconate, chloride, citrate, and hydroxide in liquid, tablet, and powder form.

Magnesium supplement for maintenance or replacement, magnesium gluconate/Magonate and magnesium-protein complex/Mg-PLUS may be ordered by the health professional.

For severe hypomagnesemia do you think the ordered magnesium replacement should be administered (orally/intramuscularly/intravenously)? _____
Why? * _____

_____

34. intravenously; It is a direct and quick method for correcting serum magnesium deficit.

35.

Magnesium sulfate is the parenteral replacement for hypomagnesemia and can be administered intramuscularly or intravenously. The drug is available in strengths of 10, 12.5, and 50%. A suggested order for adults is 10 ml of a 50% solution.

For intramuscular injections the dosage is divided and for intravenous infusion the dosage is diluted into 1 liter of solution. The two injectable routes in which magnesium sulfate can be delivered to the body are * _____.

35. intramuscular and intravenous

Hypermagnesemia Correction

36.

For a temporary correction of a serum magnesium excess, the intravenous electrolytes * _____ or * _____ may be prescribed.

36. saline (sodium chloride); calcium salt

If hypermagnesemia is due to renal failure, dialysis may be necessary. Ventilator assistance may be needed if respiratory distress occurs.

37.

Intravenous calcium is an (agonist/antagonist) _____ to magnesium; therefore, calcium can (increase/decrease) _____ the symptoms of hypermagnesemia.

37. antagonist; decrease

38.

If renal failure is the cause of severe hypermagnesemia, what is the best course to correct this imbalance? _____

38. dialysis

Drugs and Their Effect on Magnesium Balance

39.

Long-term administration of saline infusions may result in magnesium and calcium loss.

Can you explain why long-term or excessive use of saline infusions can cause magnesium and calcium deficits?
*_____

39. It expands the extracellular fluid (ECF), causes dilution, and inhibits tubular absorption of Mg and Ca.

Diuretics, antibiotics, laxatives, and digitalis are groups of drugs that promote magnesium loss (hypomagnesemia). Excess intake of magnesium salts is the major cause of serum magnesium excess (hypermagnesemia). Table 9-5 lists drugs that affect magnesium balance. Refer to the table as needed.

40.

Place MD for magnesium deficit/hypomagnesemia and ME for magnesium excess/hypermagnesemia beside the following drugs:

_____ a. Furosemide/Lasix

_____ b. Tobramycin

_____ c. Magnesium hydroxide/MOM

_____ d. Digoxin

_____ e. Magnesium sulfate for toxemia

_____ f. Laxatives

_____ g. Cortisone

_____ h. Lithium

40. a. MD; b. MD; c. ME; d. MD; e. ME; f. MD; g. MD; h. ME

Table 9-5	Drugs Affecting Magnesium Balance	
Magnesium Imbalance	**Drugs**	**Rationale**

Hypomagnesemia (serum magnesium deficit)	Diuretics
	    Furosemide/Lasix
	    Ethacrynic acid/Edecrin
	    Mannitol
		Diuretics promote urinary loss of magnesium.

	Antibiotics
	    Gentamicin
	    Tobramycin
	    Carbenicillin
	    Capreomycin
	    Neomycin
	    Polymyxin B
	    Amphotericin B
	Digoxin
	Calcium gluconate
	Insulin
		These agents can cause magnesium loss via the kidneys.

	Laxatives
	Cisplatin
	Corticosteroids
	    Cortisone
	    Prednisone
		Laxative abuse causes magnesium loss via the GI system.
		Steroids can decrease serum magnesium levels.

Hypermagnesemia (serum magnesium excess)	Magnesium salts:
	Oral and enema
	    Magnesium hydroxide/MOM
	    Magnesium sulfate/Epsom salt
	    Magnesium citrate
	    Magnesium sulfate (maternity)
		Excess use of magnesium salts can increase serum magnesium levels.
		
		Use of excess $MgSO_4$ in treatment of toxemia can cause hypermagnesemia.

	Lithium	Hypermagnesemia can be associated with lithium therapy.

41.

Excessive use of steroids (corticosteroids) can cause hypomagnesemia.

A decrease in the adrenal cortical hormone can cause (hypomagnesemia/hypermagnesemia) _____.

41. hypermagnesemia

42.

Hypomagnesemia enhances the action of digoxin and causes digitalis toxicity. Magnesium sulfate corrects hypomagnesemia and symptoms of digitalis toxicity.

Give at least three symptoms of digitalis toxicity.

*_____

What other electrolyte (cation) deficit can cause digitalis toxicity? _____

42. nausea and vomiting, anorexia, and bradycardia; potassium

● CLINICAL APPLICATIONS

Hypomagnesemia is frequently an undiagnosed problem that surfaces when the patient is hospitalized, critically ill, or not responding to correction of hypokalemia or hypocalcemia. Approximately 65% of patients with normal renal function in intensive care units (ICUs) have a low serum magnesium level. Over 40% of the patients with hypomagnesemia also have hypokalemia. Twenty percent of older adults have a decreased serum magnesium level.

43.

When a patient is being treated for hypokalemia and is not responding to therapy, the serum magnesium should be checked. If a magnesium deficit is present, hypokalemia (may/may not) _____ be completely corrected.

43. may not

44.

The kidneys regulate the concentration of magnesium in the body. When there is a slight increase in the magnesium concentration, the kidneys excrete the excess. When there is a decreased serum magnesium level, what do you think the kidneys do? *_____
_____.

If a patient has renal insufficiency and is receiving magnesium sulfate, what type of magnesium imbalance can occur? _____
Why? *_____

44. Kidneys conserve Mg or Mg is reabsorbed from the kidney tubules—not excreted; hypermagnesemia; Kidneys regulate Mg balance—do not excrete it.

45.

For patients on prolonged hyperalimentation (TPN), the serum magnesium level should be checked.

What type of magnesium imbalance can occur when magnesium is not included in the solutions for TPN?

_____

45. hypomagnesemia

46.

Magnesium is needed by the heart for myocardial contractions. It is said that magnesium slows the rate of the atrial contractions and corrects atrial flutter.

Electrocardiographic changes due to magnesium imbalances are similar to potassium imbalances. With hypomagnesemia, the T wave may be * _____ and the ST segment

_____ .

46. flat or inverted; depressed

47.

In diabetic acidosis, magnesium leaves the cells. When insulin and dextrose are given intravenously, magnesium returns to the cells.

If the diabetic condition is corrected too fast, then (hypomagnesemia/hypermagnesemia) _____ occurs. Why? * _____

_____

47. hypomagnesemia; Magnesium leaves the ECF rapidly and returns to the cells.

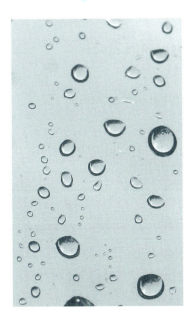

● CLINICAL CONSIDERATIONS

1. Signs and symptoms of hypomagnesemia are similar to those of hypokalemia.

2. Excess use of laxatives and antacids that contain magnesium can cause hypermagnesemia.

3. A magnesium deficit is often accompanied by a potassium and calcium deficit (40% of patients with hypomagnesemia also have hypokalemia). If a potassium deficit does not respond to potassium replacement, hypomagnesemia should be suspected.

4. Severe hypomagnesemia can cause symptoms of tetany.

5. Intravenous magnesium sulfate diluted in IV solution should be administered at a slow rate. Rapid infusion can cause hot and flushed feelings.

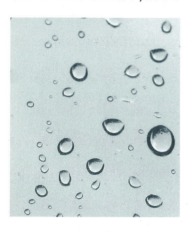

6. In emergency situations, to reverse hypermagnesemia, IV calcium gluconate is given.

7. Long-term administration of saline (NaCl) infusions can result in magnesium and calcium losses. Sodium inhibits renal absorption of magnesium and calcium.

8. A magnesium deficit enhances the action of digoxin.

9. Thiazides and loop (high-ceiling) diuretics decrease serum magnesium levels.

10. Mild to moderate hypermagnesemia is frequently asymptomatic.

CASE STUDY

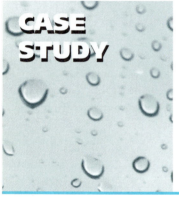

REVIEW

A 60-year-old female has experienced excessive diuresis for several days. In the hospital her diagnoses were prolonged diuresis, severe dehydration, and malnutrition. She received 3 liters of 5% dextrose in $\frac{1}{2}$ of normal saline (0.45% NaCl). Her serum magnesium was 1.3 mEq/L.

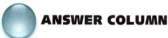

ANSWER COLUMN

1. 1.5–2.5 mEq/L

2. hypomagnesemia

3. It causes dilution of magnesium in the ECF.

4. renal insufficiency and use of Epsom salt (MgSO$_4$) as a laxative (also magnesium-containing antacids)

1. What is the "normal" serum magnesium range?
   *_____

2. Name the type of magnesium imbalance present.
   _____

3. She received fluids intravenously. Explain the relationship of IV fluids to magnesium deficit. *_____
   *_____

4. Name two clinical causes of hypermagnesemia. *_____
   _____

Her pulse was irregular, and she developed tremors and twitching of the face. The physician ordered 10 ml of magnesium sulfate IV to be diluted in 1 liter of solution. Other drugs that she was receiving included digoxin and Lasix.

5. Name her clinical signs and symptoms of hypomagnesemia.

   a. * _____

   b. * _____

   c. * _____

5. a. irregular pulse (dysrhythmia); b. tremors; c. twitching of the face

6. What cation, in a *hypo* state, causes CNS abnormalities similar to hypomagnesemia? _____

6. calcium

7. Name at least two symptoms of hypermagnesemia. * _____ _____

7. CNS depression (lethargic, drowsiness) and decrease in respiration

8. The physician ordered IV magnesium sulfate diluted in 1 liter of IV fluids. The nursing implication is to first check her urinary output. Explain the rationale. * _____ _____

8. Kidneys excrete excess magnesium and kidney impairment can cause hypermagnesemia.

9. The nurse should be assessing for digitalis toxicity while her serum magnesium is low. Explain. * _____ _____

9. Hypomagnesemia enhances the action of digitalis.

10. Lasix can cause (hypomagnesemia/hypermagnesemia) _____.

10. hypomagnesemia

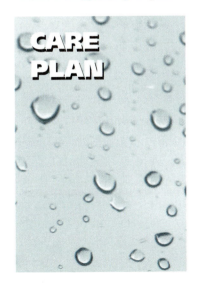

CARE PLAN

PATIENT MANAGEMENT: HYPOMAGNESEMIA

Assessment Factors

● Obtain a health history and identify which findings are associated with hypomagnesemia, such as malnutrition, chronic alcoholism, chronic diarrhea, laxative abuse, TPN with magnesium, and electrolyte imbalance (hypokalemia, hypocalcemia).

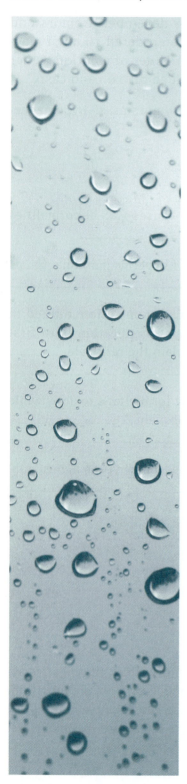

● Assess for signs and symptoms of hypomagnesemia (neuromuscular and cardiac abnormalities), i.e., tetany-like symptoms due to hyperexcitability (tremors, twitching of the face), cardiac dysrhythmias (ventricular tachycardia leading to ventricular fibrillation), and hypertension.

● Assess dietary intake and use of IV therapy without magnesium. Prolonged IV therapy including total parenteral nutrition (TPN, hyperalimentation) may be a cause of hypomagnesemia.

● Check the ECG/EKG strips for changes in the T wave (flat or inverted) and ST segment (depressed) that may indicate hypomagnesemia.

● Check serum magnesium level. Frequently the serum magnesium level is not ordered and is usually not part of the routine chemistry test. If a potassium deficit does not respond to potassium replacement, hypomagnesemia should be suspected.

Nursing Diagnosis 1

Imbalanced nutrition: less than body requirements, related to poor nutritional intake, chronic alcoholism, chronic laxative abuse, and chronic diarrhea.

Interventions and Rationale

1. Instruct the patient to eat foods rich in magnesium [green vegetables, fruits, fish and seafood, grains, and nuts (peanut butter)].

2. Report to health professionals when patients receive continuous magnesium-free IV fluids. Solutions for hyperalimentation, commonly referred to as total parental nutrition (TPN), should contain some magnesium.

3. Administer IV magnesium sulfate diluted in solution slowly unless the patient has a severe deficit. Rapid infusion can cause a hot or flushed feeling.

4. Have IV calcium gluconate available for emergency to reverse hypermagnesemia from overcorrection of a magnesium deficit.

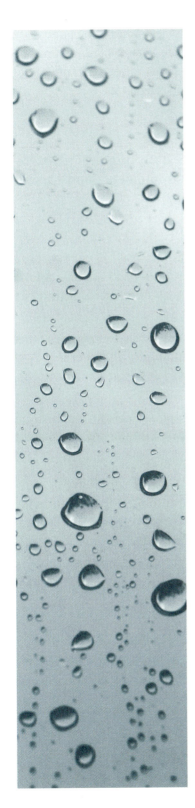

Nursing Diagnosis 2

Decreased cardiac output related to a serum magnesium deficit.

Interventions and Rationale

1. Monitor vital signs and ECG strips. Report abnormal findings to the physician.

2. Monitor serum electrolyte results. Report a low serum potassium and/or calcium level. A low serum magnesium level may be attributed to hypokalemia or hypocalcemia. When correcting a potassium deficit, potassium is not replaced in the cells until magnesium is replaced. A serum magnesium level of 1.0 mEq/L or less can cause cardiac arrest.

3. Check patients with hypomagnesemia who are taking digoxin for digitalis toxicity, e.g., nausea and vomiting, bradycardia. A magnesium deficit enhances the action of digoxin (digitalis preparations).

4. Report urine output of less than 30 ml/h or 600 ml/day when the patient is receiving magnesium supplements. Magnesium excess is excreted by the kidneys. With a poor urine output, hypermagnesemia can occur.

5. Check for positive Trousseau's and Chvostek's signs of severe hypomagnesemia. Tetany symptoms occur in both magnesium and calcium deficits.

● HYPERMAGNESEMIA

Assessment Factors

● Assess, via health history, for possible causes of hypermagnesemia, i.e., renal insufficiency or failure and chronic use of antacids and laxatives containing magnesium salts.

● Assess for signs and symptoms of hypermagnesemia, such as decreased neuromuscular activity, lethargy, decreased respiration, and hypotension.

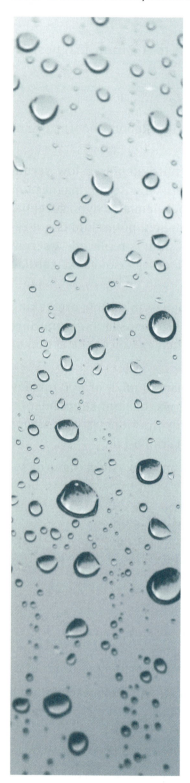

● Obtain a serum magnesium level that can be used as a baseline for comparison of future serum magnesium levels. A serum magnesium level above about 2.5 mEq/L or 3.0 mg/dl is indicative of hypermagnesemia.

Nursing Diagnosis 1

Imbalanced nutrition: more than body requirements, related to oral and IV magnesium supplements and chronic use of drugs containing magnesium.

Interventions and Rationale

1. Monitor urinary output for patients taking magnesium-containing drugs. Urine output, 600–1200 ml/day, allows for the excretion of magnesium. A poor urine output can result in hypermagnesemia.

2. Observe for signs and symptoms of hypermagnesemia, such as decreased neuromuscular activity, decreased reflexes, lethargy and drowsiness, decreased respirations, and hypotension.

3. Monitor serum magnesium levels. A serum magnesium level exceeding 10 mEq/L can precipitate cardiac arrest.

4. Monitor for ECG changes. A wide QRS complex and a prolonged QT interval can suggest hypermagnesemia.

5. Instruct the patient to avoid prolonged use of antacids and laxatives containing magnesium. Suggest that the patient check drug labels for magnesium.

6. Suggest that the patient increase fluid intake unless contraindicated. Fluids dilute the serum magnesium level and should increase urine output.

Evaluation/Outcomes

1. Confirm that the cause of the magnesium imbalance has been corrected (serum potassium level within normal range). Because potassium and magnesium are cations and have similar functions, one electrolyte imbalance affects the other electrolyte balance.

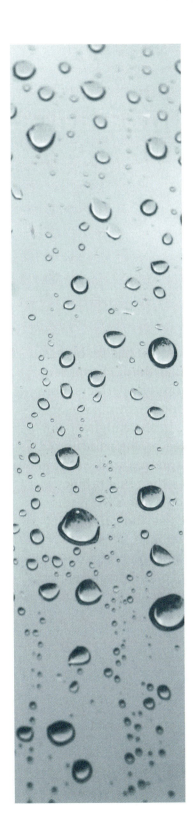

2. Evaluate the effect of the therapeutic regimen on correcting the magnesium imbalance (magnesium within normal range).

3. Remain free of clinical manifestations of hypomagnesemia and hypermagnesemia; ECG, vital signs, etc., return to the patient's normal baseline patterns.

4. Diet includes foods rich in magnesium.

5. Maintain a support system.

Phosphorus Imbalances

 INTRODUCTION

Phosphorus (P) is a major anion and has its highest concentration in the intracellular fluid. Phosphorus and calcium have similar and opposite effects. Both electrolytes need vitamin D for intestinal absorption. Phosphorus and calcium in their highest concentrations are in bones and teeth. The parathyroid hormone (PTH) acts on phosphorus and calcium differently. The PTH stimulates the renal tubules to excrete phosphorus, thus decreasing serum phosphorus levels, and it increases serum calcium levels by pulling calcium from the bone.

The ions phosphorus (P) and phosphate (PO_4) are used interchangeably. Phosphorus is measured in the serum; in the cells it appears as a form of phosphate.

● ANSWER COLUMN

1. intracellular (highest concentration)

2. hyperphosphatemia

3. 1.7–2.6; 2.5–4.5

4. cation; anion; intracellular

5. calcitriol and parathyroid hormone (PTH)

1.
Phosphorus is found in high concentration in the (extracellular/intracellular) _____ fluid.

2.
Approximately 85% of phosphorus is located in the bones and the remaining 15% is located in the intracellular fluid. The normal serum phosphorus range is 1.7–2.6 mEq/L, or 2.5–4.5 mg/dl.
   A serum phosphorus level below 1.7 mEq/L, or 2.5 mg/dl, is identified as hypophosphatemia. A serum level above 2.6 mEq/L, or 4.5 mg/dl, is labeled _____.

3.
The normal serum phosphorus range in adults is _____ mEq/L, or _____ mg/dl.
   The serum phosphorus level is usually higher in children: 4.0–7.0 mg/dl.

4.
Like potassium, 90% of the phosphorus compound is excreted by the kidneys and 10% is excreted by the gastrointestinal tract.
   Potassium is a(n) (anion/cation) _____, and phosphorus is a(n) (anion/cation) _____. Both potassium and phosphorus are most plentiful in the (extracellular/intracellular) _____ fluid.

5.
Phosphorus balance is influenced by the parathyroid hormone (PTH). PTH stimulates calcitriol, a vitamin D derivative, which increases phosphorus absorption from the gastrointestinal tract. PTH also stimulates the proximal renal tubules to increase phosphate excretion.
   The two hormones that influence phosphorus/phosphate balance are * _____.

⬤ FUNCTIONS

Phosphorus has many functions. It is a vital element needed in bone formation, a component of the cell (nucleic acids and cell membrane), and is incorporated into the molecules needed for metabolism, e.g., adenosine triphosphate (ATP) and 2,3-diphosphoglycerate (2,3-DPG), and it acts as an acid-base buffer. Table 10-1 explains the functions of phosphorus according to the body system and structure it affects. Study Table 10-1 carefully and refer to the table as needed.

6.

An important function of phosphorus is neuromuscular activity. Name at least two cations that play an important role in neuromuscular activity. *_____

7.

Phosphorus, like calcium, is needed for strong, durable teeth and _____.

8.

Intracellular ATP is needed for cellular energy.
   The red-blood-cell enzyme 2,3-DPG is responsible for *_____.

6. potassium and sodium
(answer can also be calcium and magnesium)

7. bones

8. delivering oxygen to the tissues

Table 10-1	Phosphorus and Its Functions
Body Involvement	**Functions**
Neuromuscular	Normal nerve and muscle activity.
Bones and teeth	Bone and teeth formation, strength, and durability.
Cellular	Formation of high-energy compounds (ATP, ADP). Phosphorus is the backbone of nucleic acids and stores metabolic energy.
	Formation of the red-blood-cell enzyme 2,3-diphosphoglycerate (2,3-DPG) is responsible for delivering oxygen to tissues.
	Utilization of B vitamins.
	Transmission of hereditary traits.
	Metabolism of carbohydrates, proteins, and fats.
	Maintenance of acid-base balance in body fluids.

9.

Other functions of phosphorus include which of the following:

( ) a. Utilization of vitamin A
( ) b. Utilization of B vitamins
( ) c. Metabolism of carbohydrates, proteins, and fats
( ) d. Maintenance of acid-base balance in body fluids
( ) e. Transmission of hereditary traits

9. b, c, d, e

● PATHOPHYSIOLOGY

10.

Hypophosphatemia occurs approximately 3–4 days after an inadequate nutrient intake of foods rich in phosphorus. The kidneys compensate by decreasing urinary phosphate excretion; however, a continuous inadequate intake of phosphorus results in an extracellular fluid shift to the cells in order to replace the phosphorus loss.

What happens to the serum phosphorus level with this shift?

* _____

_____

10. The serum phosphorus level decreases, resulting in hypophosphatemia.

11.

Indicate the type of phosphorus imbalance based upon the serum phosphorus level listed on the left:

_____	1. 3.0 mg/dl	a. Hypophosphatemia
_____	2. 6.8 mg/dl	b. Hyperphosphatemia
_____	3. 1.5 mg/dl	c. Normal
_____	4. 1.2 mEq/L	
_____	5. 3.2 mEq/L	
_____	6. 2.0 mEq/L	

11. 1. c; 2. b; 3. a; 4. a; 5. b; 6. c

ETIOLOGY

Table 10-2 lists the causes of hypophosphatemia and Table 10-3 lists the causes of hyperphosphatemia. Study the tables and then proceed to the questions that follow. Refer to Tables 10-2 and 10-3 as needed.

Table 10-2   Causes of Hypophosphatemia (Serum Phosphorus Deficit)

Etiology	Rationale
Dietary Changes	
Malnutrition	Poor nutrition results in a reduction of phosphorus intake.
Chronic alcoholism	Alcoholism contributes to dietary insufficiencies and increased diuresis.
Total parenteral nutrition (TPN, hyperalimentation)	TPN is usually a phosphorus-poor or -free solution. IV concentrated glucose and protein given rapidly shift phosphorus into the cells, thus causing a serum phosphorus deficit.
Gastrointestinal Abnormalities	
Vomiting, anorexia	Loss of phosphorus through the GI tract decreases cellular ATP (energy) stores.
Chronic diarrhea	
Intestinal malabsorption	Vitamin D deficiencies inhibit phosphorus absorption. Phosphorus is absorbed in the jejunum in the presence of vitamin D.
Poor Oxygenation of Tissues	Lack of 2,3-DPG, which is needed for the delivery of oxygen.
Hormonal Influence	
Hyperparathyroidism (increased PTH)	Parathyroid hormone (PTH) production enhances renal phosphate excretion and calcium reabsorption.
Cellular Changes	
Diabetic ketoacidosis	Glycosuria and polyuria increase phosphate excretion. A dextrose infusion with insulin causes a phosphorus shift into the cells; decreasing the serum phosphorus level.
Burns	Phosphorus is lost due to its increased utilization in tissue building.
Acid-base disorders Respiratory alkalosis Metabolic alkalosis	Respiratory alkalosis from prolonged hyperventilation decreases the serum phosphorus level by causing an intracellular shift of phosphorus. Metabolic alkalosis can also cause this shift.
Drug Influence	
Aluminum-containing antacids	Phosphate binds with aluminum to decrease the serum phosphorus level.
Diuretics	Most diuretics promote a decrease in the serum phosphorus level.

12. hypophosphatemia; malnutrition and chronic alcoholism (also the use of phosphorus-poor or phosphorus-free IV solutions including those used for TPN)

12.

A decreased serum phosphorus level is known as a phosphorus deficit or _____.

Name two dietary changes that can cause a decreased serum phosphorus level. *_____

_____

Table 10-3	Causes of Hyperphosphatemia (Serum Phosphorus Excess)
Etiology	**Rationale**
Dietary Changes Oral phosphate supplements	Excessive administration of phosphate-containing substances increases the serum phosphorus level.
Intravenous phosphate	
Hormonal Influence Hypoparathyroidism (lack of PTH)	Lack of PTH causes a calcium loss and a phosphorus excess.
Chemotherapy	During chemotherapy, phosphorus leaves the cells, thus, serum phosphorus level is increased.
Renal Abnormalities Renal insufficiency	Renal insufficiency or shutdown decreases phosphorus excretion.
Acid-Base Disorders Metabolic acidosis Respiratory acidosis	Acidosis is a cause of hyperphosphatemia. It prevents accumulation of cellular phosphate.
Drug Influence Laxatives containing phosphate	Frequent use of phosphate laxatives increases the serum phosphorus level.

13.

Alcoholism can cause severe hypophosphatemia. The phosphorus loss is the result of *_____ or _____.

13. a poor diet (malnutrition); diuresis

14.

Name the vitamin that is necessary for phosphorus absorption via the small intestines. _____

14. vitamin D

15.

Gastrointestinal abnormalities that may cause hypophosphatemia include _____, _____, *_____, and _____.

15. vomiting, anorexia, chronic diarrhea, intestinal malabsorption

16.

In parathyroid disorders the parathyroid hormone (PTH) influences phosphorus balance.

Increased PTH secretion causes a phosphorus (loss/excess) _____.

16. loss

17. Phosphate binds with aluminum.

18. a. Glycosuria and polyuria increase phosphorus excretion; b. Dextrose infusions with insulin cause a phosphorus shift from the serum into cells

19. Phosphorus shifts into cells (intracellular fluid); respiratory alkalosis

20. hyperphosphatemia; increases

21. decrease; loss; excess

22. Calcitriol promotes calcium absorption from the intestines.

17.
An increased calcium level is usually accompanied by a decreased serum phosphorus level.

Aluminum-containing antacids decrease the serum phosphorus level. Explain how. * _____
_____

18.
A patient in diabetic ketoacidosis may have severe hypophosphatemia. Give two reasons why the phosphorus deficit occurs.

a. * _____.

b. * _____.

19.
Explain how hypophosphatemia occurs as a result of prolonged hyperventilation.

* _____.

What type of acid-base imbalance can result from prolonged hyperventilation?

* _____

20.
An elevated serum phosphorus level is known as phosphorus excess or _____.

With a decrease in the serum calcium level, the serum phosphorus level (increases/decreases) _____.

21.
Hypoparathyroidism causes a(n) (increase/decrease) _____ in the secretion of the parathyroid hormone (PTH).

A decrease in PTH secretion causes a calcium (loss/excess) _____ and a phosphorus (loss/excess) _____.

22.
Hyperphosphatemia causes hypocalcemia by decreasing the production of calcitriol.

Do you recall the effect of calcitriol? * _____

23.

The acid-base disorders, metabolic acidosis and acute respiratory acidosis, can be causes for the occurrence of hyperphosphatemia.

Metabolic alkalosis and respiratory alkalosis cause hypophosphatemia due to a phosphorus shift to cells.

Hyperphosphatemia can occur because of which acid-base imbalances? *_____

23. metabolic acidosis and respiratory acidosis

24.

Certain groups of drugs affect phosphorus balance. Enter PD for phosphorus deficit and PE for phosphorus excess against the drug groups that can cause phosphorus imbalance.

_____ a. Aluminum antacids
_____ b. Phosphate-containing laxatives
_____ c. Thiazide diuretics
_____ d. Oral phosphate ingestion
_____ e. Intravenous phosphate administration

24. a. PD; b. PE; c. PD; d. PE; e. PE

● CLINICAL MANIFESTATIONS

25.

Clinical manifestations of hypophosphatemia and hyperphosphatemia are determined by signs and symptoms of phosphorus imbalances, particularly neuromuscular irregularities, hematologic abnormalities, and an abnormal serum phosphorus level.

The normal serum phosphorus range is *_____.

A serum phosphorus level of less than _____ mg/dl indicates hypophosphatemia, and one greater than _____ mg/dl indicates hyperphosphatemia.

25. 1.7–2.6 mEq/L, or 2.5–4.5 mg/dl; 2.5; 4.5

Table 10-4 lists the clinical manifestations of hypophosphatemia and hyperphosphatemia according to the body areas that are affected. Study Table 10-4 carefully and refer to it as needed.

Table 10-4	Clinical Manifestations of Phosphorus Imbalances	
Body Involvement	**Hypophosphatemia**	**Hyperphosphatemia**
Neuromuscular Abnormalities	Muscle weakness Tremors Paresthesia Bone pain Hyporeflexia Seizures	Tetany (with decreased calcium) Hyperreflexia Flaccid paralysis Muscular weakness
Hematologic Abnormalities	Tissue hypoxia (decreased oxygen- containing hemoglobin and hemolysis) Possible bleeding (platelet dysfunction) Possible infection (leukocyte dysfunction)	
Cardiopulmonary Abnormalities	Weak pulse (myocardial dysfunction) Hyperventilation	Tachycardia
GI Abnormalities	Anorexia Dysphagia	Nausea, diarrhea Abdominal cramps
Laboratory Values Milliequivalents per liter Milligrams per deciliter	<1.7 mEq/L <2.5 mg/dl	>2.6 mEq/L >4.5 mg/dl

26.

Indicate which of the following signs and symptoms relate to hypophosphatemia:

    ( ) a. Muscle weakness
    ( ) b. Paresthesia
    ( ) c. Bone pain
    ( ) d. Flaccid paralysis
    ( ) e. Tissue hypoxia
    ( ) f. Tachycardia
    ( ) g. Hyporeflexia

26. a (can also occur with hyperphosphatemia), b, c, e, g

27.

Indicate which of the following signs and symptoms relate to hyperphosphatemia:

    ( ) a. Muscle weakness
    ( ) b. Paresthesia
    ( ) c. Hyperreflexia
    ( ) d. Flaccid paralysis

27. a (more common with hypophosphatemia), c, d, e, f

( ) e. Tachycardia
( ) f. Abdominal cramps
( ) g. Bone pain

28.

Symptoms of phosphorus imbalance are very often vague; therefore serum values are needed. A mild to moderate phosphorus deficit is usually asymptomatic.

Hypophosphatemia is present when the serum phosphorus level is less than _____ mEq/L, or _____ mg/dl. Hyperphosphatemia is present when the serum phosphorus level is greater than _____ mEq/L, or _____ mg/dl.

28. 1.7; 2.5; 2.6; 4.5

● CLINICAL MANAGEMENT

When the serum phosphorus level falls below 1.5 mEq/L, or 2.5 mg/dl, oral phosphate, i.e., sodium or potassium phosphate tablets, or IV phosphate-containing solutions such as sodium phosphate or potassium phosphate may be ordered.

If the serum phosphorus level falls below 0.5 mEq/L, or 1 mg/dl, severe hypophosphatemia occurs. Intravenous phosphate-containing solutions are indicated.

Phosphorus Replacement

29. sodium phosphate/Phospho-Soda and potassium phosphate/Neutra-Phos K

29.

Name two drugs, oral or IV, that are administered to replace the phosphorus deficit (refer to Table 10-5 on page 231).

*
_____

30. Necrosis or sloughing of tissue. Potassium is extremely irritating to subcutaneous tissue.

30.

Concentrated IV phosphates are hypertonic and must be diluted. If IV potassium phosphate (KPO_4) is given in IV solution, the IV rate should be no more than 10 mEq/h to avoid phlebitis.

If an IV potassium phosphate solution infiltrates, what happens to the tissue? * _____

_____

31.

Foods rich in phosphorus include milk (especially skim milk), milk products, meat (beef and pork), whole-grain cereals, and dried beans.

 Phosphorus-rich foods are indicated if the serum phosphorus level is which of the following:

( ) a. 0.3 mEq/L, or 1 mg/dl
( ) b. 0.9 mEq/L, or 1.5 mg/dl
( ) c. 1.6 mEq/L, or 2.4 mg/dl

31. c

Phosphorus Correction

32.

Administration of insulin and glucose can lower the serum phosphorus level by shifting phosphorus from the extracellular fluid into the cells. The use of insulin and glucose is a (temporary/permanent) _____ treatment to correct hyperphosphatemia.

32. temporary

Drugs and Their Effect on Phosphorus Balance

The major drug group that causes hypophosphatemia is aluminum antacids; other drug groups responsible for hyperphosphatemia are phosphate laxatives, phosphate enemas, and oral and IV phosphates. Table 10-5 lists the names and rationales for drugs that affect phosphorus balance. Refer to the table as needed.

33.

Prolonged intake of aluminum antacids, with or without magnesium, decreases the serum phosphorus level. Why?
*_____

The phosphorus imbalance that results is _____.

33. Aluminum-containing antacids bind with phosphorus; hypophosphatemia

34. Aluminum binds with phosphorus to decrease the serum phosphorus level, for example, Amphojel.

34.

Aluminum antacids may be ordered for hyperphosphatemia. Do you know why? *_____
_____

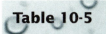

Table 10-5   Drugs That Affect Phosphorus Balance

Phosphorus Imbalance	Drugs	Rationale

Hypophosphatemia (serum phosphorus deficit)	Sucralfate
	Aluminum antacids
	  Amphojel
	  Basaljel
	Aluminum/magnesium antacids
	  Di-Gel
	  Gelusil
	  Maalox
	  Maalox Plus
	  Mylanta
	  Mylanta II
	Calcium antacids
	  Calcium carbonate
		Aluminum-containing antacids bind with phosphorus; therefore the serum phosphorus level is decreased. Calcium promotes phosphate loss.

	Diuretics
	  Thiazide
	  Loop (high-ceiling)
	  Acetazolamide
		Phosphorus can be lost when diuretics are used.

	Androgens
	Corticosteroids
	  Cortisone
	  Prednisone
	Glucagon
	Gastrin
	Epinephrine
	Mannitol
	Salicylate overdose
	Insulin and glucose
		These agents have a mild to moderate effect on phosphorus loss.

Hyperphosphatemia (serum phosphorus excess)	Oral phosphates
	Sodium phosphate/Phospho-Soda
	Potassium phosphate/Neutra-Phos K
	Intravenous phosphates
	  Sodium phosphate
	  Potassium phosphate
		Excess oral ingestion and IV infusion can increase the serum phosphorus level.

	Phosphate laxatives
	  Sodium phosphate
	  Sodium biphosphate/Phospho-Soda
	  Phosphate enema
	  Fleet sodium phosphate
	Excessive vitamin D
	Antibiotics
	  Tetracyclines
	  Methicillin
		Continuous use of phosphate laxatives and enemas can increase the serum phosphorus level.

35.

Enter PD for phosphorus deficit and PE for phosphorus excess beside the drugs that can cause a phosphorus imbalance:

_____ a. Amphojel

_____ b. Cortisone

_____ c. Phospho-Soda

_____ d. Fleet's sodium phosphate

_____ e. Epinephrine/adrenalin

_____ f. Diuretics

_____ g. IV potassium phosphate

35. a. PD; b. PD; c. PE; d. PE; e. PD; f. PD; g. PE

● CLINICAL APPLICATIONS

36.

Severe hypophosphatemia can result from hyperalimentation/TPN. Two reasons for a serum phosphorus deficit related to hyperalimentation are

a. * _____.

b. * _____.

36. a. Phosphate-poor or phosphate-free solution; b. Concentrated glucose and/or protein, given too rapidly, causes phosphorus to shift from serum into cells

37.

If a severely malnourished patient is receiving a 25% dextrose solution (TPN), the infusion rate should be (fast/slow) _____ when first administered. What type of serum phosphorus imbalance can occur if the infusion rate is faster than 80 ml/h? _____ Why? * _____

_____

37. slow; hypophosphatemia; Concentrated glucose tends to shift phosphorus into cells; the result is a serum phosphorus deficit.

38.

Any carbohydrate-loading diet can cause a phosphorus shift from the serum into the cells.

During tissue repair following trauma, phosphorus shifts into the cells. The serum phosphorus imbalance that occurs is called _____.

38. hypophosphatemia

● CLINICAL CONSIDERATIONS

1. Phosphorus is needed for durable bones and teeth, formation of ATP (high-energy compound for cellular activity), metabolism of carbohydrates, proteins, and fats, utilization of B vitamins, transmission of hereditary traits, and others.

2. Phosphorus and calcium are similar and yet differ in action. Both need vitamin D for intestinal absorption. PTH promotes renal excretion of phosphorus (phosphate) and calcium absorption from the bones.

3. Vomiting and chronic diarrhea cause a loss of phosphorus.

4. Acute hypophosphatemia may result from an abrupt shift of phosphorus into the cells. Respiratory alkalosis and metabolic alkalosis can cause shifting of phosphorus into the cells.

5. Concentrated IV phosphates are hyperosmolar and must be diluted. If IV potassium phosphate is given in IV solution, the IV rate should be no more than 10 mEq/h to avoid phlebitis and a potassium overload.

6. Aluminum-containing antacids, such as Amphojel, decrease the serum phosphorus level; phosphate binds with the aluminum.

7. Continuous use of phosphate laxatives can cause an elevated serum phosphorus level.

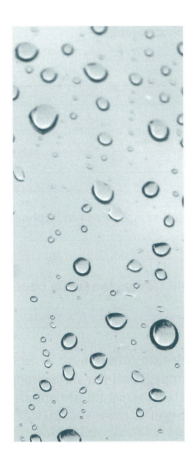

CASE STUDY

REVIEW

A 46-year-old female with a history of alcohol abuse was admitted for GI bleeding. In her own words she had not eaten a balanced diet for 2 months and had been taking Amphojel to relieve her "upset stomach." She complained of hand paresthesias and "overall" muscle weakness.

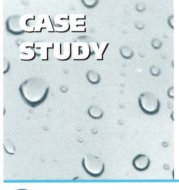

ANSWER COLUMN

1. hypophosphatemia

1. What type of phosphorus imbalance is she experiencing? _____

2. 1.7–2.6; 2.5–4.5

3. poor diet (possible malnutrition) and ingestion of aluminum hydroxide antacid, Amphojel

4. a. hand paresthesias;
b. muscle weakness

5. bone pain, tissue hypoxia, weak pulse, and hyperventilation

6. Phosphorus binds with aluminum, thus lowering the serum phosphorus level.

7. Concentrated glucose causes a shift of phosphorus from the serum into the cells.

8. monitor IV rate so she receives approximately 10 mEq/h of KPO_4; check infusion site frequently for signs of infiltration

9. sodium phosphate/ Phospho-Soda and potassium phosphate/ Neutra-Phos K

2. Give the "normal" serum phosphorus range:
_____ mEq/L, or _____ mg/dl.

3. Give two reasons for her imbalance: *_____
_____

4. What among her signs and symptoms indicated a phosphorus deficit?
a. *_____
b. *_____

5. Name four other clinical signs and symptoms of hypophosphatemia. *_____
_____

6. Explain how aluminum hydroxide lowers the serum phosphorus level. *_____
_____

She was given a 10% dextrose solution intravenously. Her serum phosphorus level was 1.5 mg/dl and her potassium level, 3.0 mEq/L. Several hours later potassium phosphate was added to her intravenous solution.

7. What effect does concentrated dextrose (glucose) solution have on the serum phosphorus level? *_____
_____

8. What is the responsibility of the nurse while the patient is receiving IV potassium phosphate diluted in this solution?
_____

9. Name two oral phosphate drugs. *_____
_____

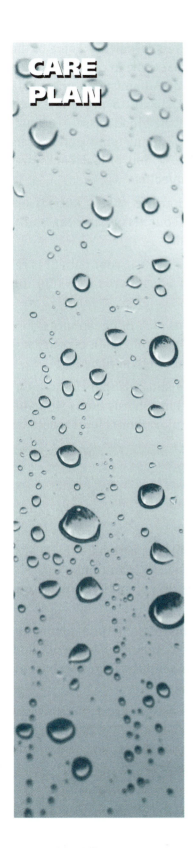

CARE PLAN

PATIENT MANAGEMENT: HYPOPHOSPHATEMIA

Assessment Factors

● Obtain a history of clinical problems. Note if the health problem is related to hypophosphatemia, i.e., malnutrition, chronic alcoholism, chronic diarrhea, vitamin D deficit, continuous use of IV solutions without a phosphate additive (including TPN), hyperparathyroidism, continuous use of aluminum-containing antacids, and alkalotic state due to hyperventilation (respiratory alkalosis).

● Assess for signs and symptoms of hypophosphatemia, i.e., muscle weakness, paresthesia, hyporeflexia, weak pulse, and over-breathing (tachypnea).

● Check serum phosphorus level. The serum phosphorus level can act as a baseline level for assessing future serum phosphorus levels.

● Check serum calcium level and, if elevated, report findings to the health care provider. An elevated calcium level causes a decreased phosphorus level.

Nursing Diagnosis 1

Imbalanced nutrition: less than body requirements, related to inadequate nutritional intake, chronic alcoholism, vomiting, chronic diarrhea, lack of vitamin D intake, intravenous fluids, including TPN with lack of phosphate additive.

Interventions and Rationale

1. Monitor neuromuscular and cardiopulmonary abnormalities related to a decreased phosphorus level, such as muscle weakness, tremors, paresthesia, hyporeflexia, bone pain, weak pulse, and tachypnea.

2. Monitor serum phosphorus and calcium levels. Report abnormal findings to the health care provider. An increase in the serum calcium level results in a decrease in the serum phosphorus level and vice versa.

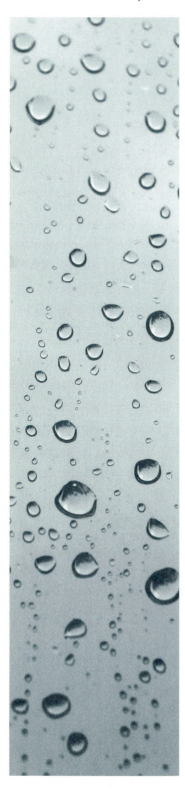

3. Monitor oral and IV phosphorus replacements. Some of the oral phosphate salts (Neutrophos) come in capsules, which are indicated if nausea is present. Administer IV phosphate [potassium phosphate (KPO_4)] slowly to prevent hyperphosphatemia and irritation of the blood vessel. The suggested amount of KPO_4 to be administered per hour is 10 mEq. Rapidly administered KPO_4 and/or high concentrations of phosphate can cause phlebitis.

4. Check for signs of infiltration at the IV site; KPO_4 is extremely irritating to subcutaneous tissue and can cause sloughing of tissue and necrosis.

5. Inform the health care provider (HCP) if your patient is receiving a phosphorus-poor or phosphorus-free solution for TPN.

6. Instruct the patient to eat foods rich in phosphorus, i.e., meats (beef, pork, turkey), milk, whole-grain cereals, and nuts. Most carbonated drinks are high in phosphates.

7. Instruct the patient not to take antacids that contain aluminum hydroxide (Amphojel). Phosphorus binds with aluminum products; a low serum phosphorus level results.

● HYPERPHOSPHATEMIA

Assessment Factors

● Obtain a history of clinical problems; associate the health problems to hyperphosphatemia, i.e., continuous use of phosphate-containing laxatives, hypoparathyroidism, and renal insufficiency.

● Assess for signs and symptoms of hyperphosphatemia, i.e., hyperreflexia, tachycardia, abdominal cramps, and tetany symptoms, which can also indicate a low serum calcium level.

● Check serum phosphorus level. A serum phosphorus level greater than 4.5 mg/dl or greater than 2.6 mEq/L indicates hyperphosphatemia. A serum phosphorus level exceeding 10 mg/dl can result in cardiac distress.

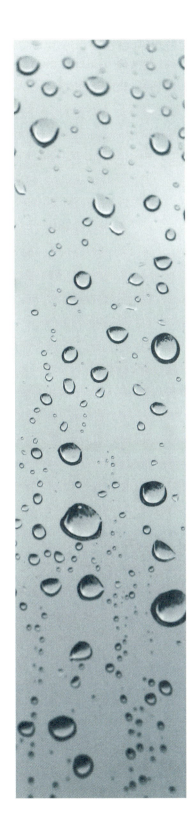

● Check urinary output. A decrease in urine output, <30 ml per hour or <600 ml per day, increases the serum phosphorus level. This is especially true if the patient is receiving a phosphate-containing product.

Nursing Diagnosis 1

Imbalanced nutrition:more than body requirements, related to excess intake of phosphate-containing compounds such as some laxatives, intravenous potassium phosphate, and others.

Interventions and Rationale

1. Monitor neuromuscular, cardiac, and GI abnormalities related to an increased phosphorus level.

2. Monitor serum phosphorus and calcium levels. A decreased calcium level can result in an increase in the phosphorus level. Report abnormal findings to the HCP.

3. Observe the patient for signs and symptoms of hypocalcemia (e.g., tetany) when phosphate supplements are being administered. An increase in the serum phosphorus level decreases the calcium level.

4. Instruct the patient to eat foods that are low in phosphorus, such as vegetables. Instruct the patient to avoid drinking carbonated beverages that contain phosphates.

5. Instruct patient with hyperphosphatemia or poor renal output to read labels on over-the-counter medications and canned foods that may contain phosphate ingredients.

6. Monitor urine output. Report inadequate urine output. Phosphorus is excreted by the kidneys and poor renal function can cause hyperphosphatemia.

Evaluation/Outcomes

1. Confirm that the cause of phosphorus imbalance has been eliminated.

2. Evaluate the effect of clinical management in correcting the phosphorus imbalance (phosphorus level within normal range).

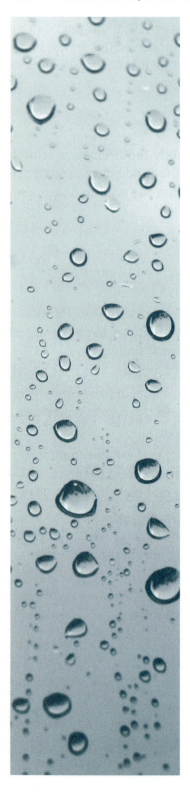

3. Determine that the signs and symptoms of phosphorus imbalance are absent. The patient is free of neuromuscular abnormalities such as muscle weakness and tetany symptoms.

4. Document compliance with prescribed drug therapy and medical and dietary regimen.

5. Maintain a support system.

ACID-BASE BALANCE AND IMBALANCE

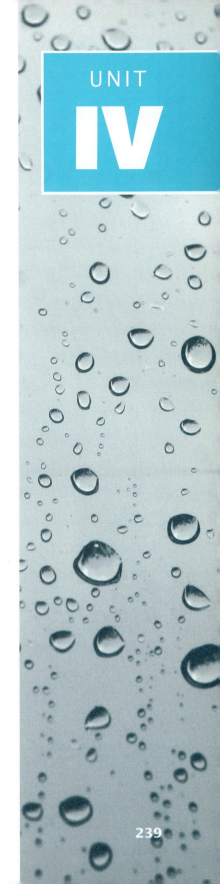

LEARNING OUTCOMES

Upon completion of this unit, the reader will be able to:
- Explain the influence of the hydrogen ion (H^+) on body fluids.
- Identify the pH ranges for acidosis and alkalosis.
- Discuss the three regulatory mechanisms for pH control and how the regulatory mechanisms can maintain acid-base balance.
- Identify metabolic acidosis and alkalosis and respiratory acidosis and alkalosis through use of arterial blood gases.
- Explain how various clinical conditions can cause metabolic acidosis and alkalosis and respiratory acidosis and alkalosis.
- Identify clinical symptoms of metabolic acidosis and alkalosis and respiratory acidosis and alkalosis.
- Discuss the body's defense action and the clinical management for acid-base balance and be able to apply this information to various clinical situations.
- Explain the health interventions for patients in metabolic and respiratory acidosis and alkalosis states.

INTRODUCTION

Our body fluid must maintain a balance between acidity and alkalinity in order for life to be maintained. *Acid* comes from the Latin word meaning "sharp," and acid is frequently referred to as being sour. According to the Bronsted-Lowry concept of acids and bases, an "*acid* is any molecule or ion that can *donate a proton* to any other substance, whereas a *base* is any molecule or ion that can *accept a proton*." The more readily an acid

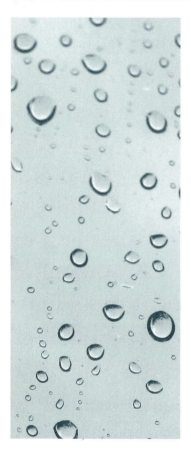

gives up its protons, the stronger it is as an acid. Acids and bases are not synonymous with anions and cations.

As you might expect from the Bronsted-Lowry concept, the concentration of hydrogen ions determines the acidity or alkalinity of a solution. The amount of ionized hydrogen in body fluids is extremely small; around 0.0000001 g/L. Instead of using this cumbersome figure, pH is used to express acidity or alkalinity. pH is the negative logarithm (exponent) of the hydrogen ion concentration. Here's how it works: the number 0.0000001 is equal to 10^{-7}. The logarithm of 10^{-7} is the exponent, -7. The negative of -7 is 7. Therefore the negative logarithm (the pH) of 0.0000001 is 7. As the hydrogen ion concentration rises (in solution), the pH value falls, indicating a more acidic solution. As the hydrogen concentration falls, the pH rises, thus indicating a more alkaline solution. An alkaline solution is also called a basic solution.

Hydroxyl ions (OH^-) can accept protons, which means they are base ions. In other words, hydroxyl ions tend to "soak up" protons, and so they tend to make a solution more alkaline—also known as more basic. Pure water has exactly equal numbers of hydrogen ions (H^+) and hydroxyl ions (OH^-), and the pH of pure water is 7. For this reason, a solution of pH 7 is said to be neutral. See Figure U4-1.

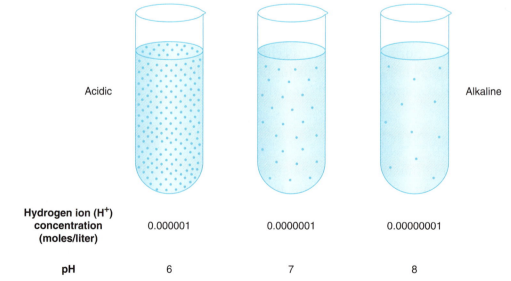

	Acidic		Alkaline
Hydrogen ion (H^+) concentration (moles/liter)	0.000001	0.0000001	0.00000001
pH	6	7	8

FIGURE U4-1   Schematic illustration of the relationship between hydrogen ion concentration, pH, and acidity and alkalinity. Dots represent hydrogen ions.

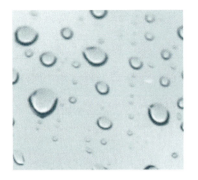

The above information helps you in the basic understanding of acidity and alkalinity. This information aids in the understanding of the regulatory mechanism for pH control; the determination of acid-base imbalances including metabolic acidosis and alkalosis; and respiratory acidosis and alkalosis.

Refer to the Introduction as needed to answer the first five frames. An asterisk (*) on an answer line indicates a multiple-word answer. The meanings for the following symbols are: ↑ increased, ↓ decreased, > greater than, < less than.

ANSWER COLUMN

1.
According to the Bronsted-Lowry concept of acids and bases, an acid is a proton (donor/acceptor) _____ and a base is a proton (donor/acceptor) _____.

1. donor, acceptor

2.
The acidity or alkalinity of a solution depends on the concentration of *_____.

An increase in concentration of the hydrogen ions makes a solution more _____ and a decrease in the concentration of hydrogen ions makes it more _____.

2. hydrogen ions; acid; alkaline

3.
The pH is used to express the _____ of a solution.

3. acidity or alkalinity

4.
As the hydrogen ion concentration increases, the pH value _____. What does this indicate? _____.

As the hydrogen ion concentration falls, the pH value _____. What does this indicate? _____

4. falls, or decreases; acidity; rises, or increases; alkalinity

5.
Another word for alkaline is _____.

5. basic/base

6.
An acidic solution has a (low/high) _____ pH.
An alkaline solution has a (low/high) _____ pH.

6. low; high

7. The number of hydrogen ions is balanced by the number of hydroxyl ions; H^+; OH^-; HCO_3; bicarbonate

8. acidosis

9. 7.35–7.45

10. acidic; d. any of the above

11. hydrogen

12. acid; alkaline or base

7.

A solution at pH 7 is neutral. Why? *_____

_____

The symbol for the hydrogen ion is _____ and the symbol for the hydroxyl ion is _____.

A hydroxyl ion and CO_2 yields _____, which is known as a _____.

8.

The pH of extracellular fluid in health is maintained at a level between 7.35 and 7.45. With a pH higher than this range (7.35–7.45), the body is considered to be in a state of alkalosis.

What would you call a state in which the pH is below 7.35?

_____.

9.

The pH norm of arterial blood plasma is 7.4; a variation of 0.4 of a pH unit in either direction can be fatal.

In a healthy individual, the pH range of arterial blood plasma is _____ .

10.

Within our bodies the pH concentration of different fluids varies. The normal pH for urine is 6.0; for gastric juice, 1.0–2.0; for bile, 5.0–6.0. These body fluids are (acidic/alkaline) _____.

The normal pH for intestinal juice is 6.5–7.6. The fluids from the intestinal tract can be which of the following:

( ) a. Acidic
( ) b. Alkaline
( ) c. Neutral
( ) d. Any of the above

11.

Whether a substance is acid, neutral, or alkaline depends on the number of _____ ions present in a given weight or volume.

12.

When the number of hydrogen ions increases in the body fluid, the body fluid becomes _____.

When the number of hydrogen ions decreases, the body fluid becomes _____.

13.

In health, there are $1\frac{1}{3}$ mEq/L of acid to each 27 mEq/L of base in extracellular fluid, which represents a ratio of 1 part of acid to 20 parts of base.

   If the ratio of 1:20 is maintained, the patient is said to be in acid-base (balance/imbalance) _____.

13. balance

Figure U4-2 demonstrates by the arrow that the body is in acid-base balance when there is 1 part acid to 20 parts base. A pH of 7.4 represents this balance. If the arrow tilts left due to a base deficit or acid excess, then acidosis occurs, and if the arrow tilts right due to a base excess or acid deficit, then alkalosis occurs. Carbonic acid is H_2CO_3.

   Study this diagram carefully. Know what happens when the arrow tilts either left or right. Refer to the figure when needed.

14.

Your patient's arterial blood pH is 7.1. Is this condition acidosis or alkalosis? _____

14. acidosis

15.

Another patient's arterial blood pH is 7.8. Is this condition acidosis or alkalosis? _____

15. alkalosis

16.

If the extracellular fluid (EFC) no longer has a 1:20 ratio of acid:base, and if the acid is increased or the base is decreased, then the patient suffers from (acidosis/alkalosis)_____.
If the base is increased or the acid is decreased, then the patient suffers from (acidosis/alkalosis)_____.

16. acidosis; alkalosis

17.

When there is acidosis, the balance shown in Figure U4-2 is tilted _____.
Which of the following occur:
   (   ) a. Base deficit
   (   ) b. Base excess
   (   ) c. Acid deficit
   (   ) d. Acid excess
   The pH is _____.

17. left; a or d or both; <7.35

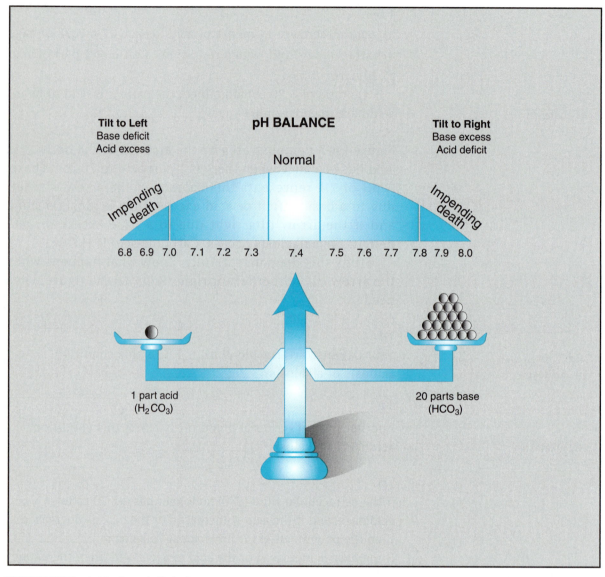

FIGURE U4-2 Acidosis and alkalosis.

18.

When there is alkalosis, the balance shown in Figure U4-2 is tilted _____.

Which of the following occur:

( ) a. Base deficit
( ) b. Base excess
( ) c. Acid deficit
( ) d. Acid excess

The pH is _____.

18. right; b or c or both;
>7.45

Regulatory Mechanisms for pH Control

William C. Rose, PhD

⬤ INTRODUCTION

There are three major mechanisms for pH control: chemical buffer systems, respiratory regulation, and renal regulation. Each regulatory mechanism is discussed individually and is accompanied with illustrations. This chapter is not a clinical chapter and does not include assessment factors, nursing diagnoses, interventions, or evaluation.

ANSWER COLUMN

1. chemical buffer systems; respiratory regulation; renal regulation

2. A compound or a group of compounds that can abosrb excessive acid or base and prevent large pH swings.

3. bicarbonate-carbonic acid buffer, phosphate buffer, ammonia buffer, and protein buffers

1.

Name the three regulatory mechanisms for pH control:
*_____, *_____, and *_____.

Chemical buffer systems are the first regulatory mechanism for pH control. A chemical buffer is a dissolved compound or group of compounds that can absorb excessive acid or base and so prevent pH from changing as much as it would have otherwise. The body has four primary chemical buffers: the bicarbonate-carbonic acid buffer, the phosphate buffer, the ammonia buffer, and protein buffers. These systems are described below.

2.

What is a chemical buffer? *_____

3.

What are the four main chemical buffers in the body?
*_____

The bicarbonate-carbonic acid buffer system operates in blood plasma. Carbonic acid (H_2CO_3) is a weak acid which can dissociate into H^+ and bicarbonate (HCO_3^-). (Remember that negatively charged compounds such as HCO_3^- are anions; positively charged compounds such as H^+ are cations.) When a strong acid (that is, a source of hydrogen ions) is added, some of the hydrogen ions combine with bicarbonate in blood plasma to make carbonic acid. Because carbonic acid is a weak acid, it does not completely dissociate into H^+ and HCO_3^-. This limits the rise in the concentration of free H^+ caused by addition of a strong acid. When a strong base (a subtance that absorbs H^+) is added, some carbonic acid (H_2CO_3) molecules dissociate into H^+ and HCO_3^-, thus partially replacing some of the "lost" H^+. This limits the fall in the concentration of H^+ caused by a strong base. So we see that a buffer system such as the bicarbonate-carbonic acid buffer minimizes the swings in hydrogen ion concentration, that is, it minimizes the swings in pH. The bicarbonate-carbonic acid buffer is the strongest of the body's chemical buffers, and it works within seconds. The other very interesting and important thing about the bicarbonate-carbonic acid buffer is that carbonic acid can dissociate in two different ways: it can turn into protons plus bicarbonate, as discussed above, but it can also turn into water (H_2O) and carbon dioxide (CO_2). The chemical equation below, with carbonic acid in the middle, shows the two ways carbonic acid can dissociate:

$$H^+ + HCO_3^- \leftrightarrows H_2CO_3 \leftrightarrows H_2O + CO_2$$
$$\text{(base)} \qquad \text{(acid)}$$

For now, it is enough to know that this creates a linkage in the body between acidity (H^+ concentration) and CO_2 level. In general, if acidity (H^+ concentration) goes up, so does the blood CO_2 level, and if the CO_2 level goes up, so does acidity. This linkage is very important for understanding the causes, symptoms, and responses to acid-base disturbances in the body. The connection between CO_2 and acidity are discussed later in this chapter and in the next three chapters.

4.

The most powerful chemical buffer system in the body is the
*_____.

4. carbonic acid-bicarbonate buffer

5.

When a strong acid enters the body, the H^+ combines with bicarbonate to form *_____. A base (a source of OH^-) added to the body is neutralized by carbonic acid (H_2CO_3) to form _____ and _____.

5. carbonic acid (H_2CO_3); water (H_2O); bicarbonate (HCO_3^-)

The phosphate buffer system operates in the kidneys. The glomerular filtrate (extracellular fluid that will eventually be excreted as urine) contains both monobasic phosphate ($H_2PO_4^-$, has one negative charge) in equilibrium with hydrogen ions (H^+) and dibasic phosphate (HPO_4^{2-}, two negative charges).

$$H^+ + HPO_4^{2-} \leftrightarrows H_2PO_4^-$$
$$\text{(base)} \qquad \text{(acid)}$$

Monobasic phosphate is a weak acid; dibasic phosphate is a weak base. Dibasic phosphate in the glomerular filtrate

(that is, in the urine-to-be) combines with excess hydrogen ions to form monobasic phosphate, and the monobasic phosphate passes out of the body in the urine, thus helping the body get rid of excess hydrogen ions when the kidneys need to excrete acid, and monobasic phosphate is a source of hydrogen ions when the kidneys need to retain acid.

Another buffer system that operates in the kidneys is the ammonia-ammonium buffer. Ammonia, NH_3, is a base, because it can combine with hydrogen ions (H^+) to form ammonium ions (NH_4^+), thus reducing the number of "free" hydrogen ions.

$$H^+ + NH_3 \leftrightarrows NH_4^+$$
$$\text{(base)} \quad \text{(acid)}$$

Ammonium ions are acidic because they are a source of hydrogen ions when they break down into NH_3 and H^+. In the kidney, ammonia (NH_3) diffuses from the cells lining the renal tubules into the lumen of the tubule, where the urine-to-be is. There the ammonia combines with H^+ to form ammonium (NH_4^+), which passes out of the body in the urine. This helps the body rid itself of hydrogen ions, that is, acid.

6.

Two buffer systems in the kidneys are the _____ buffer and the _____ buffer.

6. phosphate; ammonia-ammonium

7.

In the phosphate buffer system, _____ is a weak acid and _____ is a weak base.

7. monobasic phosphate ($H_2PO_4^-$); bibasic phosphate (HPO_4^{2-})

8.

In the ammonia-ammonium buffer system, _____ is a weak base and _____ is a weak acid.

8. ammonia (NH_3); ammonium (NH_4^+)

9.

The phosphate and ammonia-ammonium buffer systems help the (name of organ) _____ to (excrete or retain) _____ excess acid.

9. kidneys; excrete

Protein buffers operate in red blood cells, where the protein involved is hemoglobin, and in blood plasma, though plasma proteins such as albumin. All proteins are large and complex molecules containing multiple sites which can absorb or be a source of hydrogen ions. Hemoglobin, the oxygen-carrying protein in red blood cells, is the most important protein buffer. A special property of hemoglobin is that hemoglobin with oxygen attached (oxyhemoglobin, HbO_2) does not combine with hydrogen ions as well as hemoglobin without oxygen (deoxyhemoglobin, Hb). This works out very well, because when blood goes through systemic capillaries, hemoglobin "gives up" its oxygen to the tissues, and CO_2 enters the blood from the tissues. The rise in CO_2 in venous blood tends to make venous blood more acidic, due to the connection between acidity and CO_2 mentioned above. However, the deoxyhemoglobin, because it combines well with H^+, soaks up some of the acidity, and as a result, venous blood is only a little more acidic (average normal pH = 7.35) than the arterial blood (average normal pH = 7.4).

10.

10. Proteins

_____ are large molecules with sites that can donate hydrogen ions and sites that accept hydrogen ions.

11.

11. hemoglobin

The main protein found in red blood cells is _____.

12.

12. higher

Carbon dioxide levels in systemic venous blood are _____ than in systemic arterial blood.

13.

13. more

The higher level of CO_2 in venous blood tends to make venous blood _____ acidic than arterial blood.

14.

14. loses

Hemoglobin (gains/loses) _____ oxygen as it passes through capillaries.

15.

15. better

Deoxyhemoglobin (hemoglobin without oxygen) is (better/worse) _____ at soaking up hydrogen ions than oxyhemoglobin.

16.

Thanks to the ability of deoxyhemoglobin to soak up hydrogen ions, venous blood is _____ acidic than arterial blood.

16. only a little more

17.

The average normal pH of systemic arterial blood is _____; the average normal pH of systemic venous blood is _____.

17. 7.4; 7.35

The chemical buffer systems act in seconds to minimize swings in pH. However, their ability to minimize pH swings

Table 11-1

Chemical Buffer Systems in the Body

Buffer system	Location	Chemical equation: $H^+ + Base \leftrightarrows Acid$	Function
Bicarbonate-carbonic acid	Throughout the body	$H^+ + HCO_3^- \leftrightarrows H_2CO_3 \leftrightarrows CO_2 + H_2O$ (H^+ + base $\leftrightarrows$ acid $\leftrightarrows$ gas + water)	Body's most powerful buffer system. Carbonic acid (H_2CO_3) can break down to form $CO_2 + H_2O$, and the lungs can excrete CO_2. Provides a coupling between CO_2 and acidity.
Phosphate	Kidneys	$H^+ + HPO_4^{2-} \leftrightarrows H_2PO_4^-$ (H^+ + base $\leftrightarrows$ acid)	Excess H^+ combines with dibasic phosphate to form monobasic phosphate which is excreted in urine.
Ammonia-ammonium	Kidneys	$H^+ + NH_3 \leftrightarrows NH_4^+$ (H^+ + base $\leftrightarrows$ acid)	Excess H^+ combines with ammonia (NH_3) to form ammonium ion which is excreted in urine.
Proteins	Inside all cells	$H^+ + protein \leftrightarrows H$-protein	Proteins are weak acids and weak bases at the same time. They absorb excess H^+ when intracellular fluid is acidic and provide H^+ when intracellular fluid is alkaline.
Hemoglobin	Inside red blood cells	$H^+ + HbO_2 \leftrightarrows HHb + O_2$	The most important protein buffer. Oxyhemoglobin (HbO_2) gives up its oxygen and is then able to combine with H^+. Keeps venous blood from being too acidic.

is limited. Two other major regulatory mechanisms that help control pH take longer to act but have greater capacity: respiratory regulation and renal regulation. Respiratory regulation has intermediate speed (it works in one to three minutes) and intermediate capacity. Renal regulation is the slowest-acting (it takes hours to become effective) but has the largest ability to get rid of excess acid or base. A renal response to excess acid (the excretion of more acid in urine) also does not require as much physical effort as a respiratory reponse (breathing faster and more deeply).

The body's typical response to an abrupt change in pH is that the chemical buffers act first, within their limited capacity to do so. If that is not sufficient, the respiratory regulatory mechanism kicks in. Altered breathing can be tiring, however, and so the renal regulatory mechanism also starts acting to correct the problem. However, it takes hours to excrete enough urine to affect pH. As renal regulation becomes effective, the respiratory system gradually returns to normal breathing.

18.

18. seconds

Chemical buffer systems act in _____ to regulate pH.

19.

19. respiratory regulation; renal regulation

pH regulatory mechanisms that are not as fast as chemical buffers are *_____ and *_____.

20.

20. one to three minutes

Pulmonary regulation of pH takes *_____ to become effective.

21.

21. renal

The pH regulatory mechanism that is the slowest acting but has the greatest capacity is _____ regulation.

22.

22. chemical buffers; respiratory, renal

In time order, the mechanisms that respond to an abrupt change in pH are *_____ first, followed by _____, and finally _____.

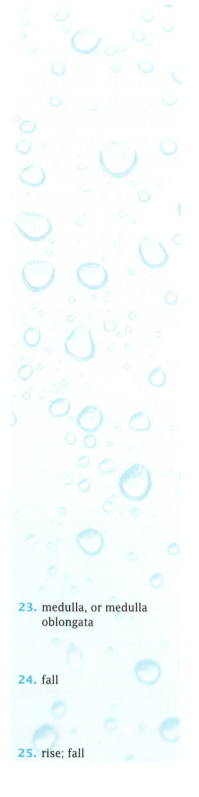

We have seen above that pH and CO_2 concentration in blood are linked due to the bicarbonate buffer system. Blood CO_2 level is expressed in terms of the partial pressure of CO_2, in millimeters of mercury (mm Hg). The partial pressure of CO_2 in arterial blood is abbreviated $PaCO_2$. As a result of the link between pH and CO_2, an increase in CO_2 causes an increase in acidity (pH down), and a decrease in CO_2 causes a decrease in acidity (increased pH). This has two important consequences. First, it means that the body can, and does, use breathing (which controls CO_2 level) to control pH. Second, it means that a problem with the respiratory system will often cause a pH problem. So the connection between pH and CO_2 can be a good thing (when the lungs are working well) or a bad thing (when the lungs are not working well). The impact of respiratory malfunctions on pH are discussed in Chapter 14, Respiratory Acidosis and Alkalosis.

Cells in the medulla oblongata (or medulla for short; it is part of the brain stem) can sense pH. The medulla also controls the respiratory muscles. When the medulla senses an abnormal pH, it responds by changing ventilation. The change in ventilation causes a change in CO_2 in the direction needed to correct the abnormal pH. We have seen that low CO_2 levels cause a decrease in acidity. We also know that an increase in ventilation causes more CO_2 to be expelled from the body, hence the $PaCO_2$ falls when ventilation increases. Therefore, when the medulla senses a low pH (acidity), it directs the respiratory muscles to increase ventilation. When the medulla senses a high pH (alkalinity), it reduces ventilation, if it can do so without compromising blood oxygen levels.

23.

23. medulla, or medulla oblongata

The part of the brain known as the _____ senses pH and controls the muscles of breathing.

24.

24. fall

An increase in ventilation causes $PaCO_2$ to _____ .

25.

25. rise; fall

An increase in ventilation causes the pH to _____ and acidity to _____ .

26.

The respiratory response to excess acidity is to _____ ventilation.

Renal regulation of pH is accomplished by adjusting the amount of acid and base (bicarbonate) excreted in the urine. The bicarbonate, phosphate, and ammonia buffers assist in this process. When the blood is acidic, some excess H^+ combines with bicarbonate to form carbonic acid, some combines with dibasic phosphate to form monobasic phosphate, and some combines with ammonia to form ammonium ions. All these compounds—carbonic acid, monobasic phosphate, and ammonium ions—are excreted in the urine more when the blood is acidic, and less when the blood is alkaline. At the same time, when the blood is acidic, bicarbonate is reclaimed more from the glomerular filtrate, before it leaves the body in urine. This reclaimed bicarbonate neutralizes acid. The increased acid excretion and increased base retention helps correct the acidosis. During alkalosis, the renal mechanism works in the opposite way to correct the problem: less acid is excreted in the urine, and less bicarboante is reclaimed, so more bicarbonate is excreted.

27.

The kidneys excrete _____ urine when pH is low.

28.

_____ bicarbonate is reclaimed from the glomerular filtrate when pH is low.

29.

The kidneys excrete _____ bicarbonate when the pH is low.

30.

When the blood is alkaline, the kidneys excrete more _____ urine.

31.

During alkalosis, _____ bicarbonate is excreted.

26. increase

27. acidic

28. More

29. less

30. alkaline

31. more

CHAPTER 12

Determination of Acid-Base Imbalances

William C. Rose, PhD

 INTRODUCTION

Accurate assessment of acid-base imbalance is identified with the use of arterial blood gases. The determinant blood gas factors used to assess the extent of acid-base imbalance include pH, $PaCO_2$, and HCO_3. Compensatory mechanisms discussed in this chapter control pH. Because this chapter describes the process for determining acid-base imbalance, assessment factors, nursing diagnoses, interventions, and evaluation are not included.

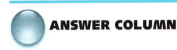

ANSWER COLUMN

1.
Carbonic acid (H_2CO_3) circulates as dissolved carbon dioxide gas (CO_2) and water (H_2O). One of the ways the body maintains acid-base balance is by controlling the excretion of the gas

_____.

1. CO_2

2.
Other acids, including lactic, pyruvic, sulfuric, and phosphoric acids, are produced by metabolic processes. These acids can be excreted from the body in water (urine). What regulatory mechanism excretes these acids? _____.

2. the kidneys or renal mechanism

Renal Regulation	Respiratory Regulation
$H^+ + HCO_3^- \Longleftrightarrow \quad [H_2CO_3]$	$\Longleftrightarrow H_2O + CO_2$

3.
The kidneys and lungs aid in acid-base balance. The kidneys excrete bicarbonate (HCO_3^-) and H^+ (in the form of ammonium and/or monobasic phosphate), while the lungs excrete CO_2. Label the chemical formula according to the organ that is responsible for acid-base regulation:

3. kidneys; lungs

_____ $H^+ + HCO_3^- \Longleftrightarrow [H_2CO_3] \Longleftrightarrow H_2O + CO_2$ _____

(organ)   (organ)

    To determine the type of acid-base imbalance, the blood tests described in Table 12-1 are essential.

4.
To determine the presence of acid-base imbalance, the pH is first checked. If the pH of the arterial blood gas is less than 7.35 (acidosis/alkalosis) _____ is present.
   If the pH of the arterial blood gas is more than 7.45 (acidosis/alkalosis) _____ is present.

4. acidosis; alkalosis

Table 12-1	Determination of Acid-Base Imbalance	
Blood Tests	**Normal Values**	**Imbalance**
Arterial pH	Adult: 7.35–7.45 Newborn: 7.27–7.47 Child: 7.33–7.43	Adult: <7.35 = acidosis >7.45 = alkalosis

$PaCO_2$ (respiratory component)	Adult and child:
	  35–45 mm Hg
	Newborn: 27–41 mm Hg
		Adult and child:
		<35 mm Hg = respiratory alkalosis
		  (hyperventilation)
		>45 mm Hg = respiratory acidosis
		  (hypoventilation)

HCO_3^-
  (metabolic and renal component)
	Adult and child:
	  24–28 mEq/L*
	Newborn: 22–30 mEq/L
		Adult and child:
		<24 mEq/L = metabolic acidosis
		>28 mEq/L = metabolic alkalosis

Base excess (BE)
  (metabolic and renal component)
	Adult and child:
	  +2 to −2 mEq/L
		Adult and child:
		<−2 = metabolic acidosis
		>+2 = metabolic alkalosis

Anion gap:
  $[Na^+] + [K^+] - [Cl^-] - [HCO_3^-]$**
	Adult and child:
	  12–20 mEq/L**
		>20 mEq/L: metablic acidosis
		  due to increased load of non-
		  carbonic acid or decreased H^+
		  secretion
		<12 mEq/L: possible hyponatremia

*Anion gap is not always reported with blood gases, because the electrolyte concentrations needed to compute it are not always measured.
**Some laboratories compute anion gap as $[Na^+] - [Cl^-] - [HCO_3^-]$, that is, they don't use $[K^+]$. In this case the normal range is 8–16 mEq/L.

5.

To determine if acidosis or alkalosis is present, the nurse should *first* check the arterial blood gas (pH/$PaCO_2$/HCO_3) _____.

6.

To determine if the acid-base imbalance is respiratory acidosis or alkalosis, the $PaCO_2$ should be checked. If the patient is acidotic and the $PaCO_2$ is normal or low, the imbalance is not respiratory. If the patient is alkalotic and the $PaCO_2$ is normal or high, the imbalance is not respiratory.

  If the $PaCO_2$ is greater than 45 mm Hg and the pH is less than 7.35, the type of acid-base imbalance is *_____.

  If the $PaCO_2$ is less than 35 mm Hg and the pH is greater than 7.45, the type of acid-base imbalance is *_____.

5. pH

6. respiratory acidosis;
    respiratory alkalosis

7.

The third step to determine the type of acid-base imbalance is to check the bicarbonate (HCO_3^-) and base excess (BE) levels of the arterial blood gas.

If the HCO_3 is less than 24 mEq/L, the BE is less than -2, and pH is less than 7.35, the type of acid-base imbalance is

* _____.

7. metabolic acidosis; metabolic alkalosis

If the HCO_3 is greater than 28 mEq/L, the BE is greater than $+2$, and pH is greater than 7.45, the type of acid-base imbalance is * _____.

8.

The normal range for pH in blood is _____. The normal range for $PaCO_2$ in arterial blood is * _____. The normal range of HCO_3^- in arterial blood is

8. 7.35–7.45; 35–45 mm Hg; 24–28 mEq/L; -2 to $+2$ mEq/L.

* _____. The normal range for base excess in arterial blood is _____.

9.

To determine acidotic and alkalotic states, the nurse must first assess the _____ level; second the _____ of arterial blood; and third the _____ of arterial blood.

9. pH; $PaCO_2$; HCO_3^- and base excess

10.

Respiratory acidosis and alkalosis are indicated by abnormal values of:

    ( ) a. pH
    ( ) b. $PaCO_2$
    ( ) c. HCO_3
    ( ) d. BE

10. a, b

11.

Metabolic acidosis and alkalosis are indicated by abnormal values of:

    ( ) a. pH
    ( ) b. $PaCO_2$
    ( ) c. HCO_3
    ( ) d. BE

11. a, c, d

12.

Place R. Ac for respiratory acidosis, R. Al for respiratory alkalosis, M. Ac for metabolic acidosis, and M. Al for metabolic alkalosis beside the following laboratory findings.

——————————, —————————— a. pH ↑

——————————, —————————— b. pH ↓

—————————— c. $PaCO_2$ ↑

—————————— d. HCO_3 ↑

—————————— e. $PaCO_2$ ↓

—————————— f. HCO_3 ↓

—————————— g. BE ↓

12. a. R. Al, M. Al; b. R. Ac, M. Ac; c. R. Ac; d. M. Al; e. R. Al; f. M. Ac; g. M. Ac

The anion gap is sometimes available in a blood gas report. Anion gap is discussed in more detail in the next chapter but we introduce it here. Anion gap is calculated as the concentrations of the major cations minus the concentrations of the major anions.

$$\text{anion gap (mEq/L)} = [Na^+] + [K^+] - [Cl^-] - [HCO_3^-]$$

The anion gap is useful for determining the cause of metabolic acidosis. When metabolic acidosis is present, anion gap may be normal (12–20 mEq/L) or high (>20 mEq/L). Metabolic acidosis with a normal anion gap is typically due to a loss of bicarbonate due to diarrhea or a GI fistula, or to renal causes such as carbonic anhydrase inhibitors or renal tubular acidosis. Metabolic acidosis with high anion gap is due to excess acid rather than a lack of bicarbonate. Possible causes of high-anion-gap metabolic acidosis include ketoacidosis; lactic acidosis; ingestion of toxins such as methanol, etheylene glycol, or aspirin; and uremic acidosis (renal failure). An abnormally low anion gap may indicate hyponatremia.

13.

Metabolic acidosis can be classified according to the

13. anion gap

————————.

14.

Anion gap equal to 12 to 20 mEq/L is ——————————; anion gap greater than 20 mEq/L is *——————————.

14. normal; abnormally high

15. metabolic acidosis;
  normal anion gap

16. metabolic acidosis; high
  anion gap

17. hyperventilating; CO_2;
  metabolic acidosis; The
  lungs compensate for the
  acidotic state by blowing
  off CO_2 (respiratory
  compensation).

15.

Conditions that cause a loss of bicarbonate, such as diarrhea, cause *_____ with *_____.

16.

Conditions which add acid other than carbonic acid to the body, such as diabetic ketoacidosis and some types of poisoning, cause *_____ with *_____.

● COMPENSATION FOR PH BALANCE

There are specific compensatory reactions in response to metabolic acidosis and alkalosis and respiratory acidosis and alkalosis. The pH returns to normal or close to normal by changing the component, e.g., $PaCO_2$ or HCO_3 and/or BE, that originally was not affected.

The respiratory system compensates for metabolic acidosis and alkalosis, and the renal system compensates for respiratory acidosis and alkalosis. With metabolic acidosis, the lungs (stimulated by the respiratory center) hyperventilate to decrease CO_2 level.

A pH of 7.33, $PaCO_2$ of 24, and HCO_3 of 15 indicate metabolic acidosis, since the pH is slightly acid and the HCO_3 is definitely low (acidosis). The $PaCO_2$ is low (less than 35 mm Hg) since the respiratory center compensates for the acidotic state by "blowing off" CO_2 (hyperventilating); thus, respiratory compensation exists. Without compensation, the pH could be extremely low, e.g., pH 7.2.

17.

For metabolic acidosis, the lungs compensate by (hypoventilating/hyperventilating) _____ to blow off _____.

With a pH of 7.32, $PaCO_2$ of 27, and HCO_3 of 14, the pH and HCO_3 indicate *_____.

The $PaCO_2$ indicates respiratory compensation. Explain.

*_____

_____

Table 12-2	Compensation for Acid-Base Imbalances	
Imbalance	**Indications**	**Compensation System and Action**
Metabolic acidosis	pH<7.35	$HCO_3^->28$ mEq/L	Respiratory: hyperventilate to lower $PaCO_2$
		BE<−2 mEq/L	
Metabolic alkalosis	pH>7.45	$HCO_3^-<24$ mEq/L	Respiratory: hypoventilate to raise $PaCO_2$
		BE>+2 mEq/L	
Respiratory acidosis	pH<7.35	$PaCO_2>45$ mm Hg	Renal (metabolic): excrete more H^+, retain HCO_3^-
Respiratory alkalosis	pH>7.45	$PaCO_2<35$ mm Hg	Renal (metabolic): excrete HCO_3^-, excrete less H^+

18. hypoventilating; CO_2; metabolic alkalosis; The lungs compensate for the alkalotic state by conserving CO_2 (respiratory compensation).

19. kidney or metabolic compensation. Without this compensation the pH is lower.

20. bicarbonate (HCO_3^-); acid (H^+); respiratory alkalosis; The kidneys compensate for the alkalotic state by excreting HCO_3 (metabolic compensation).

18.

For metabolic alkalosis, the lungs compensate by (hypoventilating/hyperventilating) _____ to conserve _____.

With a pH of 7.48, $PaCO_2$ of 46, and HCO_3 of 39, the pH and HCO_3 indicate * _____.

The $PaCO_2$ indicates respiratory compensation. Explain.

* _____

_____

19.

With respiratory acidosis, the kidneys compensate by excreting more acid, (H^+) and conserving bicarbonate (HCO_3^-).

With a pH of 7.35, $PaCO_2$ of 68, and HCO_3 of 35, the pH is low normal, borderline acidosis, and the $PaCO_2$ is highly elevated, indicating CO_2 retention—respiratory acidosis. The HCO_3 indicates * _____

_____

20.

With respiratory alkalosis, the kidneys compensate by excreting _____ ions and conserving _____ ions.

With a pH of 7.46, $PaCO_2$ of 20, and HCO_3 of 18, the pH and $PaCO_2$ indicate * _____. The HCO_3 indicates renal or metabolic compensation.

Explain how. * _____

_____

21.
a. respiratory acidosis with metabolic compensation;
b. respiratory alkalosis with NO compensation;
c. respiratory acidosis with NO compensation;
d. metabolic acidosis with NO compensation;
e. metabolic alkalosis with NO compensation;
f. normal arterial blood gases and acid-base balance;
g. respiratory acidosis with metabolic compensation;
h. metabolic acidosis with respiratory compensation;
i. metabolic alkalosis with respiratory compensation;
j. metabolic acidosis with respiratory compensation

21.

Identify the type of acid-base imbalance, and the type of compensation: metabolic, respiratory, or none. Memorize the norms for pH, $PaCO_2$, and HCO_3.

	PaCO₂	HCO₃		Compensation
pH	(mm Hg)	(mEq/L)	Imbalance	Metabolic/Respiratory/None
a. 7.33	62	32	____	____ ____ ____
b. 7.50	29	26	____	____ ____ ____
c. 7.26	59	27	____	____ ____ ____
d. 7.21	40	19	____	____ ____ ____
e. 7.53	39	36	____	____ ____ ____
f. 7.40	40	26	____	____ ____ ____
g. 7.32	79	41	____	____ ____ ____
h. 7.10	16	6	____	____ ____ ____
i. 7.57	48	40	____	____ ____ ____
j. 7.23	23	10	____	____ ____ ____

Metabolic Acidosis and Alkalosis

William C. Rose, PhD

 INTRODUCTION

Two types of metabolic acid-base imbalance are *metabolic acidosis* and *metabolic alkalosis*. With metabolic acidosis, there is either an excess acid production, e.g., excess hydrogen ions and ketone bodies, or a base (bicarbonate) deficit. With metabolic alkalosis, there is an acid (hydrogen ion) deficit or (more likely) a base (bicarbonate) excess. Metabolic acidosis and metabolic alkalosis are discussed separately in this chapter.

ANSWER COLUMN

1. pH or hydrogen ion deficit or excess

1.
Acidosis and alkalosis can be determined by the

_____.

2.
As discussed in Chapter 12, Table 12-1, the type of acid-base imbalance can be determined by the arterial blood gases,

_____, _____, and _____.

2. pH; $PaCO_2$; HCO_3^- (bicarbonate)

3.
The laboratory values most useful for identifying metabolic acidosis and alkalosis include _____ and

_____.

The laboratory value for identifying respiratory acidosis and alkalosis is _____.

3. bicarbonate; base excess; $PaCO_2$

Acid-base balance is maintained by 1 part of acid and 20 parts of base. Figure 13-1 demonstrates the normal acid-base balance, and the blood tests for pH, HCO_3^-, base excess (BE), are utilized in determining metabolic acidosis and alkalosis.

4.
When the acid-base scale tips to the left, it is an indication that an (acidotic/alkalotic) _____ state is present.

When the scale tips to the right, the type of acid-base imbalance is an (acidotic/alkalotic) _____ state.

4. acidotic; alkalotic

5.
With metabolic acidosis, the pH is _____.

With metabolic alkalosis, the pH is _____.

5. decreased; increased

6.
In metabolic acidosis, the bicarbonate and base excess are

_____.

In metabolic alkalosis, the bicarbonate and base excess are

_____.

6. decreased; increased

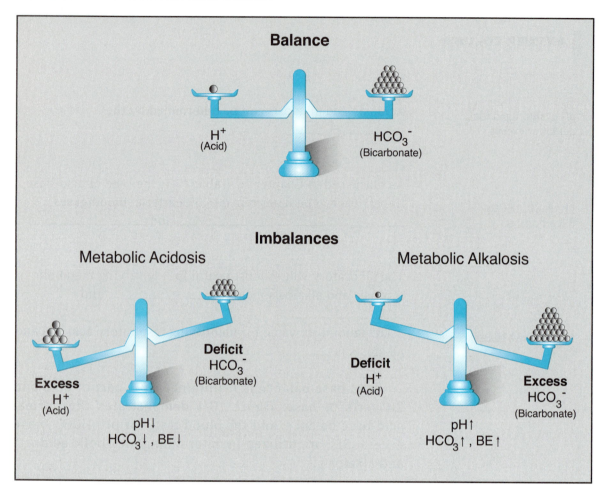

FIGURE 13-1 Acid-base balance and metabolic imbalances.

● PATHOPHYSIOLOGY

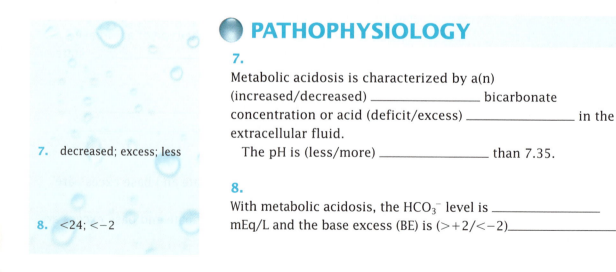

7.

Metabolic acidosis is characterized by a(n) (increased/decreased) _____ bicarbonate concentration or acid (deficit/excess) _____ in the extracellular fluid.

 The pH is (less/more) _____ than 7.35.

7. decreased; excess; less

8.

With metabolic acidosis, the HCO_3^- level is _____ mEq/L and the base excess (BE) is (>+2/<−2)_____.

8. <24; <−2

9.
Metabolic alkalosis is characterized by a(n) (increased/decreased) _____ bicarbonate concentration or loss of hydrogen ions (strong acid) in the extracellular fluid.
     The pH is *_____.

10.
With metabolic alkalosis, the bicarbonate level is _____ mEq/L and BE is _____.

● ETIOLOGY

The causes of metabolic acidosis and metabolic alkalosis are described in Tables 13-1 and 13-2. The rationale is given with each of the causes. Study the tables and then proceed to the questions. Refer to the tables as needed.

11.
With severe or chronic diarrhea, the anion that is lost from the small intestine is _____. Sodium ions are also lost in excess of the chloride ions. The chloride ions combine with the hydrogen ions to produce _____ acid.

12.
How does starvation cause metabolic acidosis?
*
_____.

13.
With uncontrolled diabetes mellitus, glucose cannot be metabolized; therefore, what occurs? *_____
_____.

14.
Shock, trauma, severe infection, and fever can cause cellular (anabolism/catabolism) _____. The acid products frequently released from the cells are *_____
_____.

---

9. increased; greater than 7.45

10. >28; >+2

11. bicarbonate; hydrochloric

12. Nonvolatile acids such as lactic acid result from cellular breakdown.

13. The liver produces fatty acids, which leads to ketone body production.

14. catabolism; nonvolatile acids such as lactic acid

Table 13-1	Causes of Metabolic Acidosis
Etiology	**Rationale**
Gastrointestinal Abnormalities Starvation Severe malnutrition	Lactic, Pyruvic, and other acids accumulate as the result of cellular breakdown due to starvation and/or severe malnutrition.
Chronic diarrhea	Loss of bicarbonate ions in the small intestines is in excess. Also, the loss of sodium ions exceeds that of chloride ions. Cl^- combines with H^+, producing a strong acid (HCl).
Renal Abnormalities Kidney failure	Kidney mechanisms for conserving sodium and water and for excreting H^+ fail.
Hormonal Influence Diabetic ketoacidosis	Failure to metabolize adequate quantities of glucose causes the liver to increase metabolism of fatty acids. Oxidation of fatty acids produces ketone bodies which cause the ECF to become more acid. Ketones require a base for excretion.
Hyperthyroidism, thyrotoxicosis	An overactive thyroid gland can cause cellular catabolism (breakdown) due to a severe increase in metabolism which increases cellular needs.
Others Trauma, shock	Trauma and shock cause cellular breakdown and the release of acids.
Excess exercise, severe infection, fever	Excessive exercise, fever, and severe infection can cause cellular catabolism and acid accumulation.

15.

Indicate which of the following conditions can cause metabolic acidosis:

    ( ) a. Starvation
    ( ) b. Gastric suction
    ( ) c. Excessive exercise
    ( ) d. Shock
    ( ) e. Uncontrolled diabetes mellitus (ketoacidosis)

15. a, c, d, e

16.

Name the anion that is lost in great quantities due to vomiting or gastric suction. _____

16. chloride

Table 13-2	Causes of Metabolic Alkalosis
Etiology	**Rationale**
Gastrointestinal Abnormalities	
Vomiting, gastric suction	With vomiting and gastric suctioning, large amounts of chloride and hydrogen ions that are plentiful in the stomach are lost. Bicarbonate anions increase to compensate for chloride loss.
Peptic ulcers	Excess of alkali in ECF occurs when a patient ingests excessive amounts of acid neutralizers such as $NaHCO_3$ to ease ulcer pain.
Hypokalemia	Loss of potassium from the body is accompanied by loss of chloride.

17. overtreated peptic ulcer, vomiting, gastric suction, and loss of potassium

17.

Name conditions that cause metabolic alkalosis. *_____, _____, *_____, and *_____

18.

For causes of metabolic acidosis and alkalosis, place M. Ac for metabolic acidosis and M. Al for metabolic alkalosis for the appropriate condition.

_____ a. Diabetic ketoacidosis
_____ b. Overtreated peptic ulcer
_____ c. Severe diarrhea
_____ d. Shock, trauma
_____ e. Vomiting, gastric suction
_____ f. Fever, severe infection
_____ g. Excessive exercise

18. a. M. Ac; b. M. Al; c. M. Ac; d. M. Ac; e. M. Al; f. M. Ac; g. M. Ac

● CLINICAL APPLICATIONS

Anion gap is a useful indicator for determining the presence or absence or metabolic acidosis.

The serum concentrations (in mEq/L) of sodium (Na^+), potassium (K^+), chloride (Cl^-), and bicarbonate (HCO_3^-) are used to compute the anion gap, as follows:

Anion gap (mEq/L) = $[Na^+] + [K^+] - [Cl^-] - [HCO_3^-]$

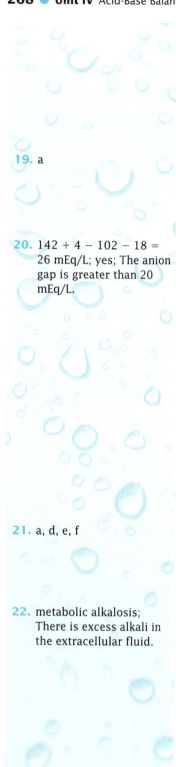

19.

If the anion gap is greater than 20 mEq/L, metabolic acidosis is suspected.

Which of the following acid-base imbalances are indicated by an anion gap that exceeds 20 mEq/L:

( ) a. Metabolic acidosis
( ) b. Metabolic alkalosis
( ) c. Respiratory acidosis

19. a

20.

A patient's serum values are Na, 142 mEq/L; K, 4mEq/L; Cl, 102 mEq/L; and HCO_3^-, 18 mEq/L.

The anion gap is *_____.

Is metabolic acidosis present? _____ Why? *_____

_____

20. $142 + 4 - 102 - 18 =$ 26 mEq/L; yes; The anion gap is greater than 20 mEq/L.

21.

Conditions associated with an anion gap that is greater than 20 mEq/L are diabetic ketoacidosis, lactic acidosis, poisoning, and renal failure.

Indicate which of the following conditions might apply to an anion gap of 25 mEq/L:

( ) a. Diabetic ketoacidosis
( ) b. Chronic obstructive pulmonary disease (COPD)
( ) c. Respiratory failure
( ) d. Renal failure
( ) e. Poisoning
( ) f. Lactic acidosis

21. a, d, e, f

22.

When a patient ingests excessive amounts of baking soda or commercially prepared acid neutralizers to ease indigestion or stomach ulcer pain, what imbalance will most likely occur?
*_____ Why? *_____

22. metabolic alkalosis; There is excess alkali in the extracellular fluid.

● CLINICAL MANIFESTATIONS

When metabolic acidosis occurs, the central nervous system (CNS) is depressed and symptoms can include apathy, disorientation, weakness, and stupor. Deep, rapid breathing is a respiratory compensatory mechanism for the purpose of decreasing acid content in the blood.

With metabolic alkalosis, excitability of the CNS occurs. These symptoms may include irritability, mental confusion, tetany-like symptoms, and hyperactive reflexes. Hypoventilation may occur, and it acts as a compensatory mechanism for metabolic alkalosis and conserves the hydrogen ions and carbonic acid.

Table 13-3 lists the clinical manifestations related to metabolic acidosis and alkalosis. Study the table and refer to it as needed when answering the questions.

23.

With metabolic acidosis, the CNS is (depressed/excited) _____.

With metabolic alkalosis, the CNS is (depressed/excited) _____.

23. depressed; excited

Table 13-3	Clinical Manifestations of Metabolic Acidosis and Metabolic Alkalosis	
Body Involvement	**Metabolic Acidosis**	**Metabolic Alkalosis**
CNS Abnormalities	Restlessness, apathy, weakness, disorientation, stupor, coma	Irritability, confusion, tetany-like symptoms, hyperactive reflexes
Respiratory Abnormalities	Kussmaul breathing: deep, rapid, vigorous breathing	Shallow breathing
Skin Changes	Flushing and warm skin	
Cardiac Abnormalities	Cardiac dysrhythmias, decrease in heart rate and cardiac output	
Gastrointestinal Abnormalities	Nausea, vomiting, abdominal pain	Vomiting with loss of chloride and potassium
Laboratory Values		
pH	<7.35	>7.45
HCO_3, BE	<24 mEq/L; <−2	>28 mEq/L; >+2

24.

Indicate which of the following CNS abnormalities are associated with metabolic acidosis (M. Ac) and metabolic alkalosis (M. Al).

_____ a. Irritability

_____ b. Apathy

_____ c. Disorientation

_____ d. Tetanylike symptoms

_____ e. Hyperactive reflexes

_____ f. Stupor

24. a. M. Al; b. M. Ac; c. M. Ac; d. M. Al; e. M. Al; f. M. Ac

25.

Metabolic acidosis results from a *_____.

In metabolic acidosis, the HCO$_3$ and BE are (decreased/increased) _____.

25. bicarbonate deficit or acid excess; decreased.

26.

With metabolic acidosis, the renal and respiratory mechanisms try to re-establish pH balance.

Explain how the renal mechanism works to re-establish balance.

*_____.

Explain how the respiratory mechanism works to re-establish balance.

*_____.

When these two mechanisms fail, what happens to the plasma pH?

*_____.

26. The kidneys excrete more H$^+$ and retain bicarbonate; As the result of the increased breathing, CO$_2$ is blown off, decreasing carbonic acid (H$_2$CO$_3$); It decreases

27.

Metabolic alkalosis results from a *_____.

In metabolic alkalosis, the HCO$_3^-$ and BE are (decreased/increased) _____.

27. bicarbonate excess; increased

28.

With metabolic alkalosis, the renal, and respiratory mechanisms try to re-establish balance.

Explain how the renal mechanism works to re-establish balance.

*_____.

Explain how the respiratory mechanism works to re-establish balance.

*_____.

When these mechanisms fail, what happens to the plasma pH?

*_____.

28. The kidneys excrete more bicarbonate and less H⁺; Pulmonary ventilation is decreased; therefore, CO_2 is retained, increasing H_2CO_3; It increases

● CLINICAL MANAGEMENT

Figure 13-2 outlines the body's normal defense actions and various methods of treatment for restoring balance in metabolic acidosis and alkalosis. Study this figure carefully, with particular attention to the cause of each imbalance, the body's defense action, the pH of the urine as to whether it is acidic or alkaline, and the treatment for these imbalances. Refer to the figure whenever you find it necessary.

29.
What is metabolic acidosis? *_____
    The urine is (acid/alkaline) _____.
    What are the body's defense actions against it?
    a. *_____.
    b. *_____.

29. bicarbonate deficit or acid excess; acid; a. Lungs blow off CO_2 or acid; b. Kidneys excrete acid or H⁺ and conserve bicarbonate

30.
Identify three treatment modalities for metabolic acidosis.

*_____

30. remove cause, administer IV alkali solution (e.g., $NaHCO_3$), and restore H_2O and electrolytes

31.
What is metabolic alkalosis? *_____
    The urine is (acid/alkaline) *_____.
    What are the body's defense actions against it?
    a. *_____.
    b. *_____.

31. bicarbonate excess; alkaline; a. Breathing is suppressed; b. Kidneys excrete HCO_3 and retain H⁺

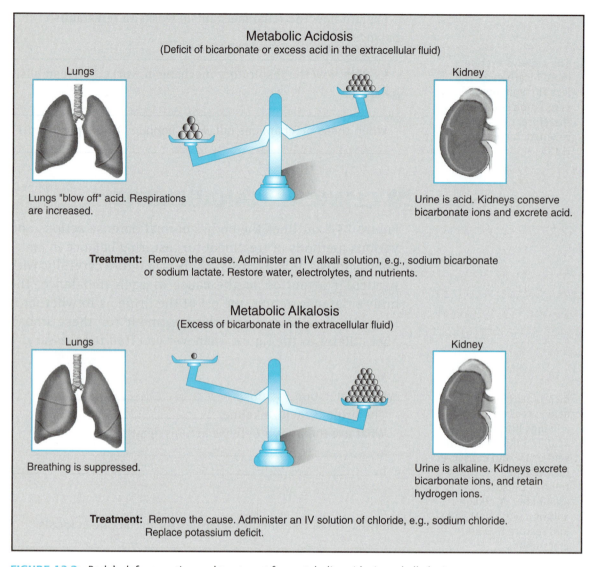

FIGURE 13-2 Body's defense action and treatment for metabolic acidosis and alkalosis.

32. remove cause, administer IV chloride solution (e.g., NaCl), and replace K deficit

32.

Identify three treatment modalities for metabolic alkalosis.

*_____

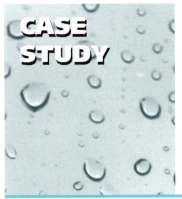

CASE STUDY

REVIEW

A 56-year-old female has chronic kidney disease. Her respirations are rapid and vigorous. She is restless. Her urine pH is 4.5 and urine output is decreased. Her arterial blood gas results are pH of 7.2, PaCO$_2$ of 38 mEq/L, and HCO$_3$ of 14 mEq/L.

ANSWER COLUMN

1. 7.35–7.45; 35–45 mm Hg; 24–28 mEq/L

2. metabolic acidosis

3. no

4. rapid, vigorous breathing and restlessness

5. b

6. rapid, vigorous breathing and excretion of acid urine

7. inadequate H$^+$ excretion

1. The "normal" arterial blood pH is _____. The normal range of PaCO$_2$ is *_____, and that of HCO$_3$ is *_____.

2. This pH and HCO$_3$ indicate imbalance that this is
*_____.

3. Is there effective respiratory compensation? _____

4. Identify two symptoms related to her acid-base imbalance.
*_____.

5. Identify the most likely source of the imbalance.
( ) a. Bicarbonate excess
( ) b. Bicarbonate deficit
( ) c. Carbonic acid excess
( ) d. Carbonic acid deficit

6. How are the patient's lungs and kidneys compensating for the acid-base imbalance? *_____ and *_____

7. Her chronic kidney disease can cause an acid-base imbalance due to
*_____.

Later her pH is 7.34, PaCO$_2$ is 31, and HCO$_3$ is 20. Fluid with sodium bicarbonate was given IV. As a nurse, you should reassess her laboratory findings.

8. metabolic acidosis

9. yes; Lungs are blowing off CO_2 and less CO_2 means less carbonic acid.

10. Sodium bicarbonate restores the bicarbonate level in ECF.

CARE PLAN

8. This pH and HCO_3 indicate *_____.

9. Is this respiratory compensation effective? _____ Explain how. *_____
_____.

10. Why are IV fluids with sodium bicarbonate administered?
*_____.

PATIENT MANAGEMENT: METABOLIC ACIDOSIS AND METABOLIC ALKALOSIS

Assessment Factors

● Obtain a patient history of clinical problems that are occurring. Recognize the patient's health problems that are associated with metabolic acidosis, i.e., starvation, severe or chronic diarrhea, kidney failure, diabetic ketoacidosis, severe infection, trauma, and shock, and with metabolic alkalosis, i.e., vomiting, gastric suction, peptic ulcer, and electrolyte imbalance (hypokalemia, hypochloremia). Poisoning, either accidental or through intentional self harm, can cause metabolic acidosis or alkalosis, depending on the substance ingested.

● Check the arterial bicarbonate and base excess levels for metabolic acid-base imbalance. Decreased HCO_3 (<24 mEq/L) and base excess (<2 mEq/L) are indicative of metabolic acidosis, and increased HCO_3 (>28 mEq/L) and base excess (2 mEq/L) are indicative of metabolic alkalosis.

● Obtain baseline vital signs for comparison with future vital signs. Note if there are any cardiac dysrhythmias and/or bradycardia that may result from a severe acidotic state. Check respirations for Kussmaul breathing. This is a sign of metabolic acidosis; such as diabetic ketoacidosis.

● Check laboratory results, especially blood sugar and electrolytes.

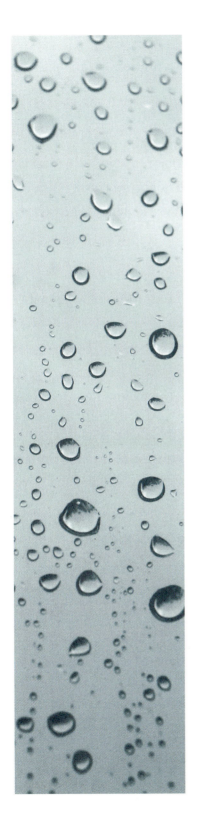

Metabolic Acidosis

Nursing Diagnosis 1

Imbalanced nutrition: less than body requirements. Nutritional intake insufficient to meet metabolic needs.

Interventions and Rationale

1. Monitor dietary intake and report inadequate nutrient and fluid intake.

2. Check the laboratory results regarding electrolytes, blood sugar, and arterial blood gases (ABGs). Some abnormal findings associated with metabolic acidosis are hyperkalemia, decreased base excess, elevated blood sugar (slightly elevated with trauma and shock and highly elevated with uncontrolled diabetes mellitus), and decreased arterial bicarbonate level and pH (HCO_3 <24 mEq/L and pH <7.35).

3. Monitor vital signs. Report the presence of Kussmaul respirations that relate to diabetic ketoacidosis or severe shock. Compare results of vital signs with baseline findings.

4. Monitor signs and symptoms related to metabolic acidosis, i.e., CNS depression (apathy, restlessness, weakness, dis-orientation, stupor); deep, rapid, vigorous breathing (Kussmaul respirations); and flushing of the skin (vasodilation resulting from sympathetic nervous system depression).

5. Administer adequate fluid replacement with sodium bicarbonate as prescribed by the healthcare provider to correct severe acidotic state.

Nursing Diagnosis 2

Deficient fluid volume related to nausea, vomiting, and increased urine output.

Interventions and Rationale

1. Monitor the heart rate closely and note any cardiac dysrhythmia. During severe acidosis, the heart rate decreases and dysrhythmias can occur causing a decrease in cardiac output.

2. Provide comfort and alleviate anxiety when possible.

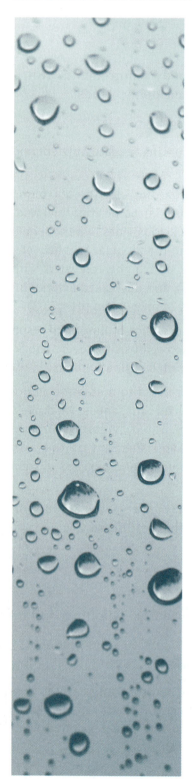

Nursing Diagnosis 3

Impaired memory related to disorientation, weakness, and stupor.

Interventions and Rationale

1. Monitor patient's sensorium and note changes, i.e., increased disorientation and stupor.

2. Provide safety measures such as bedside rails.

3. Assist the patient in meeting physical needs.

Metabolic Alkalosis

Nursing Diagnosis 1

Deficient fluid volume related to vomiting or nasogastric suctioning.

Interventions and Rationale

1. Monitor fluid intake and output. Record the amount of fluid loss via vomiting and gastric suctioning. Hydrogen and chloride are lost with the gastric secretions, which increases the pH level, causing metabolic alkalosis.

2. Administer IV fluids as ordered; fluids should contain 0.45–0.9% sodium chloride (normal saline). Encourage oral fluids if able to retain and as prescribed by the healthcare provider.

3. Monitor the serum electrolytes. If the serum chloride is decreased and the serum CO_2 is decreased, an alkalotic state is present.

4. Monitor vital signs. Note if the respirations remain shallow and slow.

5. Report if the patient is consuming large quantities of acid neutralizers that contain bicarbonate compounds, such as Bromo-Seltzer.

6. Monitor signs and symptoms of metabolic alkalosis, i.e., CNS excitability (tetany-like symptoms, irritability, confusion, hyperactive reflexes) and shallow breathing.

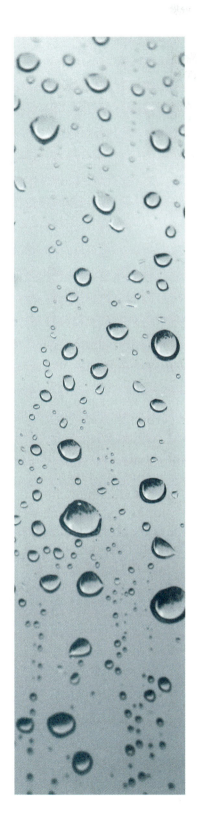

Nursing Diagnosis 2

Risk for injury related to CNS excitability secondary to metabolic alkalosis.

Interventions and Rationale

1. Provide safety measures while the patient is confused and irritable, such as bedside rails and assistance with basic needs.

2. Monitor the patient's state of CNS excitability. Report tetany-like symptoms.

Evaluation/Outcomes

1. Confirm that the cause of metabolic acidosis or metabolic alkalosis has been corrected or controlled.

2. Evaluate the therapeutic effect in correcting metabolic acidosis or metabolic alkalosis: patient's ABGs are returning to or have returned to normal range.

3. Confirm that patient remains free of signs and symptoms of metabolic acidosis and metabolic alkalosis; vital signs have returned to normal range, especially respiration.

4. Confirm that patient is able to perform activities of daily living.

5. Maintain follow-up appointments.

6. Maintain a support system for the patient.

Respiratory Acidosis and Alkalosis

William C. Rose, PhD

INTRODUCTION

Two types of respiratory acid-base imbalance are *respiratory acidosis* and *respiratory alkalosis.* Respiratory acidosis is mainly due to acid excess, particularly carbonic acid (H_2CO_3). The major problem causing respiratory acidosis is carbon dioxide (CO_2) retention due to a respiratory disorder. With respiratory alkalosis, there is a bicarbonate deficit. The result of respiratory alkalosis is mostly due to a loss of carbonic acid. Blowing off of CO_2 can be due to increased anxiety (overbreathing), excess exercise, etc. Respiratory acidosis and respiratory alkalosis are discussed separately in this chapter.

● ANSWER COLUMN

1.
The blood test for pH and $PaCO_2$ are utilized in determining respiratory acidosis and alkalosis.

The pH of arterial blood gases (ABGs) can determine the

1. acidosis; alkalosis

presence of _____ and _____.

2.
The laboratory value from the ABGs that is most useful for determining respiratory acidosis and alkalosis is

2. $PaCO_2$

_____.

3.
With respiratory acidosis, the pH is _____.

3. decreased; increased

With respiratory alkalosis, the pH is _____.

4.
In respiratory acidosis, the $PaCO_2$ is _____.

4. increased; decreased

In respiratory alkalosis, the $PaCO_2$ is _____.

● PATHOPHYSIOLOGY

5.
Respiratory acidosis is characterized by a(n) (increase/decrease) _____ of carbon dioxide (CO_2) and carbonic acid ($CO_2 + H_2O \rightarrow H_2CO_3$) concentration in the extracellular fluid.

The pH is (more/less) _____ than

5. increase; less; 7.35

_____.

6.
Respiratory alkalosis is characterized by a decrease in the
*_____ concentration in the extracellular fluid. The

6. carbonic acid; more; 7.45

pH is (more/less) _____ than _____.

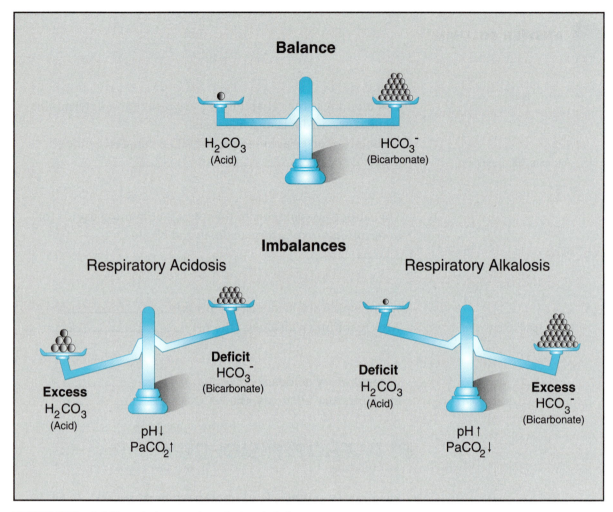

FIGURE 14-1 Acid-base balance and respiratory imbalances.

7.

With respiratory acidosis, the $PaCO_2$ is (more/less) than
_____ mm Hg.

With respiratory alkalosis, the $PaCO_2$ is (more/less) than
_____ mm Hg.

7. more; 45; less; 35

● ETIOLOGY

The causes of respiratory acidosis and alkalosis are described in Tables 14-1 and 14-2. Study the tables and then proceed to the questions. Refer to the tables as needed.

Table 14-1	**Causes of Respiratory Acidosis**

Etiology	Rationale
CNS Depressants Drugs: narcotics [morphine, meperidine (Demerol)], anesthetics, barbiturates	These drugs depress the respiratory center in the medulla, causing retention of CO_2 (carbon dioxide), which results in hypercapnia (increased partial pressure of CO_2 in the blood).
Pulmonary Abnormalities Chronic obstructive pulmonary disease (COPD: emphysema, severe asthma)	Inadequate exchange of gases in the lungs due to a decreased surface area for aeration causes retention of CO_2 in the blood.
Pneumonia, pulmonary edema	Alveolar edema inhibits effective gas exchanges resulting in a retention of CO_2.
Poliomyelitis, Guillain-Barré syndrome, chest injuries	Respiratory muscle weakness decreases ventilation, which decreases CO_2 excretion, thus increasing carbonic acid concentration.

Table 14-2	**Causes of Respiratory Alkalosis**

Etiology	Rationale
Hyperventilation Psychologic effects: anxiety, overbreathing	Excessive blowing off of CO_2 through the lungs results in hypocapnia (decreased partial pressure of CO_2 in the blood).
Pain	Overstimulation of the respiratory center in the medulla
Fever	results in hyperventilation.
Brain tumors, meningitis, encephalitis	
Early salicylate poisoning	
Hyperthyroidism	

8. It causes a retention of CO_2 in the blood: $H_2O + CO_2 \rightarrow H_2CO_3$.

8.

Explain how an inadequate exchange of gases in the lungs can cause respiratory acidosis. *_____

_____

9.

Narcotics, sedatives, chest injuries, respiratory distress syndrome, pneumonia, and pulmonary edema can cause acute respiratory acidosis. Acute respiratory acidosis results from the rapidly increasing CO_2 level and retention of CO_2 in the blood.

With chronic obstructive pulmonary disease (COPD), the body compensates for CO_2 accumulation by excreting excess hydrogen ions and conserving bicarbonate ions. The type of respiratory acidosis that occurs with COPD is (acute/chronic) _____.

9. chronic

10.
Explain how poliomyelitis and Guillain-Barré syndrome can cause CO_2 retention. * _____
_____

10. These conditions weaken the respiratory muscles, thus inhibiting CO_2 excretion.

11.
Respiratory alkalosis occurs as the result of a carbonic acid deficit due to * _____
_____

The kidneys compensate for the alkalotic state by (excreting/retaining) _____ bicarbonate ions in the plasma to maintain the bicarbonate-to-carbonic-acid ratio.

11. blowing off of CO_2, which results in a lack of H_2CO_3; excreting

12.
Indicate which of the following conditions can cause respiratory alkalosis:
_____ a. Early aspirin toxicity
_____ b. Emphysema
_____ c. Anxiety
_____ d. Encephalitis
_____ e. Narcotics
_____ f. Pneumonia
_____ g. Pain and fever

12. a, c, d, g

13.
Explain the difference between respiratory alkalosis and respiratory acidosis in terms of pH and $PaCO_2$ levels.
Respiratory alkalosis: pH _____, $PaCO_2$ _____.
Respiratory acidosis: pH _____, $PaCO_2$ _____.
*_____
_____

13. up; down; down; up

● CLINICAL APPLICATIONS

14.

For 25 years your patient has been a heavy smoker. The patient has been diagnosed as having COPD, which stands for
*_____.

15.

COPD frequently causes (acute/chronic) _____ respiratory acidosis.

16.

The patient's blood gases are pH 7.21, $PaCO_2$ 98 mm Hg, and HCO_3 40 mEq/L. The type of acid-base imbalance is *_____.
Is there metabolic (renal) compensation? _____
Explain *_____. (For acid-base compensation, see Chapter 12.)

17.

Frequently, with respiratory alkalosis, you notice that sufferers are very apprehensive and anxious. They hyperventilate due to their anxiety. Many times this occurs for a psychologic reason, e.g., giving a speech for the first time or fear of failing an exam. How do you think you might help with respiratory compensation for this imbalance? *_____
_____

● CLINICAL MANIFESTATIONS

With respiratory acidosis, hypercapnia (elevated $PaCO_2$) causes an increased pulse rate, an elevated blood pressure, and a reflex attempt to increase ventilation, which often manifests as dyspnea (difficulty in breathing). The skin may be warm and flushed due to vasodilation from the increased CO_2 concentration.

When respiratory alkalosis occurs, there is CNS hyperexcitability and a decrease in cerebral blood flow. Tetany-like symptoms and dizziness frequently result.

Table 14-3 lists the clinical manifestations related to respiratory acidosis and alkalosis. Study the table carefully. Refer to the table as needed when answering the questions.

14. chronic obstructive pulmonary disease

15. chronic

16. respiratory acidosis; Yes, there is metabolic compensation (bicarbonate is elevated).

17. Encourage the patient to breathe slowly and deeply. There is a lack of CO_2, so giving CO_2 (e.g., rebreathing CO_2 from a paper bag) can also help.

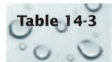

Table 14-3

Clinical Manifestations of Respiratory Acidosis and Respiratory Alkalosis

Body Involvement	Respiratory Acidosis	Respiratory Alkalosis
Cardiopulmonary Abnormalities	Dyspnea Tachycardia Blood pressure	Rapid, shallow breathing Palpitations

CNS Abnormalities	Disorientation
	Depression, paranoia
	Weakness
	Stupor (later)
		Tetany symptoms: numbness and
		  tingling of fingers and toes, positive
		  Chvostek and Trousseau signs
		Hyperactive reflexes
		Vertigo (dizziness)
		Unconsciousness (later)

Skin	Flushed and warm	Sweating may occur
Laboratory Values		

pH	<7.35 (when compensatory
	  mechanisms fail)
		>7.45 (when compensatory
		  mechanisms fail)

$PaCO_2$	>45 mm Hg	<35 mm Hg

18.

Respiratory patterns of breathing are clues to the type of respiratory acid-base imbalance.

The characteristic breathing pattern associated with respiratory acidosis is _____, and for respiratory alkalosis, the breathing pattern is *_____
_____.

18. dyspnea (labored or difficulty in breathing); rapid, shallow breathing (hyperventilating or overbreathing)

19.

Indicate which CNS abnormalities are associated with respiratory acidosis (R. Ac) and respiratory alkalosis (R. Al).

_____ a. Tetanylike symptoms
_____ b. Disorientation
_____ c. Dizziness or lightheadedness
_____ d. Depression, paranoia
_____ e. Hyperactive reflexes
_____ f. Positive Chvostek's sign

19. a. R. Al; b. R. Ac; c. R. Al; d. R. Ac; e. R. Al; f. R. Al

20.

Respiratory acidosis results from a(n) (deficit/excess) _____ of carbonic acid.

The $PaCO_2$ is (greater/less) *_____ than _____

20. excess; greater; 45 mm Hg

21. CO_2 stimulates the respiratory center to attempt to increase the rate and depth of ventilation. CO_2 is blown off, which causes the carbonic acid (H_2CO_3) level to fall. (However, usually in respiratory acidosis, the respiratory system is affected and not able to accomplish this.); More acid is excreted in the urine, and less base (bicarbonate) is excreted; It is decreased.

21.

With respiratory acidosis, the renal and respiratory mechanisms try to re-establish balance.

With an increased CO_2, explain how the respiratory mechanism works to compensate for this imbalance. *_____

_____

Explain how the renal mechanism works to compensate for this imbalance.

*_____

When these mechanisms fail, what happens to the blood pH?

*_____

22. deficit; greater 35 mm Hg

22.

Respiratory alkalosis results from a(n) (deficit/excess) _____ of carbonic acid.

The $PaCO_2$ is (greater/less) *_____ than _____.

23. an increased HCO_3 excretion and a H^+ retention; It increases.

23.

The buffer mechanism produces more organic acids, in respiratory alkalosis, which react with the excess bicarbonate ions.

How do you think the renal mechanism works to compensate for this imbalance? *_____

When these mechanisms fail, what happens to the blood pH?

*_____   .

● CLINICAL MANAGEMENT

Figure 14-2 outlines the body's normal defense actions and various methods of treatment for restoring balance in respiratory acidosis and alkalosis. Study the figure carefully, with particular attention to the factors causing the acid-base imbalances, the pH of the urine as to whether it is acid or alkaline, and the treatment for these imbalances. Refer to the figure as needed.

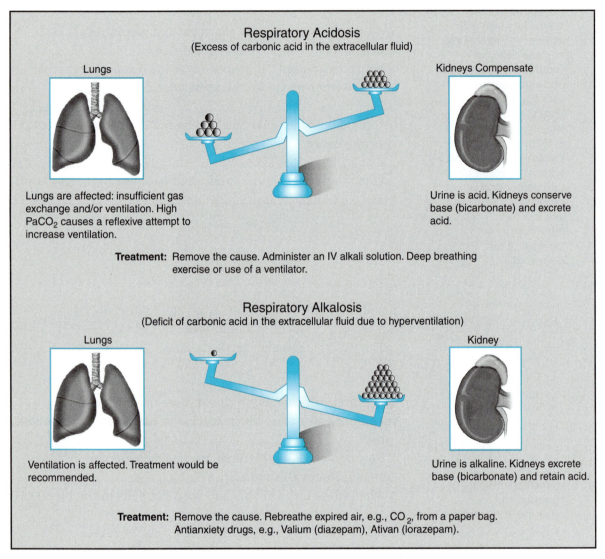

FIGURE 14-2 Body's defense action and treatment for respiratory acidosis and respiratory alkalosis.

24. carbonic acid excess; acidic; a. There is an attempt to increase ventilation.
b. Kidneys excrete acidic urine and conserve base (bicarbonate).

24.

What is the basic cause of respiratory acidosis? *_____

In compensated respiratory acidosis, the urine is (acidic/alkaline)

a. How does the respiratory system try to compensate? *_____

b. How do the kidneys compensate? *_____

25. Any three of: removal of cause, deep breathing exercise, airway management, and ventilator

26. carbonic acid deficit due to hyperventilation; alkaline; Kidneys excrete base (HCO_3) and retain acid (H^+).

27. removal of cause, rebreathing expired air, and antianxiety drugs, e.g., Ativan (lorazepam) and diazepam (Valium)

25.
Identify three treatment modalities for respiratory acidosis.
*_____

26.
What is the basic cause of respiratory alkalosis? *_____
   In compensated respiratory alkalosis, the urine is (acidic/alkaline) _____.
   Describe the renal compensation. *_____
_____

27.
Identify three treatment modalities for respiratory alkalosis.
*_____
_____

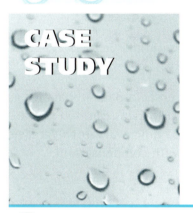

CASE STUDY

REVIEW

A 46-year-old male has a history of respiratory problems. His latest problem is pneumonia. He smokes two or three packs of cigarettes a day. His condition indicates an acid-base imbalance. Refer to Table 14-4 for a summary review, if needed.

 ANSWER COLUMN

1. hydrogen

2. hyperventilating; hypoventilating

3. hydrogen ion; bicarbonate; bicarbonate; hydrogen ion

4. lungs

1. The acidity or alkalinity of a solution depends on the concentration of the (hydrogen/bicarbonate) _____ ions.

2. The lungs help regulate acid-base balance by _____ to blow off CO_2 and by _____ to conserve CO_2.

3. The kidney maintains the acid-base balance by excreting _____ or _____ and by retaining _____ or _____.

4. Which acts faster in regulating or correcting acid-base imbalance (kidneys/lungs)? _____

5. excess; deficit

5. Respiratory acidosis has a CO_2 (excess/deficit) _____, whereas respiratory alkalosis has a CO_2 (excess/deficit) _____.

His blood gases are a pH of 7.29, $PaCO_2$ of 54 mEq/L, and HCO_3 of 25 mEq/L.

6. respiratory acidosis

6. The patients's pH and $PaCO_2$ indicate *_____.

7. no

7. Is there any renal (metabolic) compensation? _____

Two days later his blood gases had a pH of 7.34, $PaCO_2$ of 62 mEq/L, and HCO_3 of 30 mEq/L.

8. Hypoventilating. It causes CO_2 retention— respiratory acidosis.

8. The patient has been (hyperventilating/hypoventilating) _____ ?

9. Yes; If compensation was not present, the pH would be greatly decreased, causing more H^+ concentration.

9. Is there metabolic (renal) compensation? _____. Explain.*_____.

10. Complete the following chart on acid-base imbalance as to pH, $PaCO_2$, and HCO_3. Use the arrow pointed upward for increase, the arrow pointed downward for decrease, and—for not involved (except with compensation).

10. *Metabolic Acidosis*
pH↓
$PaCO_2$—
HCO_3
Metabolic Alkalosis
pH↑
$PaCO_2$—
HCO_3
Respiratory Acidosis
pH↓
$PaCO_2$↑
HCO_3
Respiratory Alkalosis
pH↑
$PaCO_2$↓
HCO_3

Metabolic Acidosis
pH
$PaCO_2$
HCO_3

Metabolic Alkalosis
pH
$PaCO_2$
HCO_3

Respiratory Acidosis
pH
$PaCO_2$
HCO_3

Respiratory Alkalosis
pH
$PaCO_2$
HCO_3

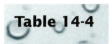

Table 14-4   **Summary of Acid-Base Imbalances**

Metabolic Acidosis	Metabolic Alkalosis
Clinical Manifestations	
Kussmaul breathing (rapid and vigorous)	Shallow breathing
Flushing of the skin (capillary dilation)	Tetany-like symptoms (numbness,
Decrease in heart rate and cardiac output	tingling of fingers)
Nausea, vomiting, abdominal pain	Irritability, confusion
Dehydration	Vomiting
Laboratory Findings	
Bicarbonate deficit	Bicarbonate excess
pH<7.35, HCO_3 <24 mEq/L,	pH>7.45, HCO_3 >28 mEq/L, BE>+2,
BE<−2, plasma CO_2 < 22 mEq/L	
Causes	
Diabetic ketoacidosis, severe diarrhea or	Peptic ulcer, vomiting, gastric suction
starvation, tissue trauma, renal and heart	
failure, shock, severe infection	

Respiratory Acidosis	Respiratory Alkalosis
Clinical Manifestations	
Dyspnea, inadequate gas exchange	Rapid shallow breathing
Flushing and warm skin	Tetany-like symptoms (numbness,
Tachycardia	tingling of fingers)
Weakness	Palpitations
	Vertigo
Laboratory Findings	
Carbonic acid excess (CO_2 retention)	Carbonic acid deficit
pH < 7.35, $PaCO_2$ > 45 mm Hg	pH > 7.45, $PaCO_2$ < 35 mm Hg
Causes	
COPD (emphysema, chronic bronchitis), severe	Anxiety, hysteria, drug toxicity, fever,
asthma, narcotics, anesthetics, barbiturates,	pain, brain tumors, early salicylate
pneumonia, chest injuries	poisoning, excessive exercise

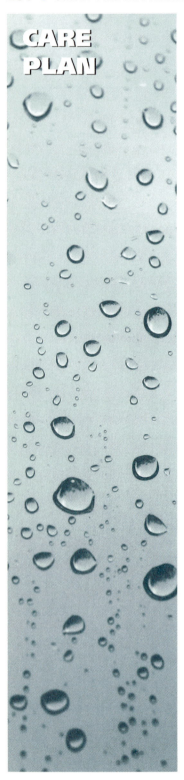

CARE PLAN

PATIENT MANAGEMENT: RESPIRATORY ACIDOSIS AND RESPIRATORY ALKALOSIS

Assessment Factors

● Obtain a patient history of clinical problems. Recognize the patient's health problems that are associated with respiratory acidosis, i.e., CNS depressant drugs (narcotics, sedatives, anesthetics), pneumonia, pulmonary edema, and chronic obstructive pulmonary disease (COPD) such as emphysema, chronic bronchitis, bronchiectasis, and severe asthma, and those associated with respiratory alkalosis, i.e., anxiety, fever, severe infection, aspirin toxicity, and deliberate overbreathing.

● Check for signs and symptoms of respiratory acidosis, i.e., dyspnea, tachycardia, disorientation, weakness, stupor, and flushed and warm skin, and signs and symptoms related to respiratory alkalosis, i.e., apprehension, rapid, shallow breathing, palpitations, tetany-like symptoms such as numbness and tingling of the toes and fingers, hyperactive reflexes, and dizziness.

● Obtain vital signs for a baseline record to compare with future vital signs.

● Check arterial blood gas report, particularly the $PaCO_2$ result. An increased $PaCO_2$ that exceeds 45 mm Hg is indicative of respiratory acidosis and a decreased $PaCO_2$ of less than 35 mm Hg is indicative of respiratory alkalosis. Report abnormal findings.

Respiratory Acidosis
Nursing Diagnosis 1

Impaired gas exchange related to alveolar *capillary membrane changes.*

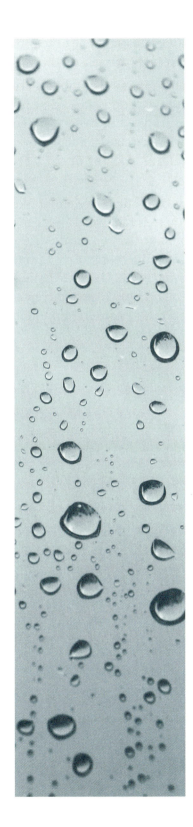

Interventions and Rationale

1. Monitor patient's respiratory status for changes in respiratory rate, distress, and breathing pattern.

2. Monitor arterial blood gases (ABGs), especially the pH, $PaCO_2$, and HCO_3. A pH of less than 7.35 indicates acidosis and a $PaCO_2$ of greater than 45 mm Hg indicates respiratory acidosis. If the bicarbonate level (HCO_3) is greater than 28 mEq/L, then there is metabolic (renal) compensation. With compensation, the respiratory acidotic state is most likely to be chronic rather than acute.

3. Auscultate breath sounds periodically to determine wheezing, rhonchi, or crackles that indicate poor gas exchange.

4. Monitor vital signs for tachycardia or cardiac dysrhythmias associated with hypercapnia and hypoxemia (oxygen deficit in the blood).

5. Monitor mechanical ventilator use for a client having respiratory distress due to impaired gas exchange.

6. Maintain adequate airway clearance by suctioning, chest physical therapy, etc., as needed.

7. Encourage pursed lips breathing and elevate head of bed.

8. Administer bronchodilators as ordered.

Nursing Diagnosis 2

Ineffective airway clearance related to thick bronchial secretions and/or bronchial spasms limiting ability to clear airway.

Interventions and Rationale

1. Assist patient with self-care.

2. Encourage patient to deep breathe and cough. This helps to eliminate bronchial secretions and improve gas exchange.

3. Assist the patient with use of an inhaler containing a bronchodilator drug. Explain the use and frequency of medications.

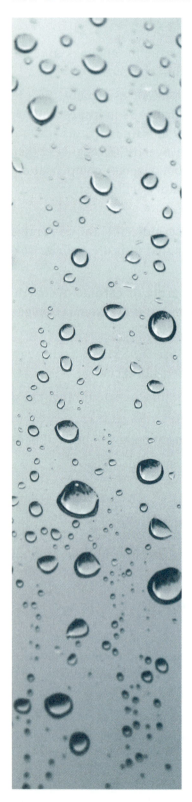

4. Administer chest clapping on COPD patients or others to break up mucous plugs and secretions in the alveoli.

5. Teach breathing exercises and postural drainage to patients with chronic obstructive pulmonary disease (COPD). Mucous secretions are trapped in overextended alveoli (air sacs), and breathing exercises and postural drainage help to remove secretions and restore gas exchange (ventilation).

6. Monitor oxygen administration. Too much oxygen intake may depress respirations and increase the severity of the respiratory acidosis. Hypercapnia (increased partial pressure of carbon dioxide) stimulates the respiratory center in the brain; however, after the $PaCO_2$ level becomes highly elevated, it is no longer a stimulus. The hypoxemia continues to stimulate the respiratory center. Too much oxygen inhibits the respiratory stimulus effect.

7. Encourage the patient to increase fluid intake in order to decrease tenacity of the secretions.

Nursing Diagnosis 3

Risk for injury related to hypoxemia and hypercapnia.

Interventions and Rationale

1. Monitor the patient's state of sensorium for signs of disorientation due to a lack of oxygen to the brain.

2. Provide safety measures, such as bedside rails when the patient is disoriented or in a stuporous state.

Nursing Diagnosis 4

Activity intolerance related to dyspnea secondary to poor gas exchange.

Interventions and Rationale

1. Assist the patient with activities of daily living.

2. Plan daily activities that follow his or her breathing exercises as indicated by the physician.

3. Encourage the patient to participate in a pulmonary rehabilitation program.

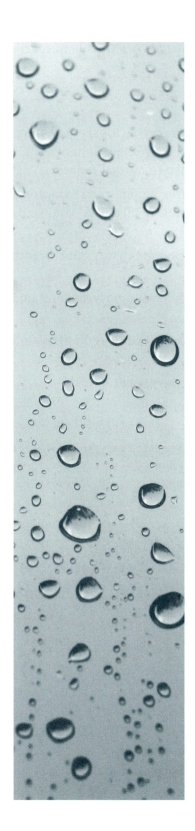

Other Diagnoses to Consider

Ineffective breathing pattern related to inadequate ventilation.

Respiratory Alkalosis
Nursing Diagnosis 1

Anxiety related to hyperventilation secondary to stressful situations.

Interventions and Rationale

1. Encourage the patient who is overanxious and hyperventilating to take deep breaths and breathe slowly. Proper breathing prevents respiratory alkalosis.

2. Listen to patient who is emotionally distressed. Encourage the patient to seek professional help for psychologic problems.

Nursing Diagnosis 2

Ineffective breathing pattern related to hyperventilation and anxiety.

Interventions and Rationale

1. Demonstrate a slow, relaxed breathing pattern to decrease overbreathing, which causes respiratory alkalosis.

2. Administer a sedative as prescribed to relax patient and restore a normal breathing pattern.

Nursing Diagnosis 3

Risk for injury related to tissue hypoxia and sensory dysfunction.

Interventions and Rationale

1. Instruct the patient to be seated when feeling dizzy or lightheaded.

2. Remove objects that may harm the patient if dizziness leads to syncope (fainting).

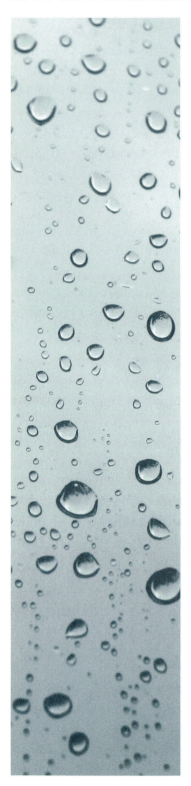

3. Provide side rails if unconsciousness occurs due to severe respiratory alkalosis.

Evaluation/Outcomes

1. Confirm that the cause of respiratory acidosis or respiratory alkalosis is corrected or is controlled. Patient's ABGs are returning to or have returned to normal ranges.

2. Confirm that patient remains free of signs and symptoms of respiratory acidosis or respiratory alkalosis; vital signs are within normal ranges.

3. Confirm that patient has a patent airway and breath sounds have improved.

4. Confirm that patient walks with little to no assistance and without breathlessness.

5. Document compliance with prescribed drug therapy and medical regimen.

6. Maintain a support system for the patient.

7. Keep scheduled follow-up appointments.

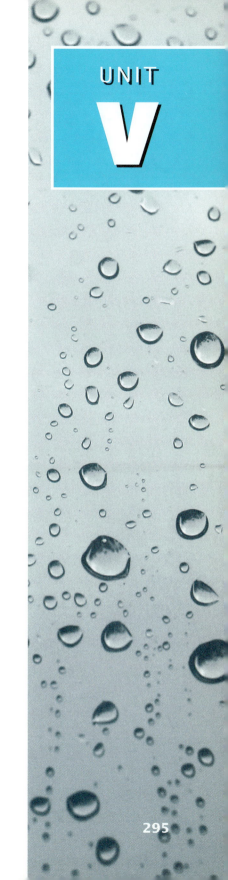

CLINICAL SITUATIONS: FLUID, ELECTROLYTE, AND ACID-BASE IMBALANCES

⬤ LEARNING OUTCOMES

Upon completion of this unit, the reader will be able to:

- Identify physiological factors that are influenced by fluid, electrolyte, and acid-base imbalances for patients across the life span.
- Identify the impact of fluid changes on normal electrolyte values for sodium, chloride, potassium, calcium, magnesium, and phosphates for patients in shock or experiencing select chronic diseases, GI surgery, and acute renal failure.
- Discuss the physiological responses to fluid volume excess in select disorders for patients of all ages.
- Discuss the physiological responses to fluid volume deficits in select disorders for patients of all ages.
- Discuss normal regulatory mechanisms for pH control for patients experiencing select chronic diseases, GI surgery, and trauma.
- Identify symptoms of acid-base imbalances for patients across the life span experiencing select chronic diseases, GI surgery, and trauma.
- Differentiate the symptoms of metabolic acidosis from the symptoms of metabolic alkalosis in select chronic diseases.
- Differentiate the symptoms of respiratory acidosis from the symptoms of respiratory alkalosis in select chronic diseases.
- Identify important assessment factors in determining fluid and electrolyte balance in patients across the life span.

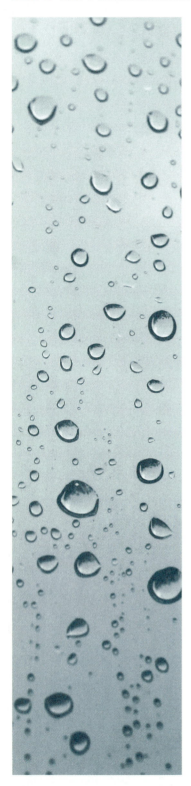

- Develop nursing diagnoses for patients across the life span who are experiencing fluid and electrolyte imbalances.
- Identify age-appropriate nursing interventions specific to select diagnoses associated with fluid balance problems.
- Understand the rationale for nursing interventions specific to fluid and electrolyte imbalances.
- Discuss the clinical management of patients across the life span with fluid and electrolyte imbalances.
- Describe potential complications associated with the management of fluid and electrolyte imbalances.

● INTRODUCTION

In clinical and home care settings health professionals provide care for persons experiencing a variety of problems related to fluid and electrolytes. Unit V addresses clinical situations. The first two chapters focus on potential developmental fluid and electrolyte issues related to infants, children, and the older adult. The remaining chapters focus on trauma and shock, gastrointestinal (GI) surgery, renal failure, and chronic diseases including heart failure, diabetic ketoacidosis, and chronic obstructive pulmonary disease (COPD). In order to assess the patient's needs and to provide the appropriate care needed for persons with selected health problems, the health professional must have a working knowledge and understanding of the concepts related to fluid and electrolyte imbalance. Knowledge of these concepts allows the health professional to assess physiologic changes that occur with fluid, electrolyte, and acid-base imbalances and to plan appropriate interventions to assist patient as they adapt to these changes.

In each clinical situation the participant will become acquainted with patients who have fluid and electrolyte imbalances. Patients are presented as part of a clinical situation. The participant in this program will gain an understanding of the physiologic changes involved in each clinical situation.

An asterisk (*) on an answer line indicates a multiple-word answer. The meanings for the following symbols are: ↑ increased, ↓ decreased, > greater than, < less than.

Fluid Problems of Infants and Children

Gail H. Wade, DNSc, RN

⬤ LEARNING OUTCOMES

Upon completion of this chapter, the reader will be able to:

- Identify three physiologic factors that influence infants' and children's responses to changes in fluid and electrolyte balance.
- Compare the total body fluid volume in infants and children to the total body fluid volume in the mature adult.
- Identify normal serum electrolyte values for sodium, potassium, and calcium in infants and children.
- Discuss how the electrolyte values for sodium, potassium, and calcium vary in response to fluid balance changes in infants and children.
- Describe a method to calculate the daily fluid and electrolyte needs of infants and children.
- Describe assessment factors important in determining fluid and electrolyte balance in infants and children.
- Develop diagnoses for infants and children experiencing fluid balance problems.
- Identify interventions specific to select diagnoses associated with fluid balance problems.

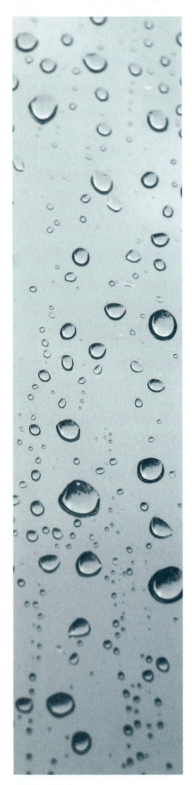

INTRODUCTION

Children are not just small adults. Many anatomic and physiologic changes occur from the neonatal period, through infancy and childhood, until the child reaches adulthood. Infancy, which lasts through the first year of life, is preceded by a neonatal period of one month. The toddler period generally begins at 12 months of age and lasts until 24 months. Childhood extends from the preschool years until adolescence, around age 12. Once the child reaches adolescence, many of the physiological and anatomic characteristics are similar to those of an adult.

The health professional's knowledge of the physiologic differences in infants and children is essential. Because these physiologic differences vary significantly throughout infancy and childhood, important regulatory factors are presented from a developmental perspective. Health professionals need to understand the implications of these developmental characteristics and the potential for fluid balance problems. This chapter addresses those factors as well as normal chemistry values and physiologic factors that influence infants' and children's rapid responses to changes in fluid and electrolyte balance.

PHYSIOLOGIC FACTORS

Physiologic differences in infant and young children's total body surface area, immaturity of renal structures, high rate of metabolism, and immaturity of the endocrine system in promoting homeostatic control predispose this age group to various fluid and electrolyte imbalances.

The physiologic differences between infants, children, and adults make infants and children more vulnerable to fluid, electrolyte, and acid-base imbalances. As body weight increases with the age of the child, the percentage of body water decreases. Premature infants have more body water then full term newborns. Newborns and infants have a proportionately higher ratio of extracellular fluid (ECF) to intracellular fluid (ICF) than do older children and adults. The proportionally larger extracellular fluid volume is because the brain and skin, both rich in interstitial fluid, occupy the

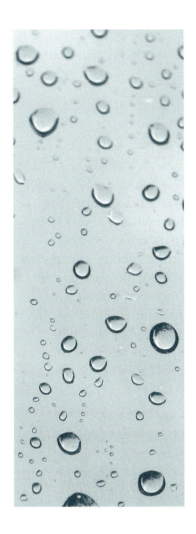

greatest portion of the developing infant's body weight (London, Ladewig, Ball, & Bindler, 2007).

Because infants and children under 2 years of age lose a greater percentage of body fluid daily than do older children and adults, they must have an adequate intake of fluid daily. Their small stomach size decreases the ability to rehydrate rapidly and a limited fluid reserve capacity inhibits adaptation to fluid losses. They also tend to have a greater insensible water loss through their skin due to their large body surface. Additional insensible water losses are related to the increased metabolic and respiratory rates of infants and young children. The kidneys act to maintain a balance between fluid loss and replacement by conserving water and needed electrolytes and excreting waste products. Children under 2, however, are unable to effectively conserve and excrete water and solutes because their renal structures are not fully developed. As more water is excreted, infants and children become more susceptible to fluid and electrolyte imbalances. Additionally, infants and young children are at risk for acid-base imbalances because the transport system for ions and bicarbonate is weaker than in older children and adults. When infants and young children become ill, it is difficult to maintain a balance between fluid and electrolyte losses and replacements. All of these factors increase the infant and young child's vulnerability to fluid and electrolyte imbalances.

ANSWER COLUMN

1.

The body is composed mostly of water. Body water in the early human embryo represents _____ % of body weight, in the newborn infant _____ %, and in the adult _____ %. (Refer to Chapter 1, question 1.)

The low-birth-weight infant's (premature infant's) body water represents 80–90% of body weight.

1. 97; 70–80; 60

2.

Complete the percentage of body weight that is representative of body water in the following:

Early human embryo _____%

Low-birth-weight infant _____%

Newborn infant _____%

Adult _____%

2. 97; 80–90; 70–80; 60

3.

Infants need proportionately more water than adults. The infant's large body surface area and immature kidneys limit the infant's ability to retain water. Their kidneys cannot concentrate urine effectively; thus, urine volume is increased. More water is lost through the infant's skin because of the increased body surface area. Since the infant cannot concentrate urine, water is needed to maintain fluid volume lost through the increased urine output and larger body surface area.

Give two reasons why the infant needs a higher percentage of total body water.

*
_____

_____

3. a large body surface (greater amounts of water loss through the skin) and inability to concentrate urine (increased urine output due to immature kidneys)

4.

Water distribution in the infant is not the same as in an adult. Water comprises 65% of the infant's body weight. Of the total body water, 25% is ECF. The percentage of water to body weight in the adult is _____ (Refer to Chapter 1.)

The ICF in the infant is 35% of body weight; whereas in the adult it is _____. (Refer to Chapter 1.) The proportionately higher ratio of ECF volume in the infant predisposes the infant to (more, less) _____ rapid losses of fluid volume; consequently, _____ develops more rapidly in infants than adults.

4. 20%; 40%; more; dehydration

5.

The percentage of the child's total body water (50%) is close in amount to the percentage of the adult's (60%) total body water; and, the proportion of ECF (10–15%) and ICF (40–45%) is also similar to that of the adult.

5. interstitial; intravascular; cellular

The extracellular fluid is composed of _____ and _____ fluid. Another name for intracellular fluid is (cellular/vascular) _____ fluid. (Refer to Chapter 1.)

6.

Increased body surface area in the infant causes excess water loss through the _____. The smaller the infant, the greater the body surface area in proportion to body weight. The infant's kidneys are (mature/immature) _____; thus, the urinary volume is (increased/decreased) _____.

6. skin; immature; increased

7.

It may take 2 years before the child's kidneys are mature.

The infant's immature kidneys decrease the glomerular filtration rate (GFR); thus, the kidney's ability to concentrate urine is (decreased/increased) _____, while the urine volume is (decreased/increased) _____.

Fluid intake in infants must be carefully monitored to insure that overhydration does not occur. With overhydration, an extracellular fluid volume excess results from too much fluid in the vascular and interstitial compartment.

Giving too much water can cause (dehydration/overhydration) _____.

7. decreased; increased; overhydration

8.

As the child grows, there is muscle growth and cellular growth. More water shifts from the ECF to the ICF compartment.

What do you think is the contributing factor when the child's ICF and ECF proportions become similar to the adult's?
*
_____

_____

8. Increased cellular and muscular growth causes water to shift from the ECF space to the ICF space.

● ETIOLOGY

9.

The infant has less body fluid reserve than the adult and is more likely to develop a fluid volume deficit.

An infant may lose one-half of ECF daily; however, under normal conditions losses are replaced simultaneously. Adults lose only one-sixth of their ECF in the same length of time.

9. large body surface area causing water to be lost through the skin (insensible perspiration) and increased urinary output (immature kidneys cannot concentrate urine); decreased

Name two reasons why an infant may lose one-half of ECF daily. * _____

_____

The infant is likely to develop dehydration more rapidly than adults who lose proportionately similar amounts of water. This increased risk for infants is the result of their (increased/decreased) _____ fluid reserve.

10.

Factors that increase insensible fluid loss are hyperthermia, increased activity, hyperventilation, radiant warmers, and phototherapy.

10. reduces

Keeping an infant covered in a neutral cool environment (reduces/increases) _____ insensible fluid loss through the body surface.

11.

Serum electrolytes do not vary greatly between infants and adults. The serum sodium level in a newborn fluctuates at birth. It may be low the first 3–6 hours after birth and then rise slightly (2–6 mEq/L increase) during the first 2 days of life.

11. 135–146 mEq/L

The infant's normal serum sodium range is 139–146 mEq/L and the child's normal serum range is 135–148 mEq/L. What is the normal adult serum sodium level? * _____

12.

Low-birth-weight infants tend to develop hypernatremia with a normal to low sodium intake. Their body surface area is (greater/lesser) _____ than an average-weight newborn's and their insensible water loss is (increased/decreased) _____.

Also, low-birth-weight infants' kidneys are more immature than the kidneys of average-weight infants; therefore, more diluted water is excreted. The loss of water is in excess of the loss of solutes. In low-birth-weight infants this increases their risk of developing _____.

12. greater; increased; hypernatremia

13.

Infant formulas come in three varieties that contain compositions of vitamins, minerals, proteins, carbohydrates, and essential amino acids. The formulas are either cow's milk protein–based; soy protein–based; or specialized, therapeutic formulas. The American Academy of Pediatrics (AAP) and the American College of Obstetricians and Gynecologists (AGOG) recommend that infants be given breast milk or iron-fortified formula instead of whole milk for the first year of life. Even with improvements in commercially prepared infant formulas, there are differences in the electrolyte composition when compared with breast milk. A 5-month-old infant who consumes infant formula and commercially prepared baby food ingests five times more sodium than a breast-fed infant.

The name for an elevated serum sodium level is

_____.

13. hypernatremia (serum sodium excess)

14.
Hyponatremia can also occur in infants and children. Another name for hyponatremia is *_____.
Three causes of hyponatremia are:
   a. Overhydration—water overloading
   b. Continuous administration of oral or parenteral electrolyte-free solutions
   c. Syndrome of inappropriate antidiuretic hormone (SIADH). This results in an excess secretion of ADH causing excess water reabsorption from the distal tubules. Factors attributing to SIADH are CNS injuries or illness (head injuries, meningitis), pneumonia, neoplasm, stress, surgery, and drugs (narcotics, barbiturates).

14. serum sodium deficit

15.
Name three causes of hyponatremia. *_____
_____

15. overhydration, continuous administration of electrolyte-free solutions, and SIADH

16.
A rapid decrease in the serum sodium, 120 mEq/L or below, can cause CNS changes such as headache, twitching, confusion, and convulsions. In infants, increased irritability or other subtle changes in mental states and feeding behavior may occur.

Observe for CNS changes when hyponatremia occurs suddenly. Give three CNS symptoms. *_____

16. headache, twitching, and confusion (also convulsions)

17. cells or ICF (In various institutions, laboratory values may vary slightly.)

18. dizziness, muscular weakness, abdominal distention, decreased peristalsis, and arrhythmia

19. hyperkalemia, or serum potassium excess

20. 139–146 mEq/L; 3.5–5.0 mEq/L

17.

The normal serum potassium range for the newborn is 300–600 mEq/L. The upper level is slightly higher than the adult's and remains in the upper level for the first few months of the infant's life.

Try to recall where the greatest concentration of potassium is found in the body. _____

18.

Infants and children may develop hypokalemia (serum potassium deficit) when cellular breakdown occurs from injury, starvation, dehydration, diarrhea, vomiting, diabetic acidosis, and the administration of steroids. Children do not conserve potassium well. The kidneys continue to excrete body potassium even with little or no potassium intake.

Give at least two signs or symptoms of hypokalemia. (Refer to Chapter 6.) * _____

19.

Eighty to 90% of body potassium loss is excreted in the urine. When oliguria (decreased urine output) occurs, what type of potassium imbalance results? _____

20.

The infant's normal serum chloride range is 96–116 mEq/L. For the first few months of the infant's life the serum sodium range is * _____ and the serum potassium range is * _____. The normal range of the child's serum chloride level is 98–111 mEq/L.

21.

The serum calcium level in the cord blood is higher than the maternal serum calcium level; however, after birth the infant's serum calcium level decreases to 3.8 mEq/L, or 7.7 mg/dL. In low-birth-weight infants, the serum calcium tends to remain lower for a longer period of time. A child's normal serum calcium range is 4.5–5.8 mEq/L, or 8–10.8 mg/dL.

Infants do not have calcium stored in their bones as do adults. If infants are fed formula, their body calcium level may remain low since infant formula has a high phosphorus content, which lowers the calcium level.

21. the breast-fed infant; Breast milk contains more calcium and less phosphorus, which gives the infant more calcium. Thus, reducing phosphorus allows the infant to retain the calcium.

   Breast-fed infants receive more calcium and retain it since breast milk contains less phosphorus.

   Which infant retains more body calcium—the infant receiving formula or the breast-fed infant?

*_____

Why? *_____

22.

Ionized calcium levels, important indicators of the child's acid-base balance, are slightly lower than serum calcium levels. The binding of calcium to protein is affected by the pH. When the pH decreases with acidosis, ionized calcium increases and calcium is removed from proteins and is available for chemical reactions. Alkalosis increases the binding of calcium to proteins and decreases the concentration of ionized calcium. Tetany symptoms occur when hypocalcemia (serum calcium deficit) is present in a normal acid-base balance or in an alkalotic state.

22. tingling of fingers and twitching around mouth (also, carpopedal spasm)

   Symptoms of tetany are *_____ and

*_____. (Refer to Chapter 8.)

23.

Newborn infants tend to have a low pH, which is indicative of metabolic acidosis. This is the result of increased acid metabolites that result from the infant's increased metabolic rate and physiologic changes during birth. The pH becomes closer to normal after the first few days or weeks of life. In low-birth-weight infants, the pH remains low for several weeks.

23. does not (Calcium is ionized in an acidotic state regardless of how low it is.)

   The low pH of infant formula combined with the low serum calcium level in infants (does/does not) _____ result in symptoms of tetany.

● CLINICAL APPLICATIONS

There are several formulas and nomograms for calculating fluid and electrolyte maintenance requirements in infants and children. Table 15-1 suggests a simple method for calculating daily fluid and electrolyte maintenance requirements for infants and children. The formula is based on the assumption that for each 100 calories metabolized, 100 mL of water is required. This method is not used with

Table 15-1	Fluid and Electrolyte Maintenance Requirements for Infants and Children According to the Holiday-Segar Method		
Body Weight (kg)	**Water (mL/kg/day)**		**Electrolytes (mEq per 100 mL H$_2$O)**
First 10 kg	100		Na$^+$3
Second 10 kg	50		Cl$^-$2
Each additional kg	20		K$^+$2

Adapted from *The Harriet Lane Handbook: A Manual for Pediatric House Officers* (17th ed.), J. Robertson, and N. Shilkofski (Eds.), 2005, Philadelphia: Elsevier Masby.

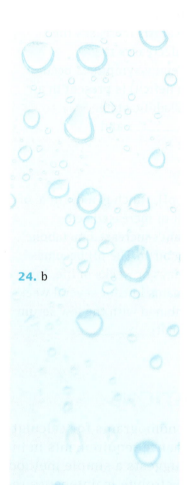

24. b

neonates less than 14 days old or with conditions of abnormal fluid losses.

To calculate the daily fluid and electrolyte needs of infants and children, first calculate the infant's/child's weight in kilograms (kg). Then use this chart to calculate the specific fluid and electrolyte needs according to the body weight in kilograms.

24.

Using Table 15-1, calculate the daily fluid requirements for an infant weighing 6 kg. The daily fluid requirements are:

( ) a. 300 mL
( ) b. 600 mL
( ) c. 900 mL

25.

Using Table 15-1, calculate the daily fluid requirements of a child weighing 30 kg:

( ) a. 1500 mL
( ) b. 1700 mL
( ) c. 1250 mL

The daily sodium requirement according to the fluid needs of this child is:

( ) d. 17 mEq
( ) e. 45 mEq
( ) f. 51 mEq

The daily potassium and chloride requirements according to the fluid needs for this child are:

( ) g. 34 mEq

( ) h. 17 mEq

( ) i. 30 mEq

In situations of minimal fluid and electrolyte imbalances, oral intake of fluids should be encouraged to maintain fluid and electrolyte balance.

26.

For fluid and electrolyte maintenance in children, soft drinks, undiluted juices, and JELL-O are not recommended. These fluids are high in glucose concentration and thus have a high osmolarity. Therefore, juices diluted with half water are more appropriate. Milk is also not considered a liquid because it forms curds when in contact with stomach renin.

Give two reasons why cola is contraindicated in the maintenance of fluid and electrolyte balance.

*_____

_____

27.

The encouragement of fluid intake in a child is often a challenge. When possible, the preferences of the child should be considered. Which of the following fluids should be encouraged in a child experiencing anorexia?

( ) a. Full-strength orange juice

( ) b. Half-strength apple juice

( ) c. Half-strength jello

( ) d. Ginger ale

● DEFICIENT FLUID VOLUME

Dehydration, a common cause of a fluid volume deficit in infants and young children, occurs when the total output of fluid exceeds the total intake. Dehydration associated with diarrhea is the number one cause of fluid and electrolyte imbalances in infants and children. When vomiting occurs with diarrhea, fluid and electrolyte losses are more severe.

25. b; f; g

26. Cola is high in glucose concentration and osmolality.

27. b

28.

The most common cause of fluid and electrolyte disturbances in infants and children is:

( ) a. Vomiting

( ) b. Diarrhea

( ) c. SIADH

28. b

( ) d. Pyloric stenosis

The most accurate way to assess a fluid volume deficit in infants and children is based on the pre-illness weight. The following formula can be used to calculate the percent of dehydration. To use this formula, the weight in pounds must be converted to kilograms (kg):

$$\% \text{ Dehydration} = \frac{\text{pre-illness weight} - \text{illness weight}}{\text{pre-illness weight}} \times 100\%$$

29.

The amount of weight loss in infants and children can indicate the degree of dehydration. A decrease in body weight of 3–5% is considered mild dehydration; moderate with a weight loss of 6–10%; and severe when the loss is over 10%. In older children, decreases of 3–5% and 6–9% represent moderate and severe dehydration.

Example: Mary weighed 30 pounds, or 13.6 kg, before she became ill. Now she weighs 26 pounds, or 11.8 kg. She has lost 4 pounds, or 1.8 kg.

The percentage of weight loss is _____ %. The degree of dehydration is (mild, moderate, severe)

29. 13; severe

_____.

30.

If a 2-year-old with diarrhea weighed 15 kg prior to the illness and 14 kg when assessed in the clinic, the percent dehydration is _____ and it is classified as

30. 6–7%; moderate

_____ dehydration.

31.

In an older child, this percent of weight loss would be an indicator of _____ dehydration.

31. severe

The degree of body fluid loss can be determined by the weight loss. Body weight loss greater than 1% per day represents loss of body water. For every 1% weight loss,

10 mL/kg of body fluid is lost. Therefore, parents should be encouraged to keep an accurate record of the child's weight. When pre-illness weight is not available, however, clinical observations as described in Table 15-2 can be used. Although

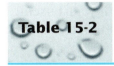

Table 15-2	Clinical Assessment of Degree of Dehydration in Infants and Children		
	% Dehydration (mL/kg)		
Degree	**Infants**	**Children**	**Clinical Assessment**
Mild	5% (50 mL/kg)	3% (30 mL/kg)	Thirst
			Slightly dry mucous membranes
			Decreased skin elasticity
			Skin color pale
			Tears present
			Fontanel flat
			Heart rate normal to slightly increased
			Urine output normal to slightly decreased
			Alert, restless
Moderate	10% (100 mL/kg)	6% (60 mL/kg)	Increased severity of symptoms
			Skin and mucous membranes dry
			Tenting
			Capillary filling 2–3 seconds
			Skin color gray
			Tears reduced
			Fontanel soft and depressed
			Deep-set eyes
			Heart rate increased
			Respirations rapid
			Urine output decreased (<1 ml/kg/hr)
			Increased specific gravity; dark urine
			Restless to lethargic
Severe	15% (150 mL/kg)	9% (90 mL/kg)	Marked severity of symptoms
			Skin clammy
			Mucous membranes parched/cracked
			Skin turgor absent
			Capillary filling > 3 seconds
			Skin color mottled
			Tears absent
			Fontanel and eyes sunken
			Heart rate rapid, weak to nonpalpable
			Blood pressure low to undetectable
			Respirations deep
			Urine output decreased or absent
			Lethargic to comatose (infants & young children); often conscious & apprehensive (older children & adolescents)

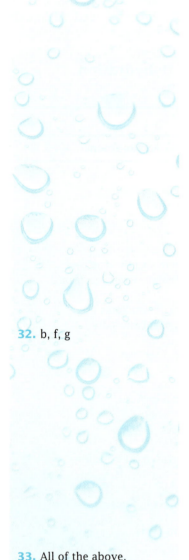

the table indicates a clear demarcation between mild and moderate dehydration, recent evidence suggests that distinguishing between mild and moderate dehydration based on clinical signs alone may be difficult. Manifestations for mild to moderate dehydration in reality may be evident over a wide range of fluid loss (i.e., from 3% to 9%). The most useful clinical signs for detecting dehydration in children are prolonged capillary refill time, abnormal skin turgor, and abnormal respiratory patterns.

32.

Evidence indicates that the most reliable clinical signs for detecting dehydration in infants and children are (check all that apply)

( ) a. increased heart rate
( ) b. decreased skin turgor
( ) c. decreased tear production
( ) d. specific gravity
( ) e. mottled skin
( ) f. prolonged capillary refill time
( ) g. abnormal respiratory patterns

32. b, f, g

33.

Indicate which symptoms are typical of moderate to severe dehydration in infants and children.

( ) a. Increased heart rate
( ) b. Decreased tears
( ) c. Sunken fontanels
( ) d. Increased specific gravity
( ) e. Sunken eyeballs
( ) f. Decreased blood pressure
( ) g. Decreased skin turgor
( ) h. Oliguria

33. All of the above.

34.

With severe dehydration, ECF and ICF are lost. With a slow, progressive fluid loss, the ICF shifts into the ECF compartment (vessels and tissue spaces) to replace the ECF loss. What do you think occurs when dehydration develops rapidly?

34. ECF loss is greater than ICF loss. ICF cannot replace ECF loss quickly.

*_____

In general, when dehydration occurs in less than 3 days, 80% of the losses are from the ECF and 20% of the losses are from the ICF. If dehydration occurs over a longer period of time, 60% of the losses are from the ECF and 40% of the losses are from the ICF.

35.

When a child develops dehydration over a period of 2 days, the percentage of ECF loss may be _____ and the percentage of ICF loss may be _____.

When dehydration occurs over a period of 1 week, the percentage of ECF loss may be _____ and the percentage of ICF loss may be _____.

35. 80%; 20%; 60%; 40%

● TYPES OF DEHYDRATION

36.

Dehydration is classified according to the serum concentration of solutes (osmolality). Sodium is the primary contributor to the serum osmolality. Dehydration has three classifications in relation to osmolality and sodium concentration: (a) iso-osmolar dehydration (isonatremic dehydration); (b) hyperosmolar dehydration (hypernatremic dehydration); and (c) hypo-osmolar dehydration (hyponatremic dehydration).

Which type of dehydration has the highest osmolality (concentration)? _____

36. hyperosmolar, or hypernatremic dehydration

37.

All degrees of dehydration are frequently associated with iso-osmolality or isonatremic dehydration. This is the most common type of dehydration, which results in proportionate losses of fluid and sodium.

Hypernatremic dehydration and hyponatremic dehydration indicate involvement of the electrolyte _____.

37. sodium

Table 15-3 lists the three types of dehydration: isonatremic, hypernatremic, and hyponatremic. For each of the dehydrations, the water and sodium loss, serum sodium level, ECF and ICF loss, causes, symptoms, and treatments are described. Study Table 15-3 carefully and refer to it as needed.

Table 15-3   Types of Dehydration: Isonatremic, Hypernatremic, and Hyponatremic

Types of Dehydration	Water and Sodium Loss	Serum Sodium Level	ECF and ICF Loss	Causes	Symptoms	Treatment
Isonatremic dehydration (iso-osmolar or isotonic dehydration)	Proportionately equal loss of water and sodium	130–150 mEq/L	Extracellular fluid volume is markedly decreased (severe hypovolemia). Since sodium and water loss are approximately the same, there is no osmotic pull from ICF to ECF. The plasma volume is significantly reduced and shock occurs from decreased circulating blood volume. ICF volume remains virtually constant.	Diarrhea, vomiting, and malnutrition (decreases in fluid and food intake) are the most common causes.	With severe fluid loss, symptoms are characteristic of hypovolemic shock: rapid pulse rate, rapid respiration; and later, a decreasing systolic blood pressure. Other symptoms are weight loss, irritability, lethargy, pale or gray skin color, dry mucous membranes, reduced skin turgor, sunken eyeballs, sunken fontanels, absence of tearing and salivation, and decreased urine output.	For mild to moderate dehydration, oral rehydration therapy (ORT) should be initiated. For mild dehydration, give 50 ml/kg over a 4 hr period; give 100 ml/kg over a 4 hr period for moderate dehydration. During the maintenance phase, infants should resume breast-feeding or formula. Children should return to their regular diet. If dehydration is severe, infants and children should be given one or more boluses (20ml/kg) of isotonic intravenous fluid (i.e., lactated ringers or 0.9% normal saline) for the first 30 minutes regardless of the type of dehydration. The boluses may be repeated for up to 40 ml/kg if child is unstable. Albumin, blood, or plasma may be prescribed if there is no response after two boluses of 20 ml/kg or if there is blood loss. Maintenance is calculated using the Holliday-Segar method (see Table 15-1). Any significant losses need to be replaced over 6 to 8 hrs. Half of the replacement therapy in addition to the maintenance needs is given over the first 8 hrs; the other half is given over the next 16 hrs.

Type	Description	Serum Sodium	Pathophysiology	Causes	Symptoms	Treatment
Hypernatremic dehydration (hyperosmolar or hypertonic dehydration) (second leading type of dehydration in children)	Water loss is greater than sodium loss; sodium excess	↑150 mEq/L	ECF and ICF volumes are both decreased. Increased ECF osmolality (solutes) results in a shift of fluid from the ICF to the ECF causing severe cellular dehydration. ECF depletion may not be as severe as ICF depletion. Loss of hypo-osmolar fluid raises the osmolality of ECF.	Diabetes insipidus; administration of IV fluids or high-protein tube feedings with high electrolyte levels; oral fluids with large amounts of solute.	Shock is less apparent since ECF loss is not as severe. Symptoms include weight loss, avid thirst, confusion, convulsions, tremors, thickened and firm skin turgor, sunken eyeballs and fontanels, absence of tearing, moderately rapid pulse, moderately rapid respirations, frequently normal blood pressure, normal to decreased urine output, and intracranial hemorrhage. Neurological symptoms such as seizures are likely to occur. This type of dehydration is the most dangerous.	Fluid replacement must be very specific to the losses. A gradual reduction in sodium over 48 hr is recommended to minimize the risk of cerebral edema. Half of the fluid deficit and the entire solute deficit may be replaced in the first 24 hrs; the remainder and maintenance fluid are replaced over the next 24 hrs. Serum sodium levels should be evaluated every 4 hrs. Dextrose 5% with 0.2% NaCl may be ordered and later lactated Ringer's solution. With normal urinary flow, potassium can be added to the solution (2–3 mEq/kg).
Hyponatremic dehydration (hypo-osmolar or hypotonic dehydration)	Sodium loss is greater than water loss; excess water	↓130 mEq/L	ECF is severely decreased, and ICF is increased. The osmolality of ECF is lower than the osmolality of ICF. Water shifts from the ECF to the ICF (lesser to the greater concentration). The cerebral cells are frequently affected first as the excess water interferes with brain cell activity.	Severe diarrhea and vomiting (sodium is lost in excess of water), excessive water intake, electrolyte-free fluid infusions (5% dextrose in water), renal disease, diuretic therapy, and burns.	Thirst, weight loss, lethargy, comatose, poor skin turgor, clammy skin, sunken and soft eyeballs, absence of tearing, shock symptoms (rapid pulse rate, rapid respirations, and low systolic blood pressure), and decreased urine output.	Rapid fluid correction with electrolytes can cause an excessive shift of cellular fluid into the plasma. The result can be over-hydration and heart failure. Half of the replacement fluids and all of the maintenance fluid should be given over the first 8 hrs and the second half over the next 16 hrs. Generally, a solution of 0.3% sodium is administered. Unless sodium deficits are extreme, sodium replacement should not exceed 2–4 mEq/L over a 4-hrs period. Ongoing electrolyte losses are calculated and replaced every 6 to 8 hrs.

38. sodium; water; 130 mEq/L; 150 mEq/L; decreased

38.

With isonatremic dehydration, there is a proportionate loss of the ions _____ and _____. The serum sodium level is between _____ and _____. The ECF volume is (increased/decreased) _____.

39. diarrhea and vomiting, also malnutrition; rapid pulse rate, rapid respiration, and decreasing systolic blood pressure (others could be gray skin color, lethargy)

39.

Two common causes of isonatremic dehydration are * _____ _____.

  With severe dehydration, shock symptoms are common. Give three shock symptoms. * _____ _____

40. water; 150↑; ICF

40.

With hypernatremic dehydration, which is lost to a greater degree: (water/sodium)? _____. The serum sodium level is _____ mEq/L. ECF and ICF volumes are decreased. Which body fluid compartment has the largest fluid loss: (ECF/ICF)? _____

41. severe diarrhea and high solute intake; are not; a, b, c, d, e

41.

Give two causes of hypernatremic dehydration. * _____ _____

  Shock symptoms (are/are not) _____ common with this type of dehydration.

  Check the symptoms found with hypernatremic dehydration:
( ) a. Avid thirst   ( ) d. Skin turgor firm and thickened
( ) b. Convulsions   ( ) e. Absence of tearing
( ) c. Tremors   ( ) f. Excess urine output

42. sodium; water; 130; decreased; increased

42.

With hyponatremic dehydration, the loss of _____ is greater than the loss of _____. The serum sodium level is _____ mEq/L. ECF is (increased/decreased) _____ and ICF is (increased/decreased) _____.

43.

Give three causes of hyponatremic dehydration. * _____ _____

43. severe diarrhea, excessive water intake, and electrolyte-free fluid infusions (others are sodium-losing nephropathy and diuretic therapy); a, c, d, e, f, g, h

Check the symptoms found with hyponatremic dehydration:

( ) a. Thirst　　　　　　　( ) e. Sunken, soft eyeballs
( ) b. Weight gain　　　　　( ) f. Rapid pulse rate
( ) c. Poor skin turgor　　　( ) g. Rapid respiration
( ) d. Clammy skin　　　　　( ) h. Low systolic blood pressure

 ## TREATMENT OPTIONS

44.

Regardless of the type of dehydration, immediate treatment of infants and children is needed to prevent hypovolemic shock. Oral rehydration is the treatment of choice for children with mild to moderate dehydration. The primary goals of rehydration therapy are to restore *_____ and to prevent *_____.

44. fluid and electrolyte balance; hypovolemic shock

For mild dehydration, parents should be urged to give the child any kind of oral fluid that the child tolerates and to continue feeding. Formula can be given to infants. If these approaches are unsuccessful, then oral rehydration solutions (ORS) should be given.

Table 15-4 contains a list of oral rehydration solutions (ORS) that are used for rehydration and maintenance. Other ORS continue to be developed. Some recent additions available in the United States are Kao Lectrolyte, Naturalyte, Oralyte, and Resol. Generic brands of the solutions are also available. When purchasing generic brands, however, it is

Table 15-4	**Composition of Oral Rehydration Solutions (ORS)**				
Solution	Carbohydrate (gm/L)	Sodium (mmol/L)	Potassium (mmol/L)	Chloride (mmol/L)	Base (mmol/L)	Osmolarity (mOsm/L)
WHO* (2002)	13.5	75	20	65	30	245
WHO (1975)	20	90	20	80	30	311
Enfalyte	30	50	25	45	34	200
Pedialyte	25	45	20	35	30	250
Rehydralyte	25	75	20	65	30	305
CeraLyte	40	50–90	20	NA	30	220

*World Health Organization
Adapted from "Managing acute gastroenteritis among children," by CDC, 2003, *Morbidity and Mortality Weekly Report, 52(RR16)*, p.1.

important to select the appropriate solution for the type of rehydration or maintenance therapy needed.

45.

The two major types of ORS are those for rehydration and those used for maintenance. Rehydration solutions contain more sodium than do maintenance solutions. The ORS that may be used for rehydration are _____ and _____.

45. Rehydralyte; ORS (WHO)

Nausea and mild vomiting are not contraindications of oral rehydration therapy. Oral rehydration solutions are given in small amounts of 5–10 mL every 5–10 minutes and increased as tolerated. Administering the solution with a tea-spoon or an oral syringe may help to monitor the amounts more accurately. Rehydration therapy for mild dehydration is 50 mL/kg given over 4 hours. For moderate dehydration, 100 mL/kg should be given over 4 hours.

46.

For a child weighing 20 kg with mild dehydration, how much rehydration fluid should be given over 4 hours? * _____ In the first Hour? * _____

46. 1000 mL; 250 mL

Once rehydration is accomplished, the child should be encouraged to resume a normal diet. Some physicians pre-scribe diluted or lactose-free formulas for infants while others believe that full-strength formula can be given. Breast-fed infants may supplement their feedings with an electrolyte solution (usually 100 mL/kg is recommended). Any ongoing losses (through stool or emesis) should also be replaced. For each loss through diarrhea stools, 10 mL/kg of child's body weight should be replaced with an electrolyte solution.

47.

Breast-fed infants on maintenance therapy are sometimes given * _____ of an ORS to supplement breast feedings. Formula-fed infants may be given * _____ or * _____ formulas.

47. 100 mL/kg; lactose-free; half-strength regular

48.

For a child weighing 15 kg that has two diarrhea stools, how much replacement solution should be given? * _____

48. 300 mL

With the resumption of a normal diet, physicians may prescribe 100 mL/kg of ORS to supplement the diet. Diets that are low in simple carbohydrates and contain easily digestible foods such as cereal, yogurt, cooked vegetables, and soups can be given to older children. Toddlers may tolerate soft or pureed foods. The BRAT diet (bananas, rice, apples, and toast or tea) is no longer recommended because of its limited nutritional value. Also, the diet is high in carbohydrates and low in electrolytes. Other foods to avoid are fried foods, soda, or jello water.

49.

A child who is recovering from dehydration should receive a _____ diet that is low in _____ and contains easily digestible foods such as *_____

*_____

49. regular (normal); carbohydrates; cooked vegetables, yogurt, cereal, soups

50.

Name two oral electrolyte solutions that might be used in the maintenance phase of rehydration therapy. *_____

_____

These solutions contain similar concentrations of glucose and important electrolytes such as _____,

_____, and _____.

50. Enfalyte and Pedialyte; sodium; potassium; chloride

Oral rehydration therapy is replaced with parenteral therapy in infants and children with severe vomiting, gastric distention, and severe dehydration.

51.

Emergency treatment of unstable children with severe dehydration is needed to prevent or correct *_____.
In emergency situations, fluids should be restored (slowly, rapidly) _____.

51. hypovolemic shock; rapidly

Careful consideration of the parameters for rehydrating children is essential. Overhydration can lead to cerebral edema with neurological symptoms such as seizures. Initial expansion of ECF volume is usually accomplished with a bolus of an isotonic solution such as 0.9% sodium chloride or lactated Ringer's solution. Recommended amount is 20 to 30 ml/kg. The bolus may be repeated if needed.

52.

For a child weighing 20 kilograms, an appropriate bolus of Ringer's lactate for immediate rehydration therapy would be between _____ and _____ ml.

52. 400; 600

    Initial expansion is to prevent shock by improving circulatory and renal function. Requirements for continued rehydration vary with the child's clinical status and the nature of the electrolyte imbalance. The amount of fluid replaced is also based on the calculated loss as well as the fluid maintenance requirements (refer to pages 4 to 7 for calculation of fluid maintenance needs).

    The type of intravenous fluid administered is determined by the type of dehydration (refer to Table 15-3).

53.

With hyponatremic dehydration, fluids are usually replaced and maintained with *_____. Sodium replacement should not exceed _____ over a _____ period.

53. 5% D/0.45% normal saline solution; 3% saline; 2–4 mEq/L; 4 hours

54.

The severity of hypernatremic dehydration is often difficult to assess because fluid shifting between the intercellular and extracellular spaces preserves the circulating volume. Therefore, the potential of giving (too much, too little) *_____ fluid is present.

54. too much

55.

The goal for correcting hypernatremic dehydration is to avoid causing what major type of fluid imbalance? *_____

55. water intoxication (overhydration)

56.

Serum Na correction in hypernatremia should not occur any more rapidly than 0.5–1.0 mEq/L/h. To ensure that serum Na levels do not decrease too rapidly or too slowly, serum Na levels should be monitored every 2–4 hours and the fluid rate adjusted accordingly. Too rapid administration of fluid may lead to *_____. When serum sodium reaches 120–125 mEq/L, fluid restrictions should be initiated.

56. cerebral edema

57.

While severe dehydration is treated with *_____,
after the fluid and electrolyte imbalances have stabilized,
*_____ is initiated.

57. intravenous therapy; oral
rehydration therapy

58.

The signs and symptoms of fluid balance deficits may vary
with the age of the child. In the hospital, children should be
assessed at least every 4 hours. Infants should be assessed
more frequently. The infant or child with an existing
imbalance should be assessed at least every hour.

  The fluid status of a child in fluid and electrolyte imbalance
should be closely monitored every *_____.

58. hour

  Table 15-5 lists the assessments with rationales for determining fluid and electrolyte imbalance in infants and
children. The table can be utilized as an assessment tool in
the hospital, community agency, or home. In the assessment
column, check or fill in the blanks. Study the table and
complete the questions that follow. Refer back to Table 15-5
as needed.

Table 15-5   **Head-to-Toe Assessment of Fluid and Electrolyte
Imbalance in Infants and Children**

Observation	Assessment	Rationale
Behavior and Appearance	Irritable/restless Anorexia Purposeless movement Unusual cry Lethargic Lethargy with hyperirritability on stimulation Unresponsive (comatose)	Early symptoms of fluid volume deficit are irritability, purposeless movements, and an unusual or high-pitched cry in infants. Young children may experience thirst with restlessness. As dehydration continues, lethargy and unconsciousness may occur.
Skin	Color _____ Temperature _____ Feel _____ Turgor _____	Skin color may be pale (mild), gray (moderate), or mottled (severe) depending on the degree of dehydration. Temperature is usually cold except with hyperosmolar dehydration where the temperature may be hot or cold. Skin feels dry with isoosmolar dehydration; clammy with hypoosmolar dehydration; and thickened and

(continues)

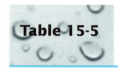

Table 15-5	Head-to-Toe Assessment of Fluid and Electrolyte Imbalance in Infants and Children—*continued*	
Observation	**Assessment**	**Rationale**
		doughy with hyperosmolar dehydration. Turgor is measured by pinching the skin on the abdomen, chest wall, or medial aspect of the thigh and assessing the rate of skin retraction (elasticity). As dehydration progresses, elasticity decreases from fair to very poor. With hypertonic dehydration, turgor may remain fair. Skin turgor on obese infants or children may appear normal even with a deficit. Undernourishment can cause poor tissue turgor with fluid balance.
Mucous Membranes	Dryness in oral cavity (cheeks and gums) _____ Dry tongue with longitudinal wrinkles _____	The mucous membranes and tongue are dry with a fluid deficit. Sodium deficit causes the tongue to appear sticky, rough, and red. A dry tongue may also indicate mouth breathing. Some medications and vitamin deficiencies cause dryness of mucous membranes. Dryness in the oral cavity membranes (cheeks and gums) is a better indicator of fluid loss.
Eyes	Sunken _____ Tears _____ Soft eyeballs _____	Sunken eyes and dark skin around them may indicate a severe fluid volume deficit. Tears are absent with moderate to severe dehydration. (Tearing is not present until approximately 4 months of age.) Soft eyeballs may indicate isonatremic or hyponatremic dehydration.
Fontanel	Sunken _____ Bulging _____	Depression of the anterior fontanel is often an indicator of fluid volume deficit. A fluid excess results in bulging fontanel.
Vital Signs Temperature	Admission Temperature_____ Time _____ (1)_____ Time _____ (2)_____	Body temperature can be subnormal or elevated. Fever increases insensible water loss. The child's extremities may feel cold because of hypovolemia (fluid volume deficit), which decreases peripheral circulation. A subnormal temperature may be due to reduced energy output.
Pulse	Admission pulse _____ Pulse rate Time _____ (1)_____ Time _____ (2)_____	A weak and rapid pulse rate (over 160 for infant and over 120 for child) may indicate a fluid volume deficit (hypovolemia) and the possibility of shock. A full, bounding, not

(continues)

Table 15-5 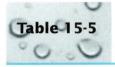	Head-to-Toe Assessment of Fluid and Electrolyte Imbalance in Infants and Children—*continued*	
Observation	**Assessment**	**Rationale**
	Pattern _____	easily obliterated pulse may indicate a fluid volume excess. An irregular pulse can be due to hypokalemia. A weak, irregular rapid pulse may indicate hypokalemia, while a weak slow pulse may indicate hypernatremia.
Respiration	Admission rate _____ Respiration Time _____ (1)_____ Time _____ (2)_____ Pattern _____	Note the rate, depth, and pattern of the infant's breathing. Dyspnea and moist crackles usually indicate fluid volume excess. Rapid breathing increases insensible fluid loss from the lungs. Rapid, deep, vigorous breathing (Kussmaul breathing) frequently indicates metabolic acidosis. Acidosis can be due to poor hydrogen excretion by the kidneys, diarrhea, salicylate poisoning, or diabetes mellitus. Shallow, irregular breathing can be due to respiratory alkalosis.
Blood Pressure	Admission BP _____ Blood pressure Time _____ (1)_____ Time _____ (2)_____	Elasticity of young blood vessels may keep blood pressure stable even when a fluid volume deficit is present. Increased blood pressure may indicate fluid volume excess. Decreased blood pressure may indicate severe fluid volume deficit, extracellular shift from the plasma to the interstitial space, or sodium deficit.
Neurological Signs	Abdominal distention _____ Diminished reflexes (hypotonia) _____ Weakness/paralysis _____ Tetany tremors (hypertonia) _____ Twitching, cramps _____ Sensorium Confusion _____ Comatose _____ Other _____	Abdominal distention and weakness may indicate a potassium deficit. Tetany symptoms can indicate a calcium and/or magnesium deficit. Serum calcium deficits occur easily in children, since their bones do not readily replace calcium to the blood. Confusion can be due to a potassium deficit and/or fluid volume imbalance.
Neurovascular Signs	Capillary filling time _____	A measure of systemic perfusion. Moderate to severe dehydration is often accompanied by delayed capillary filling time of >2–3 s.

(continues)

Table 15-5   **Head-to-Toe Assessment of Fluid and Electrolyte Imbalance in Infants and Children—*continued***

Observation	Assessment	Rationale
Weight	Preillness weight _____ Current weight _____	Weight loss can indicate the degree of dehydration (fluid loss): *Mild*—2–5% in infants and young children *Moderate*—5–10% in infants and young children; 3–6% in older children. *Severe*—10–15% in infants and young children; 6–9% in older children. Fluid loss can also be estimated by considering that 1 g of weight loss equals 1 mL of fluid loss. Edema and ascites can occur with fluid imbalances. Fluid overloads can result in hepatomegaly (enlarged liver). Weight should be taken on the same scale, at the same time each day, and with the same covering.

Urine	Number of voidings
	   in 8 hr _____
	   Amt mL/8 hr _____
	   Amt mL/hr _____
	 Urine color _____
	 Specific gravity _____
	 Urine pH _____
		Accurate measurements of intake and output from all sources is essential. Normal output ranges are:
		   Infants: 2–3 mL/kg/hr
		   Young children: 2 mL/kg/hr
		   Older children: 1–2 mL/kg/hr
		 By subtracting the weight of a saturated urine diaper from a dry diaper, output in infants and toddlers can be determined (1 g wet diaper = 1 mL urine). Because of evaporative losses, diapers must be weighed within 30 mins of the void to be accurate. Specific gravity can be obtained by refractometer or dipstick. Accurate assessment can be made within 2 hrs of the void. Oliguria (decrease in urine output) with very concentrated urine (dark yellow color) and increased specific gravity (>1.030) can indicate a moderate to severe fluid volume deficit, plasma to interstitial fluid shift, sodium deficit or severe sodium excess, potassium excess, or renal insufficiency. An elevated specific gravity is also indicative of glycosuria and proteinuria. With severe fluid

(continues)

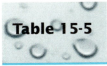

Table 15-5	Head-to-Toe Assessment of Fluid and Electrolyte Imbalance in Infants and Children—*continued*	
Observation	**Assessment**	**Rationale**
		deficit the infant may not void for 16–24 hrs and not show evidence of abdominal distention. Polyuria (increased urine output) with low specific gravity (<1.010) can indicate fluid excess, renal disease, a sodium deficit, or extracellular shift from interstitial fluid to plasma or decreased antidiuretic hormone (ADH). An acidic pH may indicate metabolic or respiratory acidosis, alkalosis with severe potassium deficit, or a fluid deficit. Alkaline urine may result from metabolic or respiratory alkalosis, hyperaldosteronism, acidosis with chronic kidney infection and tubular dysfunction, or diuretic therapy.
Stools	Number _____ Consistency _____ Color _____ Amount _____	The consistency, color, and amount of each stool should be noted. If the stool is liquid, it should be measured. Frequent liquid stools can lead to fluid volume deficit, potassium and sodium deficit, and bicarbonate deficit (acidosis).
Vomitus	Number _____ Consistency _____ Color _____ Amount _____	Vomitus needs to be described according to consistency, color, and amount. Frequent vomiting of large quantity leads to fluid loss, potassium and sodium loss, as well as hydrogen and chloride loss (alkalosis).

Other Fluid Loss	GI suction
	   Amount _____
	 Drainage tube
	   Amount _____
	 Fistula
	   Color _____
	   Amount _____
	 Other
	   Amount _____
		Fluid loss from all sources should be measured. Fluid loss from GI suctioning, drainage tubes, and fistula can contribute to severe fluid and electrolyte imbalance.

Blood Chemistry and Hematology	Electrolytes Time _____ Time _____ K _____ _____	One set of blood chemistry is not sufficient for assessment. Electrolytes should be frequently monitored when they are not in normal range.

(continues)

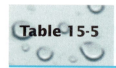

Table 15-5

Head-to-Toe Assessment of Fluid and Electrolyte Imbalance in Infants and Children—*continued*

Observation	Assessment	Rationale
	Na ___ ___	Norms are:
	Cl ___ ___	K:
	Ca ___ ___	Newborn 3.0–6.0 mEq/L
	Mg ___ ___	Infant & older 3.5–5.0 mEq/L
	BUN ___ ___	Na:
	Creatinine	Newborn 136–146 mEq/L
	___ ___	Infant 139–146 mEq/L
	Hgb ___ ___	Child 135–148 mEq/L
	Hct ___ ___	Cl:
		Newborn 97–110 mEq/L
		Child 98–111 mEq/L
		Ca:
		Newborn 7–12 mg/dL
		Child 8–10.8 mg/dL
		Mg:
		All ages 1.3–2.0 mEq/L
		BUN:
		Newborn 4–18 mg/dL
		Child 5–18 mg/dL
		Creatinine:
		Newborn 0.3–1.0 mg/dL
		Infant 0.2–0.4 mg/dL
		Child 0.3–0.7 mg/dL
		Hgb:
		Newborn 14.5–22.5 g/dL
		Infant 9–14 g/dL
		Child 11.5–15.5 g/dL
		Hct:
		Newborn 44–72%
		Infant 28–42%
		Child 35–45%
		An elevated BUN can indicate fluid volume deficit or kidney insufficiency.
		Elevated creatinine frequently indicates kidney damage.
		Elevated hemoglobin and hematocrit may indicate hemoconcentration caused by fluid volume deficit. If anemia is present, the hemoglobin and hematocrit may appear falsely normal.
	Blood gases	After the first day of life, normal range for pH is 7.35–7.45. A pH of 7.35 or less indicates acidosis. A pH of 7.45 or higher indicates alkalosis.
	pH ___	
	$PaCO_2$ ___	
	PaO_2 ___	

(continues)

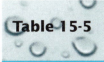

Table 15-5	**Head-to-Toe Assessment of Fluid and Electrolyte Imbalance in Infants and Children—*continued***	
Observation	**Assessment**	**Rationale**

	HCO_3^- _____
	 BE _____
		Newborns and infants have $PaCO_2$ levels that range between 27 and 41 mm Hg. After infancy, $PaCO_2$ levels range from 35 to 48 mm Hg in males and from 32 to 45 mm Hg in females. Lower values indicate respiratory alkalosis or compensation (overbreathing, hyperventilating). Higher values mean respiratory acidosis.
		 Normal range for HCO_3 in all ages is 21–28 mEq/L. BE (base excess) varies with age.
		 Normal BE ranges are:
		   Newborn $(-10)-(-2)$ mEq/L
		   Infant $(-7)-(-1)$ mEq/L
		   Child $(-4)-(+2)$ mEq/L
		 HCO_3 below 21 and BE less than the normal value for age indicates metabolic alkalosis.
		 HCO_3 above 28 and BE higher than the normal value for age indicates metabolic acidosis.

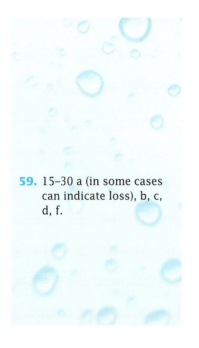

59.

Vital signs should be monitored every *_____ minutes for seriously ill infants or children. Check which of the following vital signs can indicate a fluid volume loss/deficit.

  ( ) a. Subnormal temperature
  ( ) b. Rapid, weak pulse
  ( ) c. Rapid respiration (Kussmaul)
  ( ) d. Fever
  ( ) e. Shallow breathing
  ( ) f. Systolic pressure below 80

59. 15–30 a (in some cases can indicate loss), b, c, d, f.

60.

Neurologic changes may indicate a fluid and electrolyte imbalance. Match the neurologic assessment on the left with the probable imbalance. (Refer to Table 15-5.) Some answers may be used more than once.

_____ 1. Abdominal distention   a. Potassium deficit

_____ 2. Confusion   b. Calcium deficit

_____ 3. Muscle weakness   c. Fluid volume excess

60. 1. a; 2. a, c, d; 3. a; 4. b   _____ 4. Tetany symptoms   d. Fluid volume deficit

61.

A weight loss of 12% indicates which degree of dehydration (fluid loss) in a child?

( ) a. Mild

( ) b. Moderate

61. c   ( ) c. Severe

62.

Indicate in which areas of the body skin turgor should be checked.

( ) a. Face   ( ) d. Top of thighs

( ) b. Chest wall   ( ) e. Medial aspect of thighs

62. b, c, e   ( ) c. Abdomen

63.

To determine dryness of the mucous membrane, which part of the mouth should be assessed?

( ) a. Cheeks and gums of the oral cavity

63. a   ( ) b. Teeth

64.

64. moderate to severe dehydration, or the upper range of moderate dehydration   Sunken eyeballs and fontanels frequently do not occur in infants until there is a 10% body weight loss (as fluid loss). Give the degree of dehydration that would be present with a 10% fluid loss. *_____

65.

65. moderate to severe dehydration   Delayed capillary refill time of greater than 3 seconds is most likely indicative of what degree of dehydration? *_____.

66.

Normal specific gravity for an infant is 1.002–1.010 and for a child is 1.005–1.030. A child's decreased urinary output and a specific gravity that exceeds 1.030 indicates a fluid volume

66. deficit   (deficit/excess) _____.

67. oliguria (↓ urine output)

67.

Hyperkalemia (serum potassium excess) can result from (polyuria/oliguria) _____.

68.

Frequent and increased quantities of vomitus and stools can lead to which of the following:
- ( ) a. Hypokalemia
- ( ) b. Hyperkalemia
- ( ) c. Hyponatremia
- ( ) d. Hypernatremia
- ( ) e. Acidosis
- ( ) f. Alkalosis
- ( ) g. Dehydration

68. a, c, e (↑ stools due to loss of HCO_3), f (↑ vomitus due to loss of HCl), g

69. dehydration (fluid volume deficit); potassium and sodium (important electrolytes), also hydrogen, chloride, bicarbonate, and magnesium

69.

The fluid imbalance that can result from gastrointestinal suction and from secretions from drainage tubes and fistula is

_____

Name the two important electrolytes that are lost from gastrointestinal suctioning. *_____

_____

70.

An irregular pulse (dysrhythmia) can be caused by a (potassium deficit/potassium excess) *_____.
A full bounding pulse can mean *_____.
Why are blood pressure readings in infants and young children a poor indicator of fluid imbalance? *_____

_____

70. potassium deficit; fluid volume excess; Firm elasticity of young blood vessels keeps blood pressure stable until dehydration has reached 10% or greater.

71. dehydration (fluid volume deficit) or kidney insufficiency (renal damage); kidney damage

71.

An elevated BUN (blood urea nitrogen) can indicate *_____

_____,

whereas an elevated serum creatinine indicates *_____.

72.

Arterial blood gases (ABGs) are used to assess acid-base balance. In the child:
- a. pH of 7.27 indicates *_____
- b. pH of 7.48 indicates *_____

72. a. acidosis; b. alkalosis;
c. hyperventilation due
to respiratory alkalosis
or compensation for
metabolic acidosis;
d. respiratory acidosis;
e. metabolic alkalosis;
f. metabolic acidosis

c. $PaCO_2$ of 28 indicates *_____

d. $PaCO_2$ of 60 indicates *_____

e. HCO_3^- of 34 and BE of +8 indicates *_____

f. HCO_3^- of 18 and BE of −6 indicates *_____

73.

From the following list of observations and nursing assessments, check the ones that indicate (hypovolemia or dehydration).

( ) a. BUN elevated

( ) b. Hemoglobin and hematocrit elevated

( ) c. Increased secretions from GI suction

( ) d. Increased blood pressure

( ) e. Irritability, high-pitched cry

( ) f. Confusion, disorientation

( ) g. Weight gain

( ) h. Decreased, concentrated urine

( ) i. Avid thirst

( ) j. Poor skin turgor

( ) k. Absence of tearing and salivation

( ) l. Sunken eyeballs and anterior fontanel

( ) m. Increased number and quantity of vomitus and stools

( ) n. Temperature 98.2°F or 36.8°C

( ) o. Rapid, weak pulse

( ) p. Rapid breathing

73. a, b, e, f, h, i, j, k, l, n, o, p

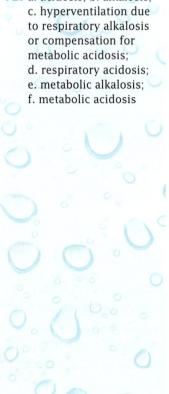

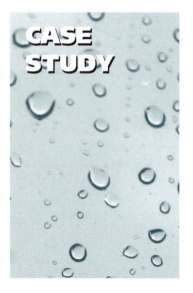

CASE STUDY

REVIEW

A 4-year-old girl has had diarrhea and anorexia for 3 days. She has taken only sips of fruit juices for the last 3 days. She weighed 38 pounds, or 17.3 kg, preillness and now weighs 35 pounds, or 15.9 kg. Her cheeks and gums are dry and her skin turgor is reduced. She is irritable. She has voided once in the last 24 hours. Vital signs: temperature 99°F, or 37.2°C, pulse rate 110, respirations 32, BP 90/60. The serum sodium level is 132 mEq/L, and the potassium level is 3.3 mEq/L. Serum calcium is 7.4 mg/dL. Results of the BUN and creatinine are pending.

ANSWER COLUMN

1. c

2. 1.4; 8%; moderate

3. 3; 60%; 40%

4. oliguria or decreased; decreased; 1.030 (or more)
5. cheeks and gums dry, reduced skin turgor, irritable, voided once (decreased urine output), and pulse rate and respiration increased
6. No; Blood pressure for that age group is normal; however, a baseline blood pressure from an office visit would be helpful.
7. rapid pulse rate, rapid respiration, and decreasing blood pressure (others—clammy skin, pale or gray color)
8. P 130 (rapid pulse rate) and R 35 (rapid respirations). Baseline vital signs are helpful.

1. Because of diarrhea, anorexia, decreased fluid intake, and weight loss, the health professional would assume the fluid imbalance to be which of the following:
( ) a. Intracellular fluid volume excess (water intoxication)
( ) b. Extracellular fluid volume excess (edema or overhydration)
( ) c. Extracellular fluid volume deficit (dehydration)

2. In kilograms, she has lost _____ kg. What percent of dehydration is present? _____ (Refer to Table 15-2 if needed.) The severity of her dehydration is (mild/moderate/severe) _____.

3. The onset of fluid loss (dehydration) has been _____ days. The percentage of fluid loss from the ECF is _____ and from the ICF is _____.

4. With moderate dehydration, the changes in the urine output and concentration are (refer to Table 15-2 if needed):
Urine volume _____
Urine osmolality _____
Urine specific gravity _____

5. List her signs and symptoms of dehydration from the health assessment. *_____
_____
_____

6. Is her blood pressure indicative of shock? _____
Explain. *_____

7. Name three shock symptoms that can occur. *_____
_____

8. Identify her vital signs that are indicative of impending shock due to hypovolemia (fluid volume loss). *_____
and *_____

9. a. 3.5–5.0 mEq/L;
b. 135–148 mEq/L;
c. 98–111 mEq/L;
d. 8–10 mg/dL

10. dizziness, soft muscles, abdominal distention, decreased peristalsis, dysrhythmia, and decreased BP

11. decreased

12. tetany; tingling of fingers and twitching of mouth (others—tremors and carpopedal spasms)

13. increased; dehydration; With a decreased urine output, there is an increase in serum solutes such as urea (due to hemoconcentration).

14. 1365; 40.8, or 41; 27.2, or 27

15. isonatremic; The serum sodium level for isonatremic dehydration is 130–150 mEq/L.

16. rapidly

---

9. The ranges of serum electrolytes for a child of this age are:
a. K * ———————————
b. Na * ———————————
c. Cl * ———————————
d. Ca * ———————————

(Refer to Table 15-5.)

10. Give some signs and symptoms of hypokalemia. * ————
————————————————————————————

11. Her serum sodium and potassium levels are (within normal limits/decreased/increased) ————————————.

12. With a serum calcium level of 7.4 mg/dL, one should observe for symptoms of ————————————. Give two of the symptoms.
————————————————————————————

13. Her BUN should be (increased/decreased) ————————————.
The most likely cause of her BUN is ————————————.
Explain.
————————————————————————————

14. Her pre-illness weight is 38 pounds, or 17.3 kg. Calculate Tonya's daily fluid maintenance requirements. ————————
mL per 24 hours. (Refer to Table 15-1 if needed.)
    Her daily sodium requirement is ————————————
mEq/L and her daily potassium requirement is
———————————— mEq/L. (Refer to Table 15-1 as needed.)

15. This type of dehydration according to her serum sodium level is (isonatremic/hypernatremic/hyponatremic)
————————————. Why? *————————————————
————————————————————————————

16. For the type of dehydration in question 15, fluids should be replaced (slowly/rapidly) ————————————.

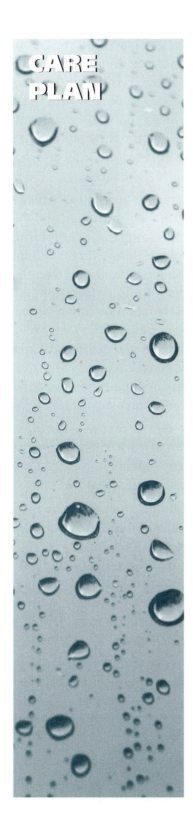

CARE
PLAN

PATIENT MANAGEMENT

Assessment Factors

● Early detection of pertinent symptoms and prompt therapeutic management of fluid and electrolyte disturbances are critical in the care of infants and children. Fluid balance is so precarious that life-threatening changes can occur rapidly with little symptomatic warning. Conditions that promote fluid imbalances in infants and children include vomiting, diarrhea, sweating, fever, burns, injury, and diseases such as diabetes, renal, and cardiac anomalies. A thorough assessment integrates the health history obtained from the parents with data from the physical examination and laboratory tests.

● Knowledge requirements and basic assessment techniques vary for infants and children. Understanding the implications of variations in laboratory studies, total body fluid volume, and developmental differences that influence the responses of infants and children to fluid problems provides a basis for data comparison. Assessment begins with observations of the infant's/child's general appearance and behavioral changes. Knowing baseline data from the infant's/child's health history is important to the assessment and interpretation of the findings.

● A baseline reading of the infant's or child's vital signs is important to the interpretation of changes. Monitor vital signs according to the severity of the illness. Seriously ill infants and children need their vital signs monitored every 15 minutes. An elevated or a subnormal temperature can indicate dehydration. With a temperature increase of one degree, the metabolic need for oxygen is increased by 7% and respiratory rate increases by four breaths per minute. Blood pressure is not a reliable sign of early fluid imbalance in young children. A rapid, weak, thready pulse is a symptom of shock associated with severe dehydration. A bounding, not easily obliterated pulse occurs with overhydration when the interstitial fluid shifts to the plasma.

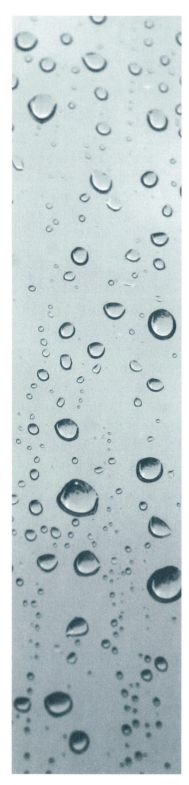

A bounding, easily obliterated pulse may indicate an impending circulatory collapse and a sodium deficit. The overall cardiac status reflects changes in levels of electrolytes. Dyspnea and moist crackles can occur with overhydration. Respiratory stridor may indicate a calcium deficit. A potassium imbalance is life threatening in a child. The skin and mucous membranes are indicators of the hydration status of children.

● Assess skin and mucous membranes; the skin is usually pale during a fluid deficit and flushed during a fluid excess. The extremities often become cold and mottled with the presence of a fever and a severe fluid volume deficit. Skin elasticity can be assessed by pinching the skin on the abdomen or inner thigh (dent test). In fluid depletion, the skin remains raised for several seconds. The skin may feel dry or cold and clammy in sodium deficits (hyponatremic dehydration). Fluid deficits cause the mucous membranes of the mouth to become dry. The tongue may have longitudinal wrinkles. A sodium excess (hyponatremic dehydration) causes a sticky, rough, red, dry tongue.

● Tears and salivation are decreased or absent with dehydration in infants and children. Dehydration causes the fontanels and eyeballs to appear soft and sunken. Conversely, in fluid excess the fontanels bulge and feel taut.

● Tingling fingers and toes, abdominal cramps, muscle cramps, lightheadedness, nausea, and thirst are important symptoms of electrolyte imbalances in infants and children. Other sensory and neurologic signs may include hypotonia and flaccid paralysis indicative of a potassium deficit. Hypertonia is evidenced as a positive Chvostek sign, tremors, cramps, or tetany, which are indicative of a calcium deficit. A magnesium deficit causes twitching.

● Knowing the variations in serum electrolyte ranges for infants and children can help prevent complications of electrolyte imbalances of sodium, potassium, chloride, calcium, and magnesium (see Table 15-1 for serum electrolyte norms).

● Even small weight changes are crucial in fluid balance problems of infants and children. Rapid loss or gain in weight indicates fluid deficits and fluid excesses in the fluid

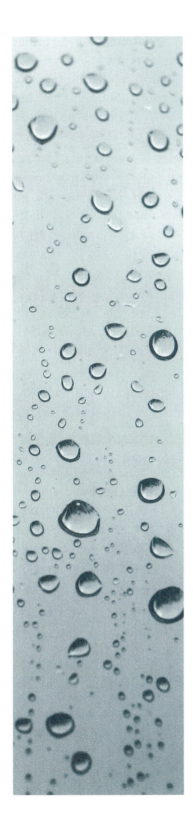

regulation process. Although baseline data on normal output is important, normal output varies with the age of the child. Normal output ranges for an infant are 2–3 mL/kg/hr and for young children it is 2 mL/kg/h. Immature kidneys limit the infant's ability to concentrate urine. Urine should be monitored for specific gravity. A specific gravity of less than 1.010 is low and indicates a fluid excess. A specific gravity of 1.030 is high and may indicate a fluid deficit with a sodium excess. An elevated specific gravity is usually accompanied by glycosuria and proteinuria. The specific gravity of infants and children can be used to monitor their hydration level. Fixed low specific gravity readings indicate renal disease.

Nursing Diagnosis 1

Deficient fluid volume related to decreased fluid reserve.

Interventions and Rationale

1. Identify source of fluid deficit. Fluid deficits result from a decreased fluid intake or an abnormal fluid loss in conditions such as diabetes insipidus, adrenocortical insufficiency, vomiting, diarrhea, hemorrhage, burns, and diabetes mellitus. Fluid deficits in infants and children are accentuated by three factors: (a) their proportionately high body surface area; (b) their high rate of metabolism; and (c) their immature renal structures. All of these factors limit the infant's ability to conserve fluid and compensate for fluid deficits.

2. The increased vulnerability of infants and children to dehydration is not easily detected in observable signs and symptoms, so try to recognize the specific symptoms of electrolyte imbalance. Monitor laboratory values for selected electrolytes (Na, Cl, K, Ca). Recognize differences between the normal values of infants and children and abnormal values in illness. Report even small changes in laboratory values.

3. Closely assess changes in general appearance and neurologic and behavioral signs. Lethargy with hyperirritability

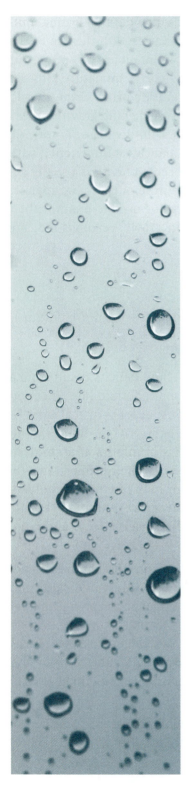

on stimulation is an early sign of deficient fluid volume (see Table 15-5). Dry mucous membranes and decreased skin turgor are often the first symptom of fluid deficits. Sunken fontanels are an indication of a fluid volume deficit in an infant. Other reliable signs are prolonged capillary refill time and abnormal respiratory patterns.

4. Monitor weight daily. The amount of weight loss is a key assessment factor for determining the severity of the fluid imbalance. Knowledge of weight in kilograms is essential to determine the degree of dehydration and to calculate the fluid replacement needs (see Table 15-1) of infants and children.

5. Monitor vital signs. A baseline value of the infant's or child's normal vital signs is important in determining the degree of the fluid deficit and assessing for hypovolemic shock (see Table 15-2). Check healthcare provider's records or ask the parents for the normal values of the child or infant.

6. Measure intake and output. The immature development of the renal structures in infants limits the kidney's ability to concentrate urine and increases the infant's risk for dehydration. A balance in intake and output is important in restoring fluid balance.

7. Integrate observations to determine the type (iso-osmolar, hypo-osmolar, or hyperosmolar) and degree of dehydration (mild, moderate, or severe). Knowledge of the type and degree of dehydration assists in identifying the ratio of ICF volume and ECF volume. This information is important in the proper selection of fluids and the regulation of the rate and volume of fluid replacement.

Nursing Diagnosis 2

Excess fluid volume related to inadequate excretion of fluid or alteration of fluid volume regulation.

Interventions and Rationale

1. Although excess fluid volume is less common than are deficits, it is important to first identify the source of the fluid volume excess. Fluid overload can be caused by rapid infusions of IV or dialysis fluid, tap water enemas,

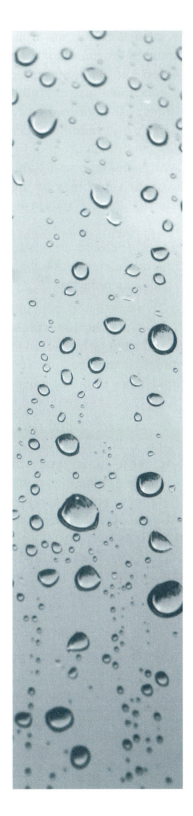

or with rapid reduction of glucose levels in diabetic ketoacidosis. Other causes that may occur in the home setting are diluted formula and water intoxication associated with swallowing pool water during swimming activities. Regulatory mechanisms in infants are not as developed as in the older child. Therefore, they are often unable to excrete a fluid overload effectively.

2. Monitor intake and output as well as laboratory values. The ingestion or infusion of excessive amounts of fluids can result in reduced sodium levels and CNS symptoms. Specific gravity measurements are used to assess urine concentration. The infant kidney's reduced ability to concentrate urine results in an excessive, diluted urine output. Urine output should be at least 1–2 mL/kg/h (refer to Table 15-5).

3. Assess neurologic symptoms. Neurologic symptoms of a fluid overload include lethargy, irritability, headache, and/or generalized seizures. These symptoms result because water moves into the brain more rapidly than sodium moves out.

4. Assess for edema. Immaturity of the kidneys and inadequate hormone production may predispose infants and young children to fluid imbalances that result in edema. Infants and young children who look well hydrated may have edema. Early recognition of edema as a consequence of fluid overload is essential. Edema may be localized to a specific body area or generalized. Common areas for assessing edema are the extremities, face, perineum, and torso.

Nursing Diagnosis 3

Diarrhea related to gastrointestinal disorder.

Interventions and Rationale

1. Identify causative factors. Compare and contrast dietary patterns 24 hours prior to the onset of diarrhea with normal dietary patterns. Assess for the possibility of allergies, contaminated foods, dietary indiscretions, bacterial or viral infections, antibiotic usage, exposure to other

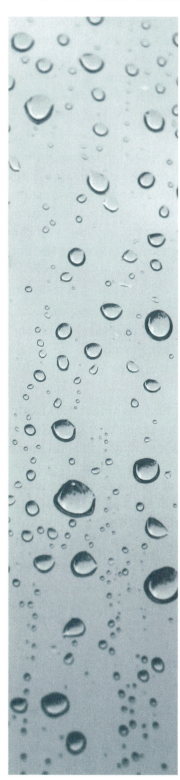

children in child care settings, or malabsorption problems. Rotavirus, the most common pathogen associated with diarrhea in hospitalized infants and children, can be identified through a stool culture. Frequent use of antibiotics may deplete the normal intestinal flora leading to colonization and toxin production by *Clostridium difficile* resulting in diarrhea and pseudomembranous colitis. Diarrhea may also be associated with upper respiratory and urinary tract infections. Although the cause may be unknown, whenever possible, causative factors should be eliminated.

2. Monitor vital signs, weight changes, and laboratory values. Determine the extent of fluid and electrolyte imbalance based on changes in these assessment factors.

3. Assess stools for frequency, consistency, blood, pH, and carbohydrate malabsorption. Liquid/diarrhealike stools contain significant fluid content and must be measured in infants and children to determine their fluid balance status. Compare frequency and consistency of bowel movements to the normal pattern.

4. If mild to moderate dehydration is suspected, oral rehydration therapy should be initiated. Oral rehydration solutions (ORSs) can be used to treat most types of dehydration in the home setting. To determine the appropriate amount of maintenance fluid requirements, refer to Table 15-1. Stool losses should be replaced with equal volumes of ORSs. Clear liquids such as fruit juices, soft drinks, and gelatin should be discouraged. These fluids are high in carbohydrates and may exacerbate the diarrhea. Caffeinated beverages act as a mild diuretic and may increase fluid and sodium losses.

5. Severe dehydration requires IV fluid replacement. Once the child is stabilized, oral rehydration therapy should be introduced.

6. A regular diet that contains easily digestible foods such as cereal, yogurt, cooked vegetables, and soups should be given. Avoid high-fiber foods as they often cause the bowel to expand and stimulate peristalsis. A BRAT diet (bananas,

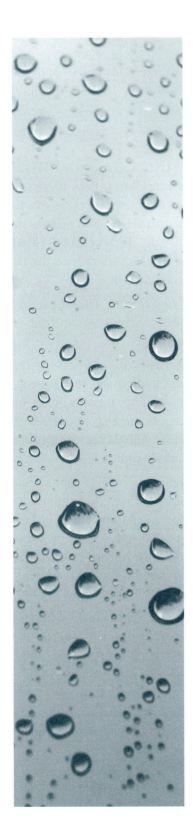

rice, applesauce, toast or tea) is no longer recommended. Formula (either half strength or lactose free) and breast feeding can be continued. Initially, there may be a higher output of stool. The benefits of a nutritionally sound diet, however, outweigh the problems with stool output. Losses are replaced with oral rehydration solutions.

7. Parental education is an important aspect of treatment. They should be taught how to recognize signs and symptoms of fluid imbalance. In addition, techniques for providing oral rehydration therapy should be discussed as well as fluids and foods to encourage and avoid. Oral rehydration therapy is very labor intensive. Small amounts of fluids (1–2 teaspoons) can provide up to 300 mL of fluid per hour.

Nursing Diagnosis 4

Imbalanced nutrition: less than body requirements, related to anorexia secondary to vomiting, diarrhea, and nausea.

Interventions and Rationale

1. Identify cause of nutritional deficit. Diarrhea and vomiting are the most common causes of fluid and electrolyte problems in infants and children. These conditions prevent the absorption of adequate nutrients and threaten the precarious fluid balance of infants and young children.

2. Initiate a regular diet as soon as possible (see 6 in Diagnosis 3). Knowledge of the nutritional requirements of various age groups is essential to adequate nutritional replacement. Changes in metabolic needs are affected by the child's physical status and pathophysiologic conditions. The health professional can help the parents plan a diet that is nutritionally sound, developmentally appropriate, and pleasing to the child.

3. Monitor weight. Weight gains or losses are indicative of nutritional status and fluid balance. Small gains or losses are significant in infants and children.

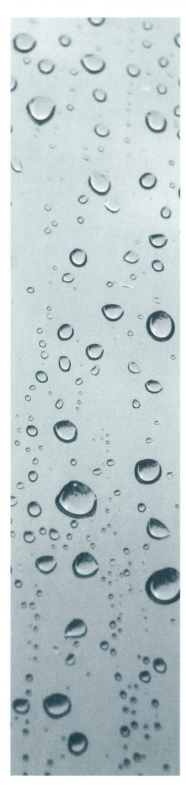

Nursing Diagnosis 5

Impaired tissue integrity related to the effects of chemical destruction or tissue deficits, secondary to diarrhea and edema.

Interventions and Rationale

1. Identify risk factors for threats to tissue integrity. Tissue destruction can occur from chemical irritants or mechanical destruction. Conditions such as diarrhea, excessive or unusual secretions, urinary incontinence, and edema increase the tissue's vulnerability to destruction. Proper identification and treatment of risk factors reduce the infant and child's vulnerability to these risks.

2. Eliminate or reduce causative factors. Diarrhea and edema are symptoms that require early interventions to reduce the risk of tissue destruction.

3. Assess nutritional status. Nutritional status affects the tissue's vulnerability to breakdown. Inadequate protein consumption reduces healing power and increases tissue vulnerability. Vitamins and minerals are also important to the health of body tissues. In fluid imbalance conditions, one's nutritional state is often compromised.

4. Promote mobility as tolerated. Many fluid imbalance problems cause lethargy and immobility. Since adequate circulation is essential to tissue nutrition and oxygenation, frequent position changes and movement promote circulation and reduce the risk of tissue breakdown. Reposition infants carefully to reduce risks related to mechanical destruction of tissues.

5. Keep the skin clean and dry. Cleanse with a mild soap and pat dry. If the skin is irritated, a hair dryer placed on the "cool" setting can be used to dry the skin. When possible, the skin should be left open to the air. Protective ointments such as zinc oxide may be applied. Most importantly, diapers should be changed frequently and the skin assessed. With diarrhea stools, skin breakdown can occur very rapidly.

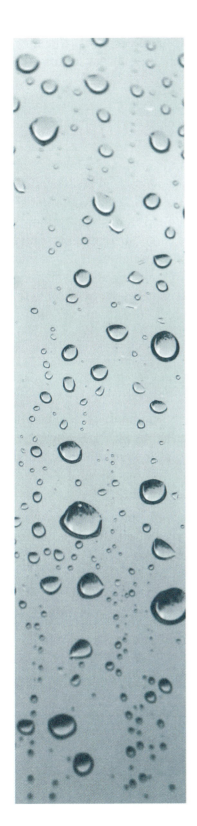

Other Nursing Diagnoses and Interventions to Consider

1. Impaired oral mucous membranes related to fluid deficit (dehydration):

    ● Apply a thin layer of a water-soluble ointment to the lips to prevent cracking (glycerin and lemon swabs have a drying effect and should be avoided).

    ● Rinse mouth with water or warm saline (do not allow swallowing if oral fluids are restricted).

    ● Clean teeth and gums with a soft sponge. Dryness may cause inflammation, bleeding, or lesions.

    ● Instruct parents to provide these interventions in situations when child is too young or unable to care for self. Maintenance of moist, adequately perfused mucous membranes is important in fluid balance problems.

2. Impaired urinary elimination related to inadequate blood volume or active losses from other sources:

    ● Monitor intake and output. Toilet-trained children and independent older children may not understand the importance of measuring intake and urinary output. This independence may pose a threat to accurate monitoring of intake and output. Altered urine output may indicate dysfunctions such as inadequate blood volume regulatory mechanisms of aldosterone and ADH, excessive fluid intake, or marked fluid loss (hemorrhage, GI bleeding). Monitor urine for presence of protein or glucose and measure the pH level. The preferred method of measuring urine output in diapered infants and children is simply to compare the dry and wet weight of the diaper. (Weight in grams corresponds to volume voided.) Urine can be aspirated from diapers or a dipstick used to obtain specific gravity readings. In children with superabsorbent diapers, the diaper should be weighed within 30 minutes of voiding to ensure accurate measurement.

    ● Monitor kidney function for early signs of renal insufficiency. The specific gravity of urine, sufficient amounts of output, BUN, serum creatinine, potassium, phosphorus, ammonia, and creatinine clearance times

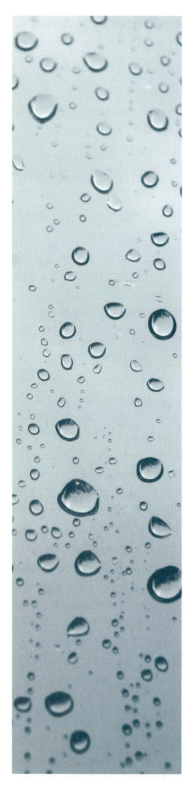

are important in the diagnosis of renal insufficiency. (Refer to Table 15-5 for normal values for infants and children.)

3. Disturbed sensory perceptions related to metabolic changes secondary to fluid and electrolyte imbalance (acidosis):

   ● Identify sensory-perceptual disturbances. Children can experience different sensory-perceptual problems depending upon the type of fluid and electrolyte imbalance. Fluid deficits promote irritability and lethargy while fluid shifts that cause cerebral edema may cause irritability and restlessness. Complaints of headaches and nausea with episodes of vomiting are not uncommon. Severe cerebral edema can cause convulsions. Selected electrolyte imbalances result in dizziness, muscle cramping or twitching, and tingling of the fingers and toes.

   ● Monitor laboratory values. An elevated BUN or serum creatinine can alter sensory-perceptual experiences.

   ● Maintain a neutral, quiet environment. To reduce unnecessary stimulation, interventions should be organized in a manner that allows for uninterrupted rest periods. Unnecessary interruptions should be prevented during these quiet times.

   ● Provide developmentally appropriate diversional activities. Asking the child and parent what activities the child enjoys during quiet times is helpful.

4. Deficient knowledge (parental) related to detection, care, and treatment of fluid and electrolyte imbalance:

   ● Teach parents basic fluid balance principles. Knowledge of basic principles of fluid and electrolyte balance can alert parents to symptoms of fluid overload and fluid deficits for early detection of potential complications.

   ● Involve parents in the infant's/child's care as much as possible. Promoting trust by involving parents enhances treatment and reduces unnecessary anxiety of parents during the infant's/child's illness.

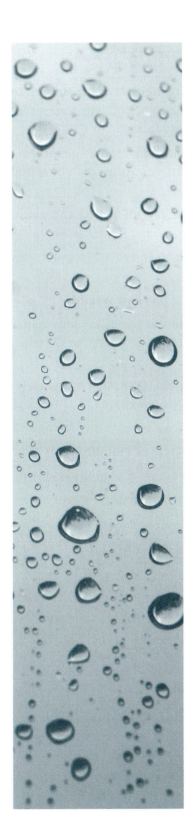

● Teach basic fluid replacement strategies. Many hospitalizations or complications from fluid problems can be prevented by early detection and appropriate fluid replacement strategies initiated at home by alert parents.

Evaluation/Outcomes

Identified below are possible outcomes for five primary nursing diagnoses.

1. Deficient fluid volume related to decreased fluid reserve.

   ● The cause of the fluid volume deficit has been eliminated (no vomiting, diarrhea, hemorrhage, etc.).

   ● Laboratory values for selected electrolytes have returned to normal for the child's age.

   ● There are no visible signs of dehydration. Skin turgor, capillary refill, and respirations have returned to normal patterns.

   ● The weight returns to stable baseline weight.

   ● The intake and output are in balance and the specific gravity is normal.

   ● Parents verbally identify signs, symptoms, and home treatment for dehydration.

2. Excess fluid volume related to inadequate excretion of fluid or alteration of fluid volume regulation.

   ● The source of the excess fluid volume is identified and eliminated.

   ● The intake and output are in balance and the specific gravity is normal.

   ● There are no visible signs of overhydration (no bulging fontanels in infants; no local or generalized edema; no weak, shrill cry; no seizures).

   ● Neurological symptoms such as lethargy, irritability, and headache are diminished or absent.

3. Diarrhea related to gastrointestinal disorder.

   ● The cause of the diarrhea has been identified and eliminated.

   ● The frequency and consistency of stools has returned to the child's normal pattern.

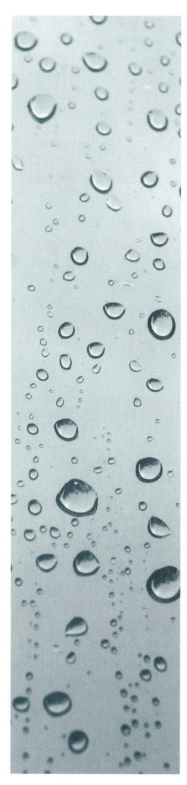

● The infant or child is able to tolerate a regular diet for age.

● Parents appropriately report their plans for a diet that is age appropriate and does not include foods that may stimulate increased peristalsis.

4. Imbalanced nutrition: less than body requirements; related to anorexia; secondary to vomiting, diarrhea, and nausea.

● The cause of anorexia has been identified and eliminated.

● The infant or child is able to tolerate a regular diet for age.

● The weight returns to stable baseline weight.

5. Impaired tissue integrity related to the effects of chemical destruction or tissue deficits, secondary to diarrhea and edema.

● There are no signs of diarrhea, excessive or usual secretions, urinary incontinence, or edema.

● The infant or child consumes a regular diet for age.

● The child returns to usual state of mobility.

● There are no signs of excoriation or skin break down.

● Parents are able to repeat instructions about maintaining skin integrity.

Fluid Problems of the Older Adult

Ingrid Aboff, PhD, RN

⬤ LEARNING OUTCOMES

Upon completion of this chapter, the reader will be able to:

- Describe structural and functional changes that occur with normal aging of the respiratory, renal, cardiac, integumentary, and gastrointestinal systems.
- Discuss the effects of normal aging (on the respiratory, renal, cardiac, integumentary, and gastrointestinal systems) that have implications for fluid and electrolyte balance.
- List risk factors, especially chronic diseases, that may cause fluid and electrolyte problems for the older adult.
- Identify common body fluid problems experienced by the older adult.
- Assess normal physiologic changes in the older patient as they relate to the signs and symptoms of fluid problems.
- Identify appropriate interventions for older patients experiencing fluid and electrolyte imbalances.

INTRODUCTION

The normal aging process has a wide range of effects on the structure and function of various organ systems. Changes in respiratory, cardiac, renal, gastrointestinal, and integumentary systems can present fluid and electrolyte problems for the older adult.

This chapter looks at the normal physiologic changes and the effects of chronic illness as they relate to the signs and symptoms of fluid and electrolyte imbalance in the older adult.

PHYSIOLOGIC CHANGES

During the normal aging process the pulmonary, renal, cardiac, gastrointestinal, and integumentary systems undergo structural changes that will ultimately decrease their functional efficiency. While these changes do not intrinsically imply that an organ system is impaired, they do explain why, in older adults, the ability to compensate for fluid and electrolyte imbalances may be decreased. In addition, risk factors such as chronic diseases increase the debilitating effects of normal functional changes in all of the body's systems and further inhibit the older adult's ability to maintain fluid and electrolyte balance.

Assessments provide information about age-related changes and factors that may place older adults at risk for fluid and electrolyte imbalances. Appropriate interventions, are needed to foster positive functional consequences and decrease the debilitating effects of risk factors and age-related changes.

Table 16-1 lists (a) age-related structural and functional changes in five major organ systems, (b) health factors increasing risk for fluid and electrolyte imbalance, (c) functional consequences, and (d) interventions to foster positive functional outcomes. Study Table 16-1 and practice stating the specific changes, risk factors, and interventions to enhance positive functional outcomes in each system.

Table 16-1   **Major Structural Changes, Risk Factors, and Functional Outcomes in Older Adults**

Organ System	Structural Changes	Risk Factors	Functional Outcomes	Nursing Interventions
Pulmonary function decreased	Loss of elasticity of parenchymal lung tissue with 20% decrease in weight Increased rigidity of chest wall and decreased recoil of lungs Fewer alveoli Decreased strength of expiratory muscles Decrease in internal surface area Decreased mucociliary transport system	Chronic diseases Emphysema Asthma Chronic bronchitis Bronchiectasis Injuries from smoking Exposure to air pollutants Occupational exposure to toxic substances Infection Decreased immune system response Medications (e.g., narcotics, benzodiazepines)	Defective alveolar ventilation Decreased gas exchange Increased work of breathing Respiratory rate may increase Baseline arterial oxygenation is lower Decreased ability to clear mucus and foreign bodies (bacteria) Decline in response to supplemental oxygen Decreased cough reflex Accumulation of bronchial secretions Increased CO_2 retention Increased difficulty in regulating pH Decreased response to hypoxia and hypercapnia Decreased tolerance for exercise Decreased vital capacity response	Increase breathing capacity to enhance the elimination of CO_2 by: 1. Breathing exercises with prolonged expiration 2. Coughing after a few deep breaths 3. Frequent position changes
Renal function decreased	Arteriosclerotic changes in large renal vessels Decrease in number of functioning cortical nephrons (begins by age 40) Reduced medullary nephron's ability to concentrate urine 30–50% less by age 70	Medications (e.g., nephrotoxic drugs, diuretics) Genitourinary diseases (e.g., infections, obstructions) Chronic renal insufficiency Hypertension Atherosclerotic vascular disease	Increased residual volume Reduced glomerular filtration rate Decreased renal blood flow Impaired ability to excrete water and solutes causing: 1. A decrease in H^+ excretion; thus metabolic acidosis can occur 2. Reduced ability to concentrate urine	Assess adaptive capacity and maintain optimal renal function by: 1. Checking fluid intake and output balance 2. Encouraging fluid intake as appropriate 3. Checking acid-base balance according to serum CO_2 or HCO_3

(continues)

Table 16-1 — Major Structural Changes, Risk Factors, and Functional Outcomes in Older Adults—*continued*

Organ System	Structural Changes	Risk Factors	Functional Outcomes	Nursing Interventions
Renal function decreased *(continued)*	Decrease in size and weight of the kidneys Increase interstitial tissue Decreased number of glomeruli Thickening of glomeruli and tubular membranes		3. Increased accumulation of waste products in body 4. Decreased ability to excrete drugs Decline in urine creatinine clearance of about 10% per decade after age 40 (Note: serum creatinine remains within normal limits) Overall decrease in adaptive capacity of the kidneys to stress Decreased thirst perception (hypodipsia) Impaired responsiveness to sodium balance	4. Testing specific gravity to determine kidneys' ability to concentrate urine 5. Tracking renal function by monitoring serum creatinine, blood urea nitrogen (BUN), and urine creatinine clearance 6. Noting drugs that may be toxic to renal function 7. Observing for side effects from drug accumulation
Circulation and cardiac function decreased	Increased rigidity and decreased elasticity of arterial walls (arteriosclerosis) Decreased elasticity of blood vessels Thickening of cardiac vessels and valves Decrease in number of conductive cells	Myocardial infarction Cardiomyopathy Obesity Smoking Dietary habits that contribute to risk factors: Hyperlipidemia, excess salt and calories Inactivity Low potassium intake Diuretic therapy Excessive alcohol consumption Stress Air pollution Hormone changes	Potential increase in blood pressure Stasis of blood causing back pressure on capillaries, which in turn causes fluid to move into tissue areas causing edema Decreased cardiac reserve (capacity of heart to respond to increased burden) slows the adaptive functions as evidenced by: 1. Heart rate same as young adults except under stress takes longer to return to normal 2. Increased incidence of edema and heart failure Diminished strength of cardiac contractions	Assess adaptive capacity of heart and maintain circulation and cardiac function by: 1. Checking blood pressure for elevations resulting from arteriosclerotic changes 2. Determining blood flow by checking peripheral pulses 3. Checking dependent extremities for edema from increased capillary pressure 4. Checking pulse rates (apical and radial) 5. Noting changes in heart rate following activity 6. Assessing lung sounds for crackles

		Decreased cardiac output and stroke volume Decreased compensatory responses to blood pressure changes Decreased maximum heart rate and aerobic capacity Decrease in maximum oxygen consumption Approximately 50% of older adults have abnormal resting electrocardiographs (EKGs)	7. Monitoring intake and output balance 8. Assessing for unexplained weight gain of 4.5 kg (10 lb), pitting edema 9. Administering diuretics as prescribed, assess effectiveness 10. Observing for signs and symptoms of hypovolemia and electrolyte depletion (namely hypokalemia) as a result of diuretic therapy 11. Monitoring serum electrolytes 12. Encouraging regular exercise, longer cooling down periods
Gastrointestinal function decreased	Atrophy of gastric mucosa Muscular atrophy and loss of supportive structures in small intestines Alcohol or medications Psychosocial factors (e.g., isolation, depression) Factors that interfere with ability to obtain, prepare, consume, or enjoy food and fluids (e.g., immobility, mental impairment) Extraintestinal disorders (diabetes, vascular disorders, and neurologic changes)	Decrease in gastric secretions, especially HCl Atrophic gastritis due to decreased HCl Weakened intestinal wall causing diverticuli Decreased motility (peristalsis) of gastrointestinal tract (may cause constipation) Decreased calcium and nutrient absorption Decreased solubility and absorption of some drugs	Assess for adaptive changes and maintain gastro-intestinal function by: 1. Discussing patient preferences for foods 2. Suggesting dietary alterations according to physiologic changes, individual preferences, and nutritional needs; may need increased calcium and vitamin D 3. Encouraging fluid intake 4. Checking frequency, consistency, and stool color in bowel elimination 5. Assessing bowel sounds and level of peristalsis

(continues)

Table 16-1

Major Structural Changes, Risk Factors, and Functional Outcomes in Older Adults—*continued*

Organ System	Structural Changes	Risk Factors	Functional Outcomes	Nursing Interventions
Liver function and endocrine gland function decreased	Liver decreases in mass of approximately 40% by age 80 Hormonal cells decrease in size and character, and outputs dwindle	Liver or endocrine diseases Medications (e.g., steroids, cardiac medications, antibiotics) Alcohol consumption	Liver: 1. Decreased hepatic capacity to detoxify drugs 2. Decreased synthesis of cholesterol and enzyme activity Hormonal: 1. Decreased overall metabolic capacity 2. Decreased endocrine gland function to react to adverse drug action	Assess adaptive liver and endocrine gland functioning by: 1. Note drugs patient is taking that may be toxic to liver 2. Observing for toxic effects of drug buildup 3. Observing for desired effects of drugs 4. Assessing alcohol consumption and teaching accordingly 5. Assessing for jaundice. 6. Assessing for fluid shift (e.g., ascites)
Skin function decreased	All three layers of the skin (epidermis, dermis, and subcutaneous) become thinner, lose elasticity and strength Blood flow—decreased Sebaceous gland—decreased production Sweat gland—decreased production Decrease in number of nerve endings	Exposure to ultraviolet rays (sunlight) Adverse medication effects Personal hygiene habits (e.g., too frequent bathing) Immobility Friction Chemical Mechanical injury Temperature—too high or low Pressure Gene influence Diabetes Peripheral vascular disease	Dryer, coarser skin Increased threshold level to pain and temperature sensitivity Decreased ability to produce sweat Impaired ability to maintain body temperature Decreased skin elasticity (making it difficult to assess skin turgor)	Maintain skin integrity and function by: 1. Maintaining hydration, monitor fluid status 2. Maintaining optimal skin temperature 3. Maintaining and encouraging mobility to enhance circulation 4. Turning patient and elevating extremities when necessary to minimize edema and skin breakdown 5. Educating about decreased sensitivity to pain and temperature 6. Providing special mattress for those at risk 7. Padding and protecting boney prominences and pressure sites as needed

ANSWER COLUMN

1. functional; structural; fluid; electrolyte imbalances

2. decreases; loss of elasticity of the parenchymal lung tissue; increased rigidity of the chest wall (also fewer alveoli)

3. defective alveolar ventilation; accumulation of bronchial secretions; a, d; emphysema, asthma, chronic bronchitis, and bronchiectasis

4. breathing exercises with prolonged expiration, coughing and deep breathing and changing positions

1.

The older adult adapts more slowly and thus has more difficulty maintaining homeostasis necessary for fluid and electrolyte balance. This factor is complicated by diminished efficiency of pulmonary, renal, cardiac, gastrointestinal, and integumentary functions.

The changes occurring in the older adult are both _____ and _____.

With diminished pulmonary, renal, cardiac, integumentary, and gastrointestinal functions, the older adult is prone to _____ and *_____.

2.

The aging process (increases/decreases) _____ the effectiveness of pulmonary ventilation and gas exchange.

The maximal breathing capacity is reduced due to *_____ and *_____.

3.

Environmental toxins and/or progressive subclinical exhaustion of internal respiratory reserve and repair mechanisms in the older adult contribute to poor diffusion of respiratory gases, which results in *_____ and *_____.

Reduced ventilation can cause which of the following:
( ) a. CO_2 retention
( ) b. CO_2 excretion
( ) c. respiratory alkalosis
( ) d. respiratory acidosis

Name four clinical diseases that cause a decrease in breathing capacity, poor diffusion, and reduced ventilation. *_____
_____

4.

Name three research-supported interventions that can increase breathing capacity and facilitate the elimination of CO_2 in the older adult.
*_____
_____

5. decreased; a reduced glomerular filtration rate; impaired ability to excrete water and solutes

6. retain; excrete; decreases; metabolic acidosis

7. reduced/decreased; a buildup (accumulation) of waste products in the body

8. decreased; increased

9. checking fluid intake and output, encouraging fluid intake, testing urine specific gravity, and noting drugs that may be toxic to renal function; also, observing lab results for signs of acid-base imbalance (according to the serum CO_2 or HCO_3), and monitoring renal function by checking BUN, serum creatinine, and urine creatinine clearance

10. decreased; an increased blood pressure

11. capillary pressure/ permeability; edema

5.
Renal function in the older adult is (increased/decreased) _____.

The persistent renal vasoconstriction and decreased numbers of functioning nephrons resulting from arteriosclerotic changes cause * _____ and * _____.

6.
Aged kidneys show evidence of a reduction in their ability to _____ or _____ water and solutes.

The kidneys' ability to excrete hydrogen (increases/decreases) _____ with age. The resulting acid-base imbalance is * _____.

7.
The aged kidneys' ability to concentrate urine is _____, resulting in * _____.

8.
Decreased renal function may result in (decreased/increased) _____ drug excretion and (increased/decreased) _____ accumulation of the drug in the body.

9.
Name at least four interventions for assessing and maintaining renal functions. * _____ _____

10.
In the aging process, circulation and cardiac function are (increased/decreased) _____.

The increased rigidity and decrease in elasticity of the arterial walls due to arteriosclerotic changes can cause * _____.

11.
Stasis of blood in the veins can cause back pressure on the capillaries, increasing * _____. The result of increased capillary pressure is _____.

12. cardiac output; blood flow

13. the capacity of the heart to respond to increased burden; quickly returns to normal; takes longer to return to normal

14. checking blood pressure for elevation or hypertension, determining blood flow in lower extremities by checking pulses (peripheral), checking for edema, checking apical and radial pulse rates for pulse deficit, and noting changes in heart rate following activities, also, assessing chest sounds for pulmonary crackles, encouraging regular exercise, assessing need for diuretic therapy, and assessing for symptoms of electrolyte depletion as a result of medical interventions

15. slowed; HCl; metabolic alkalosis

16. decrease

17. constipation

18. weakened; outpouches in the intestinal wall due to a weakened structural area

---

12.

The diminished strength of heart contractions can cause a decrease in * _____ and * _____ .

13.

The older adult has a decrease in cardiac reserve. Cardiac reserve is * _____
_____

Under stress, the heart rate increases both in the young adult and in the older adult. After stress, what happens to the heart rate in the young adult? * _____ In the older adult? * _____

14.

Name at least five interventions for assessing and maintaining circulation and cardiac function. * _____
_____
_____
_____

15.

Gastrointestinal functions are (increased/slowed) _____ in the older adult.
Atrophy of the gastric mucosa occurs with aging, causing a reduction in the important gastric secretion of _____ .
The resulting acid-base imbalance is * _____ .

16.

The muscular atrophy in the small intestine that occurs in aging can (increase/decrease) _____ gastrointestinal motility (peristalsis) when stressed.

17.

The older adult frequently has decreased motility of the gastrointestinal tract, which may result in _____ .

18.

The supportive structures in the intestinal wall (villae) are (strengthened/weakened) _____ and can cause diverticuli as a result of normal aging. Describe diverticuli.
* _____

19. discuss food preferences, suggest a diet to meet individual nutritional needs and preferences, encourage fluid intake, note color and consistency of bowel movements, and check frequency of bowel elimination and activity

20. more; slower; thinning; decreased

21. friction, chemical injury, mechanical injury, temperature, and pressure

22. monitor fluid status, maintain hydration, maintain optimal skin temperature, increase mobility (turn frequently), and elevate edematous extremities. If needed, utilize special pressure reducing mattresses to reduce skin breakdown.

19.

Name at least five interventions for assessing and maintaining gastrointestinal function. *_____
_____
_____
_____

20.

Aging skin is (more/less) _____ prone to injury and (slower/faster) _____ to heal. This occurs because of the skin's tendency toward (thinning/thickening) _____ in the older adult. These changes result in (decreased/increased) _____ elasticity and strength of the skin, which accounts for the difficulty in using skin turgor to assess fluid imbalances in the older adult.

21.

Fluid imbalances causing dehydration promote drying of the skin and make it more fragile to handle. Fluid imbalances causing overhydration and edema stretch the skin and make it thinner and more vulnerable to injury. Identify five factors that the health professional should consider to decrease the patient's risk for skin injury. *_____
_____

22.

Identify four to five interventions aimed at maintaining optimal skin integrity. *_____
_____

● ASSESSMENT FACTORS

The normal structural and functional losses that occur as a result of the aging process have important implications for assessments. The physiologic changes that alter the structure and function of the respiratory, renal, cardiac, gastrointestinal, and integumentary systems reduce the older adult's ability to adapt to changes that affect fluid and electrolyte balance. Many of these age-related changes predispose older adults to chronic diseases that further decrease their ability to adapt to fluid and electrolyte changes.

By recognizing the changes due to normal aging and additional risk factors such as chronic diseases, fluid and electrolyte problems can often be prevented or detected before major complications have occurred. A critical assessment of patients at risk for fluid imbalances requires accurate measurement of fluid intake and output, along with regularly checking the individuals weight. The magnitude of fluid problems in older adult's is often evidenced by discrepancies between their fluid intake and output or fluctuation in weight. Laboratory determinations of electrolytes and clinical assessments for edema and lung sounds provide additional information for planning and implementing care.

23.

The total body water in the healthy adult is approximately 50–60%. By age 75–80 the total body water decreases to approximately 45–50%, with even more decline in females. Changes include a slight (increase/decrease) _____ in extracellular fluid (ECF) and a(n) (increase/decrease) _____ in intracellular fluid (ICF).

23. increase; decrease

24.

Hypokalemia is a common deficit experienced by the older adult. Potassium is not conserved well at any age. Many older adults receive diuretics (potassium wasting) and steroids, which tend to (increase/decrease) _____ the serum potassium level. (Review Chapter 6, potassium with drug relationship, if needed.)

24. decrease

25.

The older adult's ECF is (increased/decreased) *_____, and the ICF is (increased/decreased) _____ because of the drop in the number of body cells (an approximate 30% decrease).

The total body water in the older adult is approximately _____%.

25. increased; decreased; 45–50

Potential fluid problems of the older adult are listed in Table 16-2, along with their related causes and suggested interventions.

Table 16-2   Body Fluid Problems in the Older Adult

Problems	Etiology	Interventions
Deficient Fluid Volume *Dehydration*	1. Insufficient water intake 2. Increased urinary output 3. Decreased thirst mechanism 4. Diminished response to ADH (antidiuretic hormone) 5. Reduced ability to concentrate urine	1. Measure fluid intake and output to assess fluid balance 2. Encourage adequate oral fluid intake 3. Assess tonicity of IV fluid intake 4. Assess for clinical signs and symptoms of hypovolemia (dehydration) 5. Monitor other types of fluid therapy and tube feeding. Adjust rate of IV fluid according to age and physiologic state 6. Monitor levels of serum electrolytes, BUN, serum creatinine, hematocrit, and hemoglobin
Excess Fluid Volume *Edema*	1. Slightly elevated ECF 2. Overhydration from IV therapy 3. Increased capillary pressure 4. Cardiac insufficiency	1. Measure fluid intake and output to assess fluid balance 2. Monitor daily weights 3. Adjust IV flow rate to prevent overhydration 4. Assess for peripheral edema in morning 5. Protect edematous skin from injury 6. Observe for signs and symptoms of hypervolemia—overhydration, which can lead to pulmonary edema such as headache, anxiety, shortness of breath, tachypnea, coughing, pulmonary crackles, and chest pain
Constipation	1. Decrease in water intake 2. Muscular atrophy of small and large intestines with a decrease in GI motility 3. Perceptual loss of bowel stimulation 4. Medications having effects on gastric motility and hydration	1. Encourage fluid intake 2. Assess bowel sounds for peristalsis 3. Administer mild laxative, and teach dangers of abuse 4. Have patient eat at regular times 5. Offer bedside commode 6. Increase roughage in diet as tolerated 7. Observe color, consistency, and frequency of stools
Diarrhea	1. Tube feedings with high carbohydrate content 2. Impaction—with small amount of liquid stools 3. Partially digested nutrients 4. Viral or bacterial infection	1. Assess for problem causing diarrhea (infectious, impaction, medications) 2. Administer drug(s), e.g., Lomotil, Imodium, Kaopectate, to decrease motility of bowel 3. Observe color, frequency, and consistency of stool 4. Monitor closely for dehydration and electrolyte imbalance (potassium, sodium) 5. Encourage clear liquids

26. decreased; insufficient water intake and increased urinary output

27. measure fluid intake and output for balance, encourage taking fluids orally, assess signs and symptoms of dehydration (hypovolemia), and assess intravenous fluid (type and rate), also, adjust replacement fluid rate according to age and condition of the patient

28. overhydration

29. refractory; nondependent

30. a. X; b. X; c. —, in the morning; d. —, chest sounds; e. —, of hypervolemia (overhydration)

26.

The thirst mechanism in the older adult is frequently (decreased/increased) _____, resulting in a decreased fluid intake.

   Name two factors that can result in dehydration for the older adult. *_____

_____

27.

Name four interventions addressing dehydration in the older adult. *_____

_____

_____

28.

Overloading the vascular system with fluids (hypervolemia) can result in heart failure (HF). The type of edema occurring in HF is pulmonary edema from (overhydration/underhydration) _____.

29.

Peripheral edema can result from dependent or refractory edema. When the feet and ankles are edematous in the morning (before getting out of bed), the type of edema present is called _____ edema. This type of edema usually results from cardiac or renal impairment/insufficiency. Another name for this type of edema is (dependent/nondependent) _____ edema.

30.

Identify selected interventions to address edema in the older adult by selecting the correct answers and adjusting the incorrect answers.

   ( ) a. Measure fluid intake and output to assess fluid balance.
   ( ) b. Adjust intravenous flow rate according to age and patient condition.
   ( ) c. Assess for peripheral edema in the evening for refractory or nondependent edema.
   ( ) d. Assess bowel sounds.
   ( ) e. Observe for signs and symptoms of hypovolemia.

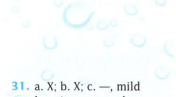

31.

Identify appropriate interventions related to constipation and adjust the incorrect answers:

( ) a. Encourage fluid intake.

( ) b. Assess bowel sounds for peristalsis.

( ) c. Administer harsh cathartics.

( ) d. Offer bedside commode.

( ) e. Have meals at regular times.

32.

Name four causes of diarrhea in the older adult. *_____

_____

What is the most important intervention for correcting diarrhea? *_____

_____

31. a. X; b. X; c. —, mild laxatives or stool softeners; d. X; e. X

32. tube feedings with high carbohydrate content, impaction with small liquid stools, partially digested nutrients, and viral or bacterial infections; identification of the problem causing diarrhea

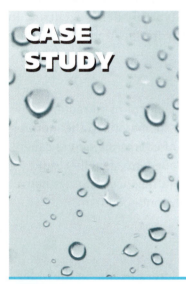

CASE STUDY

REVIEW A

A 76-year-old woman with hypertension hospitalized for treatment of heart failure exhibits a blood pressure of 174/102, a pulse of 104, and respirations of 16. Her lung exam reveals decreased air movement with crackles noted bilaterally at the bases. She has significant lower extremity edema and her urine output has been 500 mL in the past 24 hours. She reports a recent weight gain of approximately 10 lb. She is having some shortness of breath and complains of constipation. Laboratory studies revealed an elevated serum creatinine of 2.3 and BUN of 31.

ANSWER COLUMN

1. pulmonary; renal; cardiac; gastrointestinal; integumentary

1. As an older adult her organ systems most prone to changes are _____, _____, _____, _____, and _____.

2. a. loss of elasticity of the parenchymal lung tissue; b. increased rigidity of the chest wall
3. CO_2; respiratory acidosis
4. breathing exercise with prolonged expiration, coughing after a few deep breaths, and changing positions
5. increased rigidity of the arterial walls due to arteriosclerotic changes
6. increased capillary pressure forcing fluid into the tissues
7. check blood pressure, determine blood flow in lower extremities by checking pulses, assess fluid balance, and assess effectiveness of diuretics and antihypertensives
8. 30; 720; inadequate; a. inadequate fluid intake; b. kidneys unable to excrete water and solute (you could have answered: reduced glomerular filtration rate and decrease in number of functioning nephrons)
9. check intake and output, track renal function by monitoring serum creatinine, BUN, electrolytes, and monitor drugs' effects on renal function
10. reduced motility of the gastrointestinal tract and loss of perception for bowel elimination
11. suggest diet (foods) to meet nutritional needs and maintain bowel function; also, check frequency of bowel elimination and determine the presence of peristalsis (bowel sounds)

2. The patient's decreased air movement may be due to the following structural changes seen in the older adult:
   a. *_____
   b. *_____

3. Hypoventilation can result in _____ retention, which may cause an acid-base imbalance called *_____.

4. Identify at least three interventions that can improve her pulmonary function. *_____
   _____

5. Her blood pressure is elevated due to *_____
   _____
   _____

6. The physiologic reason for edema in her lower extremities is
   *_____
   _____

7. Identify at least three interventions regarding blood pressure and edema.

8. Urine output should be _____ mL/hr or _____ mL/24 hr to maintain adequate renal function. Urine output of 500 mL in 24 hours, is (adequate/inadequate) _____. Identify two possible reasons for her poor urinary output.
   a. *_____
   b. *_____

9. Identify at least three interventions in regard to her renal function. *_____
   _____

10. What two physiologic factors can cause constipation?
    *_____
    _____

11. Two interventions aimed at alleviating constipation are
    *_____.

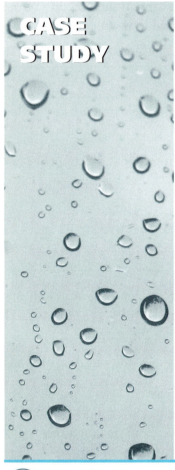

CASE STUDY

REVIEW B

A 77-year-old single man who until recently lived alone in his own house now lives in an intermediate-care unit of a continuing care facility where his meals are provided. He is independent in activities of daily living but requires help with shopping and money management. He was a financial analyst who led an active social life that included almost nightly "happy hours" with work associates until his retirement 5 years ago. After his retirement he started to drink alone. He quit going to the dining room for his meals and gradually stopped drinking fluids other than his beer and wine. The day shift recorded his vital signs as blood pressure 130/74, temperature 99°F, pulse 104, and respirations 28. His laboratory studies revealed an elevated BUN, hemoglobin, and hematocrit. Other laboratory studies revealed an elevated prothrombin time of 16.2; decreased albumen; serum potassium, 3.4 mEq/L; serum Na, 147; and Cl, 105 mEq/L (review Chapters 6–10 for normal electrolyte ranges). His exam revealed peripheral edema, ascites, and very dry skin and mucous membranes. He complained of constipation.

ANSWER COLUMN

1. dehydration, edema, constipation, and ascites

2. insufficient water intake (you might have answered that a decreased thirst mechanism was present)

3. a. vital signs: temperature slightly elevated, pulse and respirations elevated; b. Hgb, Hct, and BUN elevated; c. serum sodium elevated; d. skin and mucous membranes very dry

1. From this history, identify four fluid problems. *_____
_____

2. What is the clinical source of his dehydration?
*
_____
_____

3 Identify four clinical signs and symptoms of dehydration experienced by him.
a. *_____
b. *_____
c. *_____
d. *_____

4. Yes. Frequently a person can have edema and be dehydrated due to hypovolemia in the vascular system with increased fluids in the interstitial space.

5. The nurse should assess fluid intake and output balance and daily weights.

6. hypervolemia or overhydration (pulmonary edema); elevated blood pressure and pulse, increased venous pressure (venous distention, engorged neck veins), headache, anxiety, shortness of breath, tachypnea, coughing, pulmonary crackles, and chest pain

7. diarrhea

8. poorly conserved; deficit; hypokalemia

9. increased

4. Is it possible to have dehydration and edema at the same time? _____ Explain why. *_____
_____

He was given IV fluids for several days.

5. Identify at least two interventions aimed at maintaining an appropriate fluid balance for patients receiving IV fluids. *_____
_____

6. If the intravenous fluids were administered too rapidly, what type of fluid imbalance is most likely to develop? *_____. Identify at least three symptoms of this imbalance.
*_____

He continued to deteriorate and was unable to eat, so continuous tube feedings were initiated.

7. Tube feedings high in carbohydrate content can cause what type of a fluid problem? _____.

8. The normal potassium level in the older adult is *_____, and therefore fluid balances often result in a potassium (deficit/excess) _____ called _____.

9. Fluid imbalances can cause an (increased/decreased) _____ risk for skin breakdown.

Nursing Diagnoses and Related Interventions and Rationale

The purpose of assessing patients is to form nursing diagnoses based on the assessment data.

As you formulate a nursing care plan, consider the major organ systems affected and what additional risk factors for fluid and electrolyte imbalances exist. Now you should be ready to formulate the most important nursing diagnosis related to fluid and electrolyte balances for both of these patients.

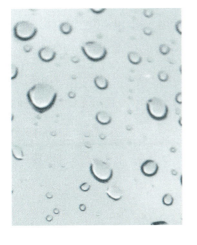

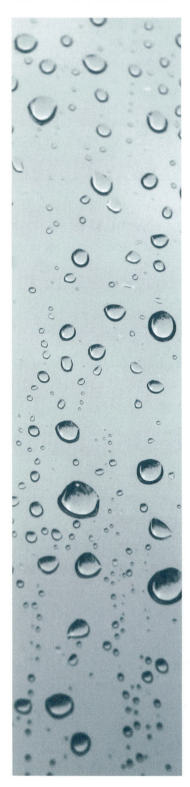

Nursing Diagnosis 1

Excess fluid volume (edema) related to decreased cardiac output as evidenced by weight gain of 10 pounds, lower extremity edema, and pulmonary crackles.

Interventions and Rationale

1. Monitor intake and output, body weight, vital signs, and neck veins for distension. Checking for signs and symptoms of overhydration is important for assessing the condition of the patient as well as for measuring the effectiveness of medical treatment and interventions.

2. Monitor hemoglobin (Hb) and hematocrit (Hct), serum creatinine, BUN, and electrolytes. These labs are important in assessing fluid balance changes. A decrease in Hb and Hct levels can indicate fluid overload.

3. Administer diuretics as prescribed. Diuretics promote fluid loss and decrease edema. Be careful to monitor electrolytes as many diuretics can cause potassium loss.

Nursing Diagnosis 2

Impaired gas exchange related to ineffective breathing patterns.

Interventions and Rationale

1. Assess chest for adventitious sounds. Crackles indicate fluid volume overload related to cardiac reasons.

2. Observe for cough. A cough may indicate pulmonary edema; it may also be an early sign of fluid overload.

3. Teach breathing exercises (such as purse-lip breathing) to foster prolonged expiration. This type of breathing assists in the removal of excess CO_2. Also teaching the patient to cough after a few deep breaths will enhance gas exchange ($O_2 + CO_2$).

4. Encourage patient to change position frequently as this assists in lung expansion and aids in loosening mucus.

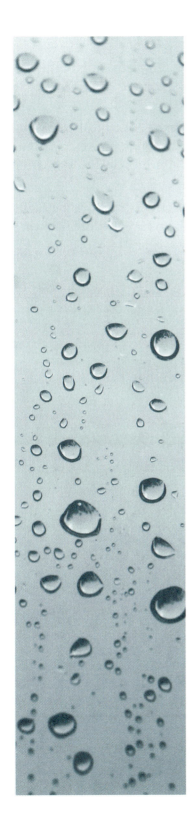

Nursing Diagnosis 3

Excess fluid volume related to renal insufficiency as evidenced by decreased urine output and increased serum creatinine and BUN.

Interventions and Rationale

1. Assessing the intake and output of the patient will allow you to determine the amount of excess fluid loss or retention. Weighing daily and assessing for edema provides valuable information in terms of fluid status. While all of these indicators are important to observe, daily weight is the best indicator of fluid status.

2. Auscultate lung and heart sounds. Fluid overload may lead to pulmonary edema and heart failure.

3. Assess urine specific gravity. Increased urine specific gravity indicates inadequate fluid intake or decreased renal function.

4. Monitor serum creatinine and BUN. Assess progression and management of renal dysfunction.

5. Monitor serum sodium, Hb, and Hct. These may decrease in value as a result of hemodilution.

6. Monitor potassium, as lack of renal excretion may lead to hyperkalemia.

7. Administer diuretics as indicated to promote diuresis.

Nursing Diagnosis 4

Constipation related to decreased fluid volume, age-related changes, and immobility.

Interventions and Rationale

1. Assess bowel sounds, check frequency of bowel elimination and consistency of stools in order to determine function status of the GI system.

2. Increase mobility as tolerated. Mobility promotes proper bowel elimination.

3. Encourage proper diet to ensure elimination. A balanced diet with fiber enhances bowel elimination.

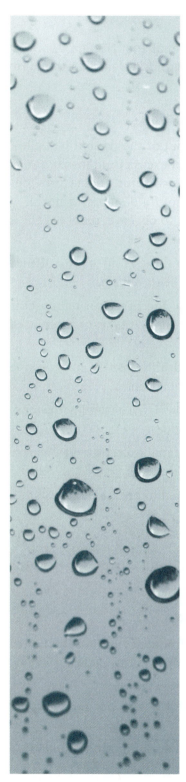

Nursing Diagnosis 5

Impaired skin integrity related to edema and immobility.

Interventions and Rationale

1. Avoid friction, prolonged pressure, chemical irritation, mechanical injury, and excessive temperature variations to the skin. These measures help protect the skin from breakdown.

2. Encourage mobility to enhance circulation. Good circulation improves skin repair and helps prevent breakdown.

3. Elevate edematous extremities. This will improve circulation and reduce edema in limbs.

4. Implement interventions for excess fluid volume. Fluid balance reduces risks to integumentary system.

Evaluation/Outcomes

1. Evaluate weight and intake and output for fluid balance.

2. Evaluate effectiveness of medications and fluid replacement in treatment.

3. Monitor nutritional intake to ensure fluid balance.

4. Evaluate body weight and vital signs for return to normal patient values.

5. Evaluate skin turgor, sensitivity, circulation, temperature, and moisture to reduce effects of risk factors.

6. Monitor lab results for Hgb, Hct, Na, Cl, K, and serum bicarbonate, serum creatinine, and BUN until findings are within normal range.

7. Monitor reduction of signs and symptoms related to fluid imbalance.

8. Maintain a support system.

A website that may be helpful in understanding fluid and electrolyte balance, but not necessarily specific to the older population: http://www.nlm.nih.gov/medlineplus/fluidandelectrolytebalance.html

Trauma and Shock

Linda Laskowski-Jones, RN, MS, APRN, BC CCRN, CIEN CEN

● LEARNING OUTCOMES

Upon completion of this chapter, the reader will be able to:

- Discuss the physiologic changes in fluids and electrolytes that occur as a result of traumatic injuries and shock.
- Describe the clinical manifestations associated with traumatic injuries and shock.
- Discuss the assessment guidelines for fluid, electrolyte, and acid-base imbalances in the traumatically injured patient.
- Identify the four types of shock and the physiologic basis for specific clinical symptoms.
- Discuss the clinical management of traumatic injuries as they relate to the four types of shock.
- Identify the assessment factors for evaluating shock and trauma patient.
- Develop nursing diagnoses and interventions with rationales appropriate in the clinical treatment of trauma and shock patient.

● INTRODUCTION

There are numerous physiologic changes in fluids and electrolyte imbalances that occur as a result of

traumatic injuries and shock. Swift and accurate assessment and intervention are necessary to protect the life of the injured patient. This chapter is divided into two sections relating to fluid and electrolyte changes, trauma and shock.

● TRAUMA

Fluid, electrolyte, and acid-base changes occur rapidly in the acutely traumatized patient. Quick assessments and actions are needed for the best chance of survival.

In trauma (acute injury), the sodium shifts into cells, potassium shifts out, and the fluid shifts from the vascular to the interstitial spaces and cells. These shifts can result in severe fluid and electrolyte imbalances.

● ANSWER COLUMN

1. potassium and sodium; Fluid shifts from the vascular to the interstitial spaces and cells.

1.

The two electrolytes that change spaces during trauma are

* _____.

  Explain the fluid shifts during trauma. *_____

*
_____

Pathophysiology

Following a severe traumatic injury, there is cellular break-down due to cell damage and hypoxia. The physiologic changes that occur during trauma are described in Table 17-1. The information in Table 17-1 will help you to accurately assess traumatic injuries.

2.

2. a. potassium is lost from the cells; b. sodium shifts into the cells; c. chloride shifts into the cells; d. water shifts into the cells

Explain what happens to the following electrolytes and water:
  a. Potassium *_____
  b. Sodium *_____
  c. Chloride *_____
  d. Water *_____

| Table 17-1 | Physiologic Changes Associated with Trauma |

Physiologic Changes	Causative Factors
Potassium, sodium, chloride, bicarbonate	Potassium is lost from cells due to catabolism (cellular breakdown). As potassium leaves, sodium and chloride with water shift into the cells. The sodium pump does not function properly (see Chapter 7).
Fluid changes	Fluids along with sodium shift into cells and to the third space (interstitial space—at the injured site). The increased cellular and third-space fluids cause a vascular fluid deficit (dehydration) and hyponatremia.
	Serum osmolality may be normal or increased due to the fluid deficit and excess solutes other than sodium, such as potassium and urea. Remember, sodium influences the osmolality of plasma (see Chapter 1).
	The volume and composition of extracellular fluid (ECF) fluctuates depending on the number of cells injured and the body's ability to restore balance. Two to three days following injury, fluid shifts from the third space at the injured site back into the vascular space.
Protein changes	Trauma results in nitrogen loss due to increased protein catabolism, decreased protein anabolism, and/or a protein shift with water to the interstitial space. The colloid osmotic pressure is decreased in the vascular fluid and increased in the interstitial fluid (tissues), which causes fluid volume deficit (vascular) and edema.
Capillary permeability	Increased capillary permeability causes water to flow into and out of the cells and into tissue spaces. This contributes to hypovolemia (fluid volume deficit).
Hormonal influence	ADH and aldosterone help to restore the ECF. A vascular fluid deficit and/or increased serum osmolality stimulates ADH secretion, which causes water reabsorption from the distal tubules of the kidneys. In certain traumatic situations (surgery, trauma, pain), SIADH (syndrome of inappropriate ADH) occurs and causes excess water reabsorption from the kidneys.
	Aldosterone is secreted from the adrenal cortex due to hyponatremia and stress. Aldosterone promotes sodium reabsorption from the renal tubules and is reabsorbed with water. Potassium is excreted.
Kidney influence	Kidney activity is altered during and after a severe traumatic injury. Sodium, chloride, and water shift to the injured site, which causes hypovolemia. Decreased circulatory flow can decrease renal arterial flow, which can cause temporary or permanent kidney damage. Impaired kidney function results in hyperkalemia.
Acid-base changes	With cellular breakdown and hypoxia from decreased perfusion, nonvolatile acids (acid metabolites), e.g., lactic acid, increase in the vascular fluid, causing metabolic acidosis.
	Kidneys conserve or excrete the hydrogen ion to maintain the acid-base balance. Decreased kidney function can cause hydrogen retention and acidosis.
	The lungs try to compensate for the acidotic state by blowing off excess CO_2—hyperventilation. Blowing off CO_2 decreases the formation of carbonic acid.

3. To maintain cellular activity, sodium shifts into the cells and potassium shifts out of the cells. Or, sodium shifts into the cell and depolarization occurs, and then potassium shifts back into the cell and repolarization occurs.

4. cells and injured site(s) or cells and interstitial (third) space; Fluids shift to the interstitial space at the injured site. Fluid in the third space is considered physiologically useless or nonfunctional fluid

5. increased; it increases

6. ADH promotes water absorption from the distal tubules of the kidneys due to hypovolemia and/or the increased serum osmolality; Aldosterone causes sodium to be reabsorbed from the distal tubules of the kidney when hyponatremia or stress is present.

7. a

8. aldosterone; excretion

3.

The sodium pump is necessary for cellular activity (see Chapter 7).

Explain the sodium pump action. *_____

_____

4.

During and after an acute injury, fluids shift to _____ and *_____.

Do you know what is meant by fluids shifting to the third space? *_____

_____.

5.

With vascular fluid deficit (loss), the serum osmolality is (increased/decreased) _____.

What happens to the permeability of capillaries as a result of injury? *_____.

6.

Explain how ADH and aldosterone restore water balance.
ADH *_____
Aldosterone *_____

7.

The syndrome of inappropriate antidiuretic hormone secretion (SIADH) frequently occurs following surgery, trauma, stress, pain, and CNS depressants (narcotics). The water reabsorption can be continuous for several days.

The nurse should assess for what type of fluid imbalance:
( ) a. Overhydration (hypervolemia)
( ) b. Dehydration (hypovolemia)

8.

Kidneys are the chief regulators of sodium and water balance. Kidneys conserve sodium when there is a sodium deficit. The hormone that is responsible for sodium reabsorption is _____. This hormone also causes potassium (excretion/retention) _____.

9.

A decrease in circulation from trauma, stress, or shock can cause a decrease in renal arterial blood flow. What effect does this have on the kidney? *_____

_____

For circulating blood to perfuse the kidneys, the systolic blood pressure should be _____ mm Hg or greater. (Refer to Chapter 2, ECFV deficit.)

10.

Severe trauma resulting in inadequate tissue perfusion with hypoxia releases nonvolatile acids (acid metabolites), such as lactic acid, from cells. What type of acid-base imbalance can occur? *_____.

How do the lungs compensate for this imbalance?

*_____.

11.

From the following list of fluid, electrolyte, and acid-base changes, check those that are affected by trauma, and correct the incorrect responses.

( ) a. Cellular loss of potassium

( ) b. Sodium shifts into cells

( ) c. Hypervolemia or overhydration

( ) d. Fluid shifts to the cells and injured site(s)

( ) e. Protein loss

( ) f. Decreased capillary permeability

( ) g. ADH secretion promoting reabsorption of water from the kidneys

Clinical Manifestations

The health care professional assesses injured sites, orders fluid replacements, and performs medical or surgical interventions as needed.

Responsibility for care is ongoing assessment and monitoring of fluid electrolyte and acid-base imbalances as they occur.

12.

The three imbalances that the health professional should assess are *_____

Sidebar answers:

9. temporary or permanent kidney damage; 70

10. metabolic acidosis; by blowing off CO_2 (reducing carbonic acid)

11. a, b, d, e, g; Corrections: c. hypovolemia or dehydration; f. increased capillary permeability

12. fluids, electrolytes, and acid-base

The clinical manifestations that frequently occur in traumatic injuries depend upon the type of imbalance (fluid, electrolyte, or acid-base) and include changes in vital signs, behavioral changes, cardiac conduction changes, venous changes, renal changes, neuromuscular changes, integumentary changes, and laboratory findings. Table 17-2 lists the signs and symptoms that may occur as the result of trauma. For further clarification of these changes and rationale, refer to Table 17-3 on assessment.

Table 17-2	Clinical Manifestations Related to Trauma
Clinical Manifestations	**Signs and Symptoms**
Vital Signs	Increased pulse rate (tachycardia)
Pulse	Irregular pulse rate
	Weak, thready pulse
Blood Pressure	Blood pressure decreases when severe fluid loss occurs
	Pulse pressure narrows
Respiration	Increased breathing (tachypnea)
	Dyspnea
	Deep, vigorous breathing (Kussmaul breathing)
Temperature	Hypothermia commonly associated with shock
Behavioral Changes	Irritability, restlessness, and confusion
Cardiac Conduction Changes	ECG: T-wave changes (inverted or peaked), ST-segment changes, and cardiac dysrythmias
Venous Changes	Neck vein engorgement with cardiac tamponade or tension pneumothorax
	No vein engorgement with fluid loss
Renal Changes	Hourly urine output decreases
Neuromuscular Changes	Muscular weakness
Integumentary Changes	Poor skin turgor
	Dry mucous membrane
	Edema at injury site(s)
	Diaphoresis
	Draining wound, exudate
Laboratory Findings	
Electrolytes ↓ or ↑	Serum potassium, sodium, magnesium, chloride may be decreased or increased
Serum CO_2	Decreased CO_2 indicates metabolic acidosis; increased CO_2 indicates metabolic alkalosis or respiratory acidosis
BUN ↑	Increased BUN: fluid loss or decreased renal function
Serum creatinine ↑	Increased serum creatinine indicates impaired renal function
Arterial blood gases: pH, $PaCO_2$, HCO_3	Decreased pH and HCO_3 indicate metabolic acidosis

13. a. tachycardia, irregular pulse rate, or weak, thready pulse;
b. decreased blood pressure, narrow pulse pressure with severe fluid loss; c. tachypnea, dyspnea, or deep vigorous breathing;
d. hypothermia is commonly associated with shock
14. irritability and confusion (also restlessness, disorientation)

13.

Indicate the typical effects of trauma on the vital signs:
a. Pulse *_____
b. Blood pressure *_____
c. Respiration *_____
d. Temperature *_____

14.

Behavioral changes are frequently observed with fluid and electrolyte imbalances.
   Name two behavioral changes that can occur following severe trauma. *_____

15.

Trauma usually results in loss of body fluid. When elevated above the heart level the neck veins become (engorged/flat) _____.

15. flat

16.

Urine output following trauma may be _____.
   Following trauma, urine output should be checked (every hour/every 8 hours/once a day) _____.

16. decreased; every hour

17.

Integumentary changes may not be noted immediately following severe trauma with fluid losses. However, after several hours or a day, the skin turgor can be affected and mucous membranes become (dry/wet) _____.
   These signs indicate (hypovolemia/hypervolemia) _____.

17. dry; hypovolemia

18.

Many abnormal laboratory results occur in severe trauma.
   Cellular breakdown and poor urine output (increase/decrease) _____ the serum potassium level.
   Poor renal function causes the BUN and serum creatinine to (increase/decrease) _____.

Frequently, metabolic acidosis results following severe trauma due to cellular breakdown and poor tissue perfusion. Which arterial blood gas changes are indicative of metabolic acidosis?

( ) a. pH decreased

( ) b. $PaCO_2$ increased

( ) c. HCO_3 decreased

18. increase; increase; a, c

Clinical Applications

Accurate assessment is vitally important when planning and implementing care. Table 17-3 is a guide that may be used when assessing the patient for fluid, electrolyte, and acid-base imbalances. The table includes key observations, assessment factors, and rationale. To understand the significance of the assessment, the rationale helps to identify the type of imbalance that is present. Use Table 17-3 in clinical assessments.

19.

Vital signs should be constantly monitored following an acute injury. Tachycardia or pulse rate greater than 120 can indicate _____ and should be reported.

19. hypovolemia or fluid volume deficit

20.

Blood pressure does not immediately fall after an injury. With a fluid volume deficit, the pulse rate increases first, and later the blood pressure drops if fluid loss is not replaced.

A pulse pressure of less than 20 can indicate _____.

20. shock

21.

A respiratory rate greater than 32 can indicate _____.

Deep, rapid, vigorous breathing occurring after cellular damage or shock due to acute injury can indicate (metabolic acidosis/metabolic alkalosis) *_____. Why?

*_____

21. hypovolemia or fluid volume deficit; metabolic acidosis; Acid metabolites, such as lactic acid, are released from cells due to anaerobic metabolism from inadequate perfusion.

22.

Temperature changes frequently do not occur immediately after injury. When there is a slight temperature elevation, this can indicate _____.

If a high temperature elevation occurs 2–5 days after the injury, what might it indicate? _____.

22. hypovolemia or a fluid volume deficit or dehydration; infection

| Table 17-3 | Assessment of Fluid, Electrolyte, and Acid-Base Imbalances in the Traumatically Injured Patient |

Observation	Assessment		Rationale
1. Vital signs: Pulse	Pulse rate Volume Pattern	_____ _____ _____	Changes in vital signs (VS) are indicators of patient's physiologic status. Several VS should be taken and the first reading acts as the baseline for comparison. Pulse rate and pattern should be monitored frequently. Pulse rate >120 may indicate hypovolemia and the possibility of shock. Full, bounding pulse can mean hypervolemia and an irregular pulse can mean hypokalemia.
Blood pressure	Admission BP Time Time	 _____ _____	Decrease in BP (systolic and diastolic) may not occur until severe fluid loss has occurred. Several BP readings should be taken, and the first BP reading acts as the baseline for comparison. A drop in systolic pressure can indicate hypovolemia. Pulse pressure (systolic minus diastolic) of <20 can indicate shock.
Respiration	Respiration Pattern	_____ _____	Note changes in rate, depth, and pattern. A rate >32 can indicate hypovolemia. Deep, rapid, vigorous breathing can indicate acidosis as a result of cellular damage and shock. Hyperventilating (fast, shallow breathing) can be due to anxiety or hypoxia. Head injury can produce a wide variety of respiratory patterns.
Temperature	Temperature on admission	_____	Hypothermia is a common finding in shock; an elevated temperature can indicate infection.
2. Behavioral changes	Irritable Apprehensive Restless Confused Delirious Lethargic	_____ _____ _____ _____ _____ _____	Irritability, apprehension, restlessness, and confusion are indicators of hypoxia and later of fluid and electrolyte imbalances (hypovolemia, water intoxication, and potassium imbalance).

3. Neurologic and neuromuscular signs	Sensorium
	  Confused
	  Semiconscious
	  Comatose
	Muscle weakness
	Pupil dilation
	Tetany
	  Tremors
	  Twitching
	Others
		
		_____
		_____
		_____
		_____
		_____
		
		_____
		_____
		_____
			Changes in sensorium can be indicative of fluid imbalance. Tetany can indicate a calcium and magnesium deficit. Hypocalcemia can occur with multiple transfusions of banked blood.

(continues)

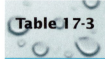

Table 17-3 **Assessment of Fluid, Electrolyte, and Acid-Base Imbalances in the Traumatically Injured Patient—*continued***

Observation	Assessment		Rationale
4. Fluid loss	Wound(s)	_____	Note the presence of an open draining wound. Kidneys regulate fluids and electrolytes. Monitoring the urine output hourly is most important. Oliguria can indicate a lack of fluid intake or renal insufficiency due to decreased circulation/circulatory collapse or hypovolemia.
	Urine		
	Number of voidings	_____	
	Amount	_____	
	mL/hr	_____	
	mL/8 hr	_____	
	mL/24 hr	_____	
	Color	_____	
	Specific gravity	_____	
	Vomitus		Frequent vomiting in large quantities leads to fluid, electrolyte (potassium, sodium, chloride), and hydrogen losses. Metabolic alkalosis can occur.
	Number	_____	
	Consistency	_____	
	Amount	_____	
	Nasogastric tube		Gastrointestinal secretions should be measured. Large quantity losses of GI secretions can cause hypovolemia.
	Amount—mL/8 hr	_____	
	Amount—mL/24 hr	_____	
	Drain(s)		Excess drainage contributes to fluid loss and should be measured if possible.
	Number	_____	
	Amount	_____	
5. Skin and mucous membrane	Skin color		Pale and/or gray-colored skin can indicate hypovolemia or shock. Flushed skin can be due to hypernatremia, metabolic acidosis, or early septic shock.
	Pale	_____	
	Gray	_____	
	Flushed	_____	
	Skin turgor		Poor skin turgor can result from hypovolemia/dehydration. This may not occur until 1–3 days after the injury.
	Normal	_____	
	Poor	_____	
	Edema—pitting peripheral		Edema indicates sodium and water retention. Sodium, chloride, and water shift into the cells and to the injury site(s) (interstitial or third space).
	Feet	_____	
	Legs	_____	
	Dry mucous membranes	_____	Dry, tenacious (sticky) secretions and dry membranes are indicative of dehydration or fluid loss. This may not occur until 1–3 days after the injury.
	Sticky secretions	_____	
	Diaphoresis	_____	Increased insensible fluid loss can result from diaphoresis (excess perspiration). Amount of fluid loss from skin can double.
6. Chest sounds and vein engorgement	Pulmonary crackles	_____	The chest should be checked for pulmonary crackles due to overhydration (pulmonary edema) following fluid administration/resuscitation.

(continues)

Table 17-3 **Assessment of Fluid, Electrolyte, and Acid-Base Imbalances in the Traumatically Injured Patient—*continued***

Observation	Assessment		Rationale
	Neck vein engorgement	_____	Neck and hand vein engorgement are indicators of fluid excess. Crackles and vein engorgement can occur from excess IV fluids or rapid IV administration.
	Hand vein engorgement	_____	
7. ECG (EKG)	T wave		Flat or inverted T waves indicate cardiac ischemia and/or a potassium deficit. Peaked T waves indicate a potassium excess.
	Flat	_____	
	Inverted	_____	
	Peaked	_____	
8. Fluid intake	Oral fluid intake		Oral fluids should not be given until the injury(s) can be assessed. If surgery is indicated, the patient should be NPO.
	Amount		
	mL/8 hr	_____	
	mL/24 hr	_____	
	Types of IV fluids		Crystalloids, i.e., normal saline, lactated Ringer's, are normally ordered first to restore fluid loss, correct shocklike symptoms, restore or increase urine output, and serve as a lifeline to administer IV drugs.
	Crystalloids	_____	
	Colloids	_____	
	Blood	_____	
	Amount		Five percent dextrose in water can cause water intoxication (ICF volume excess) and is contraindicated as a resuscitation fluid in shock states.
	mL/8 hr	_____	
	mL/24 hr	_____	
	mL/hr	_____	
9. Previous drug regimen	Diuretics	_____	A drug history should be taken and reported to the physician. Potassium-wasting diuretics taken with a digitalis preparation can cause digitalis toxicity in the presence of hypokalemia. Steroids cause sodium retention and potassium excretion.
	Digitalis	_____	
	Steroids	_____	
	Beta blockers	_____	
	Calcium channel blockers	_____	
			Long-term steroid use can impair adrenal function in shock states and impair the patient's ability to mount a stress response. A steroid bolus or "stress dose" is indicated for steroid-dependent patients. Beta blockers and calcium channel blockers block the effects of the sympathetic nervous system. They may block the compensatory mechanisms for shock.

(continues)

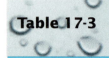

Table 17-3	**Assessment of Fluid, Electrolyte, and Acid-Base Imbalances in the Traumatically Injured Patient—*continued***

Observation	Assessment		Rationale
10. Chemistry, hematology, and arterial blood gas changes	Electrolytes *Serum* K ____ Na ____ Cl ____ Ca ____ Mg ____	*Urine/24 hr* K ____ Na ____ Cl ____	Electrolytes should be drawn immediately after a severe injury and used as a baseline for future electrolyte results. (See Chapters 6, 7, 8, and 9 for normal values.) Urine electrolytes are compared to serum electrolytes. Normal range for urine electrolytes are: K 25–120 mEq/24 hr Na 40–220 mEq/24 hr Cl 150–250 mEq/24 hr
	Serum CO_2	_____	Serum CO_2 >32 mEq/L indicates metabolic alkalosis and <22 mEq/L indicates metabolic acidosis.
	Osmolality Serum Urine	_____ _____	Serum osmolality >295 mOsm/kg indicates hypovolemia/dehydration and <280 mOsm/kg indicates hypervolemia. Urine osmolality can be 100–1200 mOsm/kg with a normal range of 200–600 mOsm/kg.
	BUN Creatinine		An elevated BUN can indicate fluid volume deficit or kidney insufficiency. Elevated creatinine indicates kidney damage. Normal range: BUN 10–25 mg/dL Creatinine 0.7–1.4 mg/dL
	Blood glucose	_____	Blood sugar increases during stress (up to 180 mg/dL, or higher in diabetics).
	Hbg ____	Hct ____	Elevated hemoglobin and hematocrit can indicate hemoconcentration caused by fluid volume deficit (hypovolemia).

(continues)

Table 17-3	Assessment of Fluid, Electrolyte, and Acid-Base Imbalances in the Traumatically Injured Patient—*continued*

Observation	Assessment	Rationale

	Arterial blood gases (ABGs)
	  pH ————
	  $PaCO_2$ ————
	  HCO_3 ————
	  BE ————
		pH: <7.35 indicates acidosis and >7.45 indicates alkalosis.
		$PaCO_2$ (respiratory component):
		 Norms 35–45 mm Hg
		Respiratory acidosis ($\downarrow$ pH, $\uparrow$ $PaCO_2$) may occur due to inadequate gas exchange. A $\uparrow$ pH and $\downarrow$ $PaCO_2$ indicate respiratory alkalosis from hyperventilation.
		HCO_3 (renal component):
		 Norms 24–28 mEq/L
		A $\downarrow$ HCO_3 and $\downarrow$ pH means metabolic acidosis, which is the most common acid-base imbalance following injury from inadequate perfusion and lactic acid production. (See Table 17-1.)
		A $\uparrow$ HCO_3 and $\uparrow$ pH means metabolic alkalosis.
		BE (base excess)
		 Norms +2 to −2. Same as bicarbonate.
		A base excess of < −2 (also termed base deficit) is an indication of poor perfusion/inadequate resuscitation.

23.

Irritability, apprehension, restlessness, and confusion are usually the result of hypoxia and of fluid and electrolyte imbalances. Name two fluid and one electrolyte imbalance associated with the stated behavioral changes.

Fluid imbalances: *_____

Electrolyte imbalances: _____

23. hypovolemia or fluid volume deficit and water intoxication; hypokalemia

24.

Match the neurologic and neuromuscular signs on the left with fluid and electrolyte imbalances on the right:

_____ 1. Decreased sensorium   a. Hypokalemia

_____ 2. Muscle weakness   b. Hypovolemia

_____ 3. Tetany—tremors and twitching   c. Hypocalcemia

24. 1. b; 2. a; 3. c

25. hypovolemia, or a lack of fluid intake; dehydration/ hypovolemia, or lack of fluid intake

26. hypovolemia; 1. a; 2. a; 3. b

27. hypovolemia or shock; dehydration or fluid loss

28. overhydration, or ECFV excess (extracellular fluid volume excess); chest crackles and neck or hand vein engorgement (also constant irritating cough or dyspnea)

29. hypokalemia or potassium deficit or cardiac ischemia; hyperkalemia or potassium excess

30. should not; The patient may need surgery and would be NPO (nothing by mouth).

25.

Oliguria is not uncommon following an acute injury. Decreased urine output can be due to *_____.

Do you recall what elevated specific gravity (>1.030) indicates? *_____.

26.

Vomitus, nasogastric tubes, and diarrhea can cause what type of fluid imbalance? _____.

Indicate which acid-base imbalance listed on the right occurs with the causes of fluid loss listed on the left:

_____ 1. Vomiting   a. Metabolic alkalosis
_____ 2. Nasogastric tubes (loss of   b. Metabolic acidosis
           stomach secretions)
_____ 3. Diarrhea

27.

Pale or gray-colored skin can indicate _____.

Poor skin turgor, dry mucous membranes, and tenacious or sticky mucous secretions are indicative of _____.

28.

When the patient is receiving IV therapy at an increased flow rate to correct fluid loss, the patient should be assessed for potential signs of overhydration.

Excess and/or rapidly administered IV fluids can cause what type of fluid imbalance? _____

Name two symptoms associated with this imbalance. (Refer to Chapter 3, section on ECFVE.) *_____

29.

A flat or inverted T wave can indicate _____, and a peaked T wave can indicate _____.

30.

Immediately after an acute injury, oral fluids (should/should not) _____ be given. Why? *_____
_____

31. d, e; to restore fluid loss and correct shocklike symptoms (correction may be temporary) (also, increase urine output); Water intoxication (ICFV excess). In early shock/trauma massive infusions of D_5W can also cause hyperglycemia. Dextrose 5% in water should never be used as a replacement fluid in shock states.

32. c, d

33. increase (release of potassium from severe tissue damage; if urine output is poor, serum K can also increase); decrease

34. hypovolemia; hypervolemia; It is caused from overhydration or hemodilution (excess water in proportion to solutes).

35. fluid volume deficit or renal insufficiency; renal insufficiency; hypovolemia or fluid volume deficit

31.

Indicate which of the following are crystalloids used in IV therapy for shock states:
( ) a. Dextrose 5% in water (D_5W)
( ) b. Dextran 40, 6%
( ) c. Plasmanate
( ) d. Normal saline (0.9% NaCl)
( ) e. Lactated Ringer's
Give two reasons for using crystalloids. *_____
_____.

What type of fluid imbalance occurs when using 5% dextrose in water as a resuscitation fluid? *_____

32.

Identify the drugs that cause sodium retention or potassium excretion.
( ) a. Diuretics
( ) b. Digoxin
( ) c. Cortisone
( ) d. Diuretics (potassium wasting)

33.

After severe tissue injury, serum potassium levels _____. If lactic acid is released from the cells due to a cellular breakdown, the serum CO_2 would (increase/decrease) _____. Serum CO_2 is a bicarbonate determinant.

34.

A serum osmolality greater than 295 mOsm/kg indicates (hypovolemia/hypervolemia) _____.

A serum osmolality less than 280 mOsm/kg indicates (hypovolemia/hypervolemia) _____. Why? *_____
_____

35.

An elevated BUN can indicate *_____ or *_____.
After hydration, if the BUN does not return to normal, the elevated BUN indicates *_____.

An elevated hemoglobin and hematocrit level can indicate hemoconcentration caused by _____.

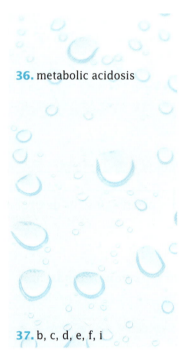

36. metabolic acidosis

36.

What type of acid-base imbalance is present if the patient's arterial blood gases are: pH 7.25; $PaCO_2$ 35 mm Hg; and HCO_3 18 mEq/L? *_____

37.

From the following list of observations and assessments, mark the ones that indicate fluid volume deficit (hypovolemia).

( ) a. Pulse 76
( ) b. Blood pressure 86/68
( ) c. Irritability, restlessness, confusion
( ) d. Specific gravity 1.034
( ) e. Excess GI drainage (>2 liters)
( ) f. Dry mucous membrane and dry, tenacious mucous
    secretions
( ) g. Chest crackles
( ) h. Peaked T waves
( ) i. Elevated BUN and Hgb

37. b, c, d, e, f, i

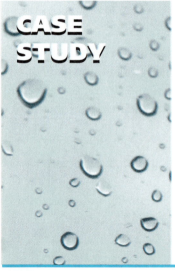

CASE STUDY

REVIEW

A 58-year-old female was in a motor vehicle crash and was taken by ambulance to the emergency department of a large medical center. Her vital signs on admission are blood pressure 134/88, pulse rate 106, respiration 30, and temperature 98.8°F (37.1°C). She complained of pain in her abdomen and leg. A liter of 0.9% normal saline solution (NSS) is started. Blood chemistry, x-rays (leg), and CT scan (abdomen) are ordered. Abdominal area appears distended, and there are diminished bowel sounds. A nasogastric tube is inserted and attached to low continuous suction.

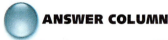

ANSWER COLUMN

1. fluid loss or hypovolemia
   or impending shock

1. The patient's pulse rate indicates tachycardia (mild to moderate) and can be indicative of *_____.

2. normal; heart rate (pulse) was compensating for fluid loss and in response to injury. Later, if heart rate does not compensate, blood pressure will fall.
3. crystalloids. This group of solutions increases fluid volume and acts as a lifeline for emergency IV drugs.
4. Intra-abdominal injury (most likely a traumatized or injured area)
5. to remove accumulated stomach and intestinal fluid (secretions) that resulted from an abdominal injury; gastric decompression

6. a. tachycardia from fluid volume deficit (hypovolemia); b. drop in BP and pulse pressure 20 indicate hypovolemia and shock (impending); c. tachypnea from hypovolemia and stress

7. a. N; b. L; c. N; d. N

8. to monitor urine output (common practice following a traumatic injury); adequate

9. GI injury or abdominal injury

10. hypovolemia and/or hypoxemia

2. Her blood pressure is (normal/high/low) _____ and may mean * _____.

3. Name the solution category for normal saline. * _____

4. A distended abdomen and decreased peristalsis can indicate
*_____

5. The purpose for the nasogastric tube connected to suction would be * _____.

The x-rays showed a fractured right femur and the CT scan of the abdomen revealed possible free abdominal fluid. Vital signs 1 hour later were blood pressure 106/86, pulse rate 128, respiration 34. The patient was apprehensive and restless and had periods of confusion. Blood chemistry results were K 3.7 mEq/L, Na 134 mEq/L, Cl 99 mEq/L, serum CO_2 24 mEq/L. A Foley catheter was inserted, and 350 mL of urine was obtained. The secretions from GI suction were "bloody."

6. Changes in the vital signs indicate:
   a. Pulse *_____
   b. Blood Pressure *_____
   c. Respiration *_____

7. Indicate whether the results from the blood chemistry are normal (N), low (L), or high (H).
   ( ) a. Potassium
   ( ) b. Sodium
   ( ) c. Chloride
   ( ) d. Serum CO_2

8. Why is a Foley catheter inserted? *_____
   Was the amount of urine obtained (adequate/inadequate)?
   _____

9. Bloody GI secretions can indicate *_____.

10. Apprehension, restlessness, and bouts of confusion can indicate _____.

Two hours after admission, her vital signs are blood pressure 84/66, pulse rate 136, respiration 36. Her skin color is gray and she is diaphoretic. Urine output is averaging 15–20 mL/hr. Blood chemistry, type, and cross-match and blood gases are ordered. A second liter of normal saline to run wide open is ordered.

11. hypovolemia (severe) and shock

12. Fluid shifts from the vascular fluid to the cells and to the injured sites (third spaces—abdominal area and injured leg tissue area). Fluids are also lost from GI suction, hemorrhage or blood loss, and from diaphoresis.

13. No. It is less than 25 mL/h.

14. No. Dextrose 5% in water (D₅W) is not an appropriate solution and can cause water intoxication if used in large quantities.

11. Vital signs are indicative of *_____.

12. Explain why there is a fluid volume deficit. *_____
_____

13. Is the hourly urine output adequate? *_____
Why? *_____

14. Is 5% dextrose in water an appropriate IV solution to be used in this case? _____ Why? *_____
_____

She is immediately scheduled for the OR. The second laboratory results are K 5.0 mEq/L, Na 130 mEq/L, Cl 94 mEq/L, serum CO$_2$ 18 mEq/L, blood sugar 166 mg/dL, BUN 32 mg/dL, ABG—pH 7.32, PaCO$_2$ 35 mm Hg, HCO$_3$ 19 mEq/L.

15. a. normal;
b. hyponatremia;
c. hypochloremia;
d. metabolic acidosis;
e. stress; f. hypovolemia/dehydration; g. acidosis;
h. low normal;
i. metabolic acidosis

15. Her lab results indicate:
a. Potassium _____
b. Sodium _____
c. Chloride _____
d. Serum CO$_2$ *_____
e. Blood sugar _____
f. BUN _____
g. pH _____
h. PaCO$_2$ _____
i. HCO$_3$ *_____

● SHOCK

The state of inadequate perfusion, known as *shock,* occurs when the hemostatic circulatory mechanism, which regulates circulation, fails to maintain adequate circulation. With shock, the cardiac output is insufficient to provide vital organs and tissues with blood. There are four categories of shock: (1) hypovolemic, which includes hematogenic from hemorrhage; (2) cardiogenic; (3) septic; and (4) neurogenic.

38.

Shock is a state of *_____.

Shock occurs when the hemostatic circulatory mechanism fails to *_____.

39.

A common feature of shock, regardless of the cause, is a low circulating blood volume in relation to the vascular capacity. There is a loss of blood, not necessarily from hemorrhaging, but from "pooling" in body areas so that adequate blood does not circulate. This causes inadequate tissue perfusion.

A low blood volume is known as _____.

A disproportion between the volume of blood and the capacity (size) of the vascular chamber is the essential feature of _____.

40.

A common feature of shock is *_____.

With shock, is hypovolemia always due to hemorrhaging? _____

Explain. *_____

Pathophysiology

The physiologic changes resulting from shock include a decrease in blood pressure, an increase in vasoconstriction of the blood vessels, an increase in heart rate, a decrease in metabolism (inadequate oxygenation of the blood, electrolyte changes, metabolic acidosis, and a decline in liver glycogen), and a decrease in renal function. Table 17-4 describes these physiologic changes. Study the table, noting if there is an increase or decrease in action or function. Refer to Table 17-4 as needed as you proceed to the questions.

41.

Place I for increase and D for decrease beside the physiologic factors as they occur with shock.

_____ a. Arterial blood pressure

_____ b. Kidney function

_____ c. Heart rate

_____ d. Anaerobic metabolism

_____ e. Vasoconstriction

Table 17-4	Physiologic Changes Resulting from Shock
Physiologic Changes	**Rationale**
Arterial blood pressure: decreased	Reduced venous return to heart decreases cardiac output and arterial blood pressure (BP). Decrease in BP is sensed by baroreceptors in carotid sinus and aortic arch, which leads to immediate reflex increase in systemic vasomotor activity. (This center is found in medulla.) Cardiac acceleration and vasoconstriction occur in order to maintain homeostasis with respect to blood pressure. This may be sufficient for early or impending shock.
Vasoconstriction of blood vessels: increased	Increased sympathetic nervous system activity causes vasoconstriction. Vasoconstriction tends to maintain blood pressure and reduce discrepancy between blood volume and vascular capacity (size). Vasoconstriction is greatest in skin, kidneys, and skeletal muscles and not as significant in cerebral vessels. Coronary arteries actually dilate with a decrease in blood volume. This is a compensatory mechanism to provide sufficient blood to the heart muscle (myocardium) for heart function.
Heart rate: increased	Heart rate is increased to overcome poor cardiac output and to increase circulation. Rapid, thready pulse is often one of the first identifiable signs of shock.
Metabolism: decreased	Unopposed plasma colloid osmotic pressure draws interstitial fluid into vascular bed. Blood loss results in loss of serum potassium, phosphate, and bicarbonate. Inadequate oxygenation of cells prevents their normal metabolism and leads to anaerobic metabolism and the formation of nonvolatile acids (acid metabolites), thus lowering serum pH values. With a fall in serum pH and a decrease in HCO_3, metabolic acidosis results. A rise in blood sugar is first seen due to release of epinephrine; later, blood sugar may fall due to a decline in liver glycogen.
Kidney function: decreased	Fall in plasma hydrostatic pressure reduces urinary filtration. Low blood pressure causes inadequate circulation of blood to the kidneys. Renal ischemia is the result of a lack of O_2 to the kidneys. Renal insufficiency follows prolonged hypotension. Systolic blood pressure must be 70 mm Hg and above to maintain kidney function. One of the body's compensatory mechanisms in shock is to shunt blood around kidney to maintain intravascular fluid. Deficient blood supply makes tubule cells of kidneys more susceptible to injury. Urine output of less than 30 mL/hr may be indicative of shock and/or decrease in renal function.

42.

When there is a low blood pressure, the baroreceptors in the carotid sinus and aortic arch cause an increase in the systemic vasomotor activity that leads to what two activities in order to maintain homeostasis? *_____

42. vasoconstriction and cardiac acceleration; homeostasis

Increased systematic vasomotor activity occurs in order to maintain _____.

43.

Increased sympathetic activity results in (vasoconstriction/vasodilation) _____.

43. vasoconstriction; skin, kidneys, and skeletal muscles; dilate

Vasoconstriction is greatest in what three parts of the body?
* _____.

The coronary arteries (dilate/constrict) _____ with a decrease in blood volume.

44.

Heart rate in shock is (increased/decreased) _____ to overcome poor cardiac output and to increase circulation.

The pulse rate is _____ and _____.

44. increased; rapid and thready; tachycardia

A person with a pulse rate above 120 has (bradycardia/tachycardia) _____.

45.

The following metabolic changes occur with shock:

Fluid is drawn from the interstitial space into the vascular space due to what kind of pressure? * _____

Inadequate oxygenation of cells leads to the formation of nonvolatile acids (acid metabolites), causing the pH to (rise/fall) _____.

A fall in pH and HCO_3 leads to (metabolic acidosis/metabolic alkalosis) * _____.

45. colloid osmotic pressure; fall; metabolic acidosis; rise; fall

In shock, there is a release of epinephrine, which causes the blood sugar to (rise/fall) _____. Later, there may be a (rise/fall) _____ in blood sugar due to a decline in liver glycogen.

46.

In shock, the compensatory mechanisms shunt the blood around the kidney in order to maintain the volume of * _____.
This results in a lack of oxygen in the kidneys known as
* _____, causing a decrease in kidney function.

The systolic blood pressure for kidney function must be at least * _____.

46. intravascular fluid; renal ischemia; 70 mm Hg; 30 mL/hr

An indication of shock related to kidney dysfunction is a urine output of less than * _____.

47.

Extracellular fluid volume shifts occur during shock. In *early* shock, fluid is shifted from the interstitial space to the intravascular space to compensate for the fluid deficit in the vascular system. More fluid in the vascular system increases the venous return to the heart; thus it increases cardiac output.

As the interstitial fluid becomes depleted, tissue (dehydration/edema) _____ occurs.

47. dehydration

48.

In *late* shock, fluid is forced from the intravascular space (blood vessels) back into the interstitial space (tissues).

In *early* shock, fluid is shifted from the *_____ to the *_____. Why? *_____

48. interstitial space; intravascular space; This shift compensates for fluid deficit in the vascular system.

Etiology

The clinical symptoms and related physiologic basis for each of the four types of shock—hypovolemic, cardiogenic, septic (also known as endotoxic or vasogenic), and neurogenic—are presented. Table 17-5 describes the four types of shock, the clinical causes, and the rationale and physiologic changes that occur with each type.

Study the table carefully, noting the causes (etiology) for each type of shock. Refer to the glossary for unfamiliar terms and refer to Table 17-5 as needed.

Table 17-5	Types and Clinical Causes of Shock	
Type of Shock	**Clinical Causes**	**Rationale and Physiologic Results**
Hypovolemic: Hematogenic (from hemorrhage)	Severe vomiting or diarrhea—acute dehydration Burns, intestinal obstruction, fluid shift to third space Hemorrhage that results from internal or external blood loss	Blood, plasma, and fluid loss from decreased circulating blood volume *Physiologic Results* 1. Decreased circulation 2. Decreased venous return 3. Reduced cardiac output 4. Increased afterload 5. Decreased preload 6. Decreased tissue perfusion

(continues)

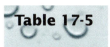

Table 17-5	**Types and Clinical Causes of Shock—*continued***	
Type of Shock	**Clinical Causes**	**Rationale and Physiologic Results**
Cardiogenic	Myocardial infarction Severe arrhythmias Heart failure Cardiac tamponade Pulmonary embolism Blunt cardiac injury (formerly "cardiac contusion")	Because of these clinical problems, the pumping action of the heart is inadequate to maintain circulation. (Pump failure of myocardium.) *Physiologic Results* 1. Decreased circulation 2. Decreased stroke volume 3. Decreased cardiac output 4. Increased preload 5. Increased afterload 6. Increased venous pressure 7. Decreased venous return 8. Decreased tissue perfusion
Septic: Endotoxic Vasogenic	Severe systemic infections Septic abortion Peritonitis Debilitated conditions Immunosuppressant therapy	Septic shock is characterized by increased capillary permeability that permits blood, plasma, and fluid to pass into surrounding tissue. Often caused by a gram-negative organism. *Physiologic Results* 1. Vasodilatation and peripheral pooling of blood 2. Decreased circulation 3. Decreased preload, early shock and increased preload, late shock 4. Decreased afterload, early shock and increased afterload, late shock 5. Decreased tissue perfusion
Neurogenic	Mild to moderate neurogenic shock: Emotional stress Acute pain Drugs: narcotics, barbiturates, phenothiazines High spinal anesthesia Acute gastric dilation Severe neurogenic shock: Spinal cord injury	Neurogenic shock is caused by loss of vascular tone. *Physiologic Results* 1. Decreased circulation 2. Vasodilatation and peripheral pooling of blood 3. Decreased cardiac output 4. Decreased venous return 5. Decreased tissue perfusion

49. hypovolemic, cardiogenic, septic, and neurogenic

49.

The four types of shock are *_____

_____.

50.

Match the following types of shock with the appropriate clinical causes.

    a. Hypovolemic shock

    b. Cardiogenic shock

    c. Septic shock

    d. Neurogenic shock

    _____ 1. High spinal anesthesia, emotional factors, or spinal cord injury

    _____ 2. Hemorrhaging from surgery or injury, burns, or GI bleeding

    _____ 3. Severe bacterial infection, immunosuppressant therapy

50. 1. d; 2. a; 3. c; 4. b

    _____ 4. Myocardial infarction, cardiac failure, and cardiac tamponade

51.

Match the following types of shock with the appropriate rationale.

    a. Hypovolemic shock

    b. Cardiogenic shock

    c. Septic shock

    d. Neurogenic shock

    _____ 1. Failure of the myocardium causes a decrease in the circulating blood volume

    _____ 2. Loss of vascular tone with vasodilation

    _____ 3. Decrease in blood volume due to loss of blood and plasma

51. 1. b; 2. d; 3. a; 4. c

    _____ 4. Increase in capillary permeability resulting from an infection

52.

Match the following types of shock with the physiologic results. Your response may be used more than once.

    a. Hypovolemic shock

    b. Cardiogenic shock

    c. Septic shock

    d. Neurogenic shock

   ____ , ____ , ____ , ____   1. Decreased circulation

         ____ , ____ , ____   2. Decreased cardiac output

         _____ , ____   3. Vasodilatation

       _____ , ____ , ____   4. Decreased venous return

   ____ , ____ , ____ , ____   5. Decreased tissue perfusion

Clinical Manifestations

The clinical manifestations of shock are listed in Table 17-6 with the types of shock and rationale that are related to the signs and symptoms. Immediate medical action needs to be taken when shock occurs so that it can be reversed. Therefore, the health professional should frequently check for signs and symptoms of shock when impending shock is suspected.

    Study Table 17-6 carefully and be able to explain the signs and symptoms that frequently occur in shock.

53.

Two early mental changes occurring in shock are *_____.

  They generally result from *_____.

54.

The central venous pressure (CVP), pulmonary artery pressure (PAP), and pulmonary capillary wedge pressure (PCWP) are decreased in which types of shock?

    ( ) a. Hypovolemic

    ( ) b. Cardiogenic

    ( ) c. Septic

    ( ) d. Neurogenic

55.

Increased rate and depth of respirations are present in shock. Why? *_____.

52. 1. a, b, c, d; 2. a, b, d;
    3. c, d; 4. a, b, d;
    5. a, b, c, d

53. apprehension and restlessness; cerebral hypoxemia

54. a, c, d

55. Increased hydrogen ion concentration stimulates the respiratory center in the medulla; OR nonvolatile acids (acid metabolites) from anaerobic metabolism increase respiratory rate and depth; Note: The purpose of increased rate and depth of respiration is to decrease the acidotic state.

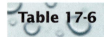

Table 17-6

Clinical Manifestations of Shock

Signs and Symptoms	Types of Shock	Rationale
Skin: pale and/or cold and moist (except when caused by a spinal cord injury)	Hypovolemic Cardiogenic Neurogenic Septic (late)	Pale, cold, and/or moist skin results from increased sympathetic action. Peripheral vasoconstriction occurs and blood is shunted to vital organs. Skin is warm and flushed in early septic shock. Skin is warm and dry in neurogenic shock due to spinal cord injury.
Tachycardia (pulse fast and thready)	Hypovolemic Cardiogenic Septic	Increased pulse rate is frequently one of the early signs, except in neurogenic shock, in which the pulse is often slower than normal. Norepinephrine and epinephrine, released by the adrenal medulla, increase the cardiac rate and myocardial contractibility. Tachycardia, pulse >100, generally occurs before arterial blood pressure falls.
Apprehension, restlessness	Hypovolemic Cardiogenic Septic Neurogenic	Apprehension and restlessness, early signs of shock, result from cerebral hypoxemia. As the state of shock progresses, disorientation and confusion occur.
Muscle weakness, fatigue	Hypovolemic Cardiogenic Septic Neurogenic	Muscle weakness and fatigue, which occur early in shock, are the result of inadequate tissue perfusion.
Arterial blood pressure: early, a rise in or normal BP; late, a fall in BP	Hypovolemic Cardiogenic Septic Neurogenic	In early shock blood pressure rises or is normal as a result of increased heart rate. As shock progresses, blood pressure falls because of a lack of cardiac and peripheral vasoconstriction compensation.
Pulse pressure: narrowed, <20 mm Hg		Narrowing of pulse rate occurs because the systolic BP falls more rapidly than the diastolic BP.
Pressures: CVP, PAP, PCWP— decreased in hypovolemic, septic, neurogenic; increased in cardiogenic	Hypovolemic Cardiogenic Septic Neurogenic	Normal values: 1. Central venous pressure (CVP): 5–12 cm H_2O. With decreased blood volume CVP <5 cm H_2O. 2. Pulmonary artery pressure (PAP): 20–30 mm Hg systolic, 10–15 mm Hg diastolic. With blood volume depletion or pooling of blood PAP in hypovolemic <10 mm Hg, septic <10 mm Hg, neurogenic <10 mm Hg. In cardiogenic shock PAP >30 mm Hg. 3. Pulmonary capillary wedge pressure (PCWP): 8–15 mm Hg. With blood volume depletion or peripheral pooling the PCWP in hypovolemic, septic, and neurogenic <8 mm Hg and in cardiogenic >15 mm Hg.
Respiration: increased rate and depth (tachypnea)	Hypovolemic Cardiogenic Septic Neurogenic	Increased hydrogen ion concentration in the body stimulates the respiratory centers in the medulla, thus increasing the respiratory rate. Acid metabolites, e.g., lactic acid from anaerobic metabolism increases the rate and depth of respiration. Rapid respiration acts as a compensatory mechanism to decrease metabolic acidosis.
Temperature: subnormal	Hypovolemic Cardiogenic Neurogenic	Body temperature is subnormal in shock because of decreased circulation and decreased cellular function. In early septic shock the temperature is elevated.
Urinary output: decreased	Hypovolemic Cardiogenic Septic Neurogenic	Oliguria (decreased urine output) occurs in shock because of decreased renal blood flow caused by renal vasoconstriction. Blood is shunted to the heart and brain. Urine output should be >30 mL/hr.

56. Decreased urinary output is the result of decreased renal blood flow caused by renal vasoconstriction.

57. increase; It will first rise and then fall

58. a. Arterial blood pressure rises, then falls;
b. Bradycardia occurs in neurogenic shock. Tachycardia is common in other forms of shock;
c. Fast and deep; d. X;
e. Not in early septic shock; f. Decreased output; g. It is low in hypovolemic (hematogenic) shock; h. Pale or cold and moist, or both

59. shock

56.

Frequently the urinary output is decreased in all types of shock. Why? *_____

_____

57.

In shock, tachycardia is frequently seen before the arterial blood pressure begins to fall.

The heart beats faster to (increase/decrease)

_____ the circulating blood volume. This is an early compensatory mechanism to overcome shock.

With shock, what happens to the arterial blood pressure?

*_____.

58.

Some signs and symptoms follow. Check the ones that are true about shock. Correct the false ones.

( ) a. Arterial blood pressure low
( ) b. Bradycardia
( ) c. Respiration slow and deep
( ) d. Apprehension, restlessness
( ) e. Temperature low in all types of shock
( ) f. Urine output increased
( ) g. Central venous pressure high in cardiogenic shock and in hypovolemic shock
( ) h. Skin pale and hot

Clinical Applications

59.

Normal blood pressure is the usual level of blood pressure in a person and varies to some extent from person to person.

A systolic blood pressure of less than 90 mm Hg is significant for shock in most people.

A systolic pressure of 70 mm Hg is necessary to maintain the coronary circulation and renal function (urinary output). A person with a systolic pressure of 50–60 mm Hg is said to be in _____.

60.

A low pulse pressure, which is the difference between the systolic and diastolic pressures, is indicative of shock. The systolic blood pressure usually decreases before the diastolic.

To maintain coronary circulation and renal function, the systolic pressure should be at least *_____.

A pulse pressure of 20 mm Hg is indicative of

_____.

60. 70 mm Hg; shock

61.

Blood supply to the organs most susceptible to acute anoxia (absence or lack of oxygen), i.e., the brain and the heart, is maintained as long as possible at the expense of the less vital organs and tissues.

The two organs most susceptible to anoxia are the *_____

_____.

61. heart and brain

The brain can survive 4 minutes in an anoxic state before cerebral damage occurs.

62.

Which of the following physiologic symptoms indicate shock?
( ) a. Arterial blood pressure less than 90
( ) b. Pulse pressure of 55 mm Hg
( ) c. Pulse pressure of 20 mm Hg
Which two organs are most susceptible to acute anoxia?
( ) a. Heart
( ) b. Brain
( ) c. Intestines
The organ that cannot survive anoxia longer than 4–6

62. a, c; a, b; brain

minutes without permanent damage is the _____.

Clinical Management

To maintain body fluid volume and particularly the intravascular fluid, fluid resuscitation must begin immediately for patients who are in shock or impending shock. Improvement of blood volume is needed to maintain tissue perfusion and oxygen delivery. The types of solutions for fluid replacement include crystalloids or balanced salt solutions and colloid solutions.

Crystalloids

Crystalloids expand the volume of the ECF (intravascular and interstitial spaces). The two common types of crystalloids used for fluid replacement are normal saline solution (0.9% sodium chloride) and lactated Ringer's solution. Lactated Ringer's solution contains the electrolytes sodium, potassium, calcium, and chloride with their milliequivalents, which are similar to the plasma values.

Table 17-7 lists examples of crystalloids that can be used for fluid replacement.

63. 0.9% NaCl (normal saline solution) and lactated Ringer's solution

63.

Name two commonly prescribed crystalloids that are used for fluid resuscitation. * _____

64.

Normal saline solution (0.9% NaCl) is a popular IV solution used for fluid resuscitation because it is iso-osmolar (isotonic) (approximately the same milliosmoles as plasma). Excess use of normal saline can increase the serum sodium level and can cause (hypochloremia/hyperchloremia) _____.

64. hyperchloremia; increase

If metabolic acidosis is present, the chloride level can (increase/decrease) _____ the acidotic state.

65.

The lactate of the lactated Ringer's solution acts as a buffer to increase the pH, thus decreasing the acidotic state. Large quantities of lactated Ringer's solution might cause metabolic (acidosis/alkalosis) _____.

65. alkalosis

Table 17-7	Crystalloids for Fluid Replacement						
	mEq/L						
Crystalloids	**Na**	**K**	**Ca**	**Mg**	**Cl**	**Lactate**	**Gluconate**
0.9% NaCl (normal saline)	154	—	—	—	154	—	—
Lactated Ringer's	130	4	3	—	109	28	—

66.

If the patient has a liver disorder, the lactate is not metabolized into bicarbonate; therefore lactic acid can result.

If large quantities of lactated Ringer's solution are administered to a patient with a liver disorder, the metabolic acidotic state can be (intensified/lessened) _____.

Alternating the crystalloid solutions, such as normal saline solution and lactated Ringer's solution, usually (maintains/ disturbs) _____ the electrolyte and acid-base balance.

66. intensified; maintains

67.

Intravenous solutions containing calcium should NOT be administered with blood transfusions. The calcium in the solution precipitates when it comes in contact with blood.

Indicate which of the following solutions can be administered through the same IV line with blood.

( ) a. 0.9% NaCl (normal saline solution)
( ) b. Lactated Ringer's solution
( ) c. D_5W
( ) d. $D_5$0.45 normal saline

67. a

68. hypotonic; The dextrose is rapidly metabolized, leaving water, a hypotonic solution. Use of D_5W can lead to intracellular fluid volume excess (water intoxication) or cellular swelling.

68.

The crystalloid 5% dextrose in water (D_5W) should never be ordered for total fluid replacement during shock. Dextrose 5% in water is an isotonic solution, but if it is used in large volumes, it becomes a (hypotonic/hypertonic) _____ solution. Why? *_____
_____

Colloids

Colloids are substances that have a higher molecular weight than crystalloids and therefore cannot pass through the vascular membrane. Colloids increase the intravascular fluid volume. When colloid therapy is used, less fluid is needed to re-establish the fluid volume in the vascular space.

Table 17-8 lists the colloids that may be used for fluid replacement.

Colloids	Brand Names	Comments
Blood products	Packed RBCs Whole blood	Used to replace blood loss.
Albumin, 5% or 25%	Albuminar Plasbumin	Not used in acute shock; 1–4 mL/min.
Plasma protein fraction, 5%	Plasmanate	Rapid infusion rate can decrease blood pressure.
Hetastarch	Hespan	Synthetic starch similar to human glycogen. Very expensive.
Dextran 40	Dextran	Low-molecular-weight dextran 40 may prolong bleeding time.

Table 17-8 — Colloids

69.

In comparison with crystalloids, colloids are (more/less) _____ expensive. Colloid therapy requires (more/less) _____ solution replacement than needed with crystalloid solutions for fluid replacement.

69. more; less

70.

Colloid solutions are useful in replacing fluid losses from which of the following:
( ) a. Intravascular space (blood vessels)
( ) b. Interstitial space (tissue area)
( ) c. Cellular space (cells)

70. a

71.

Prior to a blood transfusion, what two crystalloid solutions can be used to manage shock? * _____

71. lactated Ringer's and normal saline solution

72.

Which crystalloid solution is the only one compatible to infuse in the same line as blood? * _____

72. 0.9% normal saline solution

73.

The colloids albumin 5%, plasma protein fraction (Plasmanate), and hetastarch increase the vascular volume to approximately the same amount that is infused. With the low-molecular-weight dextran (40), the vascular fluid is expanded by one to two times the amount that is infused. With albumin 25%, the vascular volume is expanded four times the amount that is infused.

To increase the vascular volume more than the amount of colloid that is infused, which of the following colloid solutions might be used?

( ) a. Albumin 5%
( ) b. Albumin 25%
( ) c. Plasmanate
( ) d. Dextran 40
( ) e. Hetastarch

73. b, d

Crystalloids are the first choice for treating hypovolemic shock. Crystalloids can restore fluid volume in the vascular and interstitial spaces and improve renal function; however large quantities of crystalloids are needed. Excessive infusions of crystalloids might cause fluid overload in patients who are elderly or who have heart disease. Frequently, a combination of crystalloids and colloids is used for fluid replacement. If severe blood loss occurs, blood transfusion may be necessary after infusion of 1–2 liters of crystalloids. Each fluid replacement situation differs and each individual situation must be evaluated separately.

There are many suggested formulas for restoring fluid loss, especially for patients in hypovolemic shock who have lost massive amounts of blood and/or body fluid. The simplest formula for fluid replacement is the 3:1 rule: for every 1 mL of blood lost, 3 mL of crystalloid solution is necessary to restore fluid volume (to a point that if hypotension persists despite 2 liters of crystalloid solution replacement, a blood transfusion should be considered). Table 17-9 outlines the calculation of blood loss and fluid replacement for three states of hypovolemic shock from hemorrhage.

74.

If a patient is in Class I shock due to hemorrhage, blood volume loss is *_____ and systolic blood pressure is probably _____. The replacement fluid for this blood volume loss is _____. This shock state is considered _____.

74. up to 750 mL (up to 15% BV); normal; crystalloid; mild

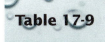

Table 17-9	**Calculation of Blood Loss and Fluid Replacement for Four States of Hypovolemic Shock from Hemorrhage**			
	Class I	**Class II**	**Class III**	**Class IV**
Blood loss (mL)	Up to 750 mL	750–1500 mL	1500–2000 mL	2000 mL or more
Blood loss (%BV)	Up to 15%	15%–30%	30%–40%	40% or more
Heart rate	<100	>100	>120	>140
Blood pressure	Normal	Normal	Decreased	Decreased
Fluid replacement (3:1 rule)	Crystalloid	Crystalloid	Crystalloid and blood	Crystalloid and blood
	Mild Shock State	Moderate Shock State	Severe Shock State	Severe Shock State

75.

If a patient is in Class II hypovolemic shock, blood volume loss is *_____, and systolic blood pressure is probably _____. The replacement fluid for this blood volume loss is _____. The heart rate is probably _____.

75. 750–1500 mL (15–30% BV); normal; crystalloid; >100

76.

If a patient is in Class III or IV hypovolemic shock, the shock state is considered _____. Blood volume loss is *_____; systolic blood pressure is _____; heart rate is *_____. Replacement fluid will consist of _____ and _____.

76. severe; 1500–2000 mL or more (30–40% BV or more); decreased; >120–140; crystalloid and blood

Table 17-10 outlines the clinical management for alleviating four types of clinical shock: hypovolemic, cardiogenic, septic, and neurogenic. Many years ago the first and foremost treatment of shock was to administer a vasopressor drug. The drug constricts the dilated blood vessels that occur with shock and raises the blood pressure. Vasopressors act as a temporary treatment for shock, and the shock continues to increase if the cause is not alleviated or removed. Today vasopressors are only used for severe shock and types of shock nonresponsive to treatment. Note that vasopressors are *not* effective in the treatment of hypovolemic shock, since

Table 17-10		Clinical Management for Various Types of Shock States	
Hypovolemic Shock	**Cardiogenic Shock**	**Septic Shock**	**Neurogenic Shock**
1. O_2	1. O_2	1. O_2	1. O_2
2. IV fluids, such as	2. IV therapy is limited	2. IV therapy crystalloids	2. IV therapy
a. Lactated Ringer's	when pulmonary	3. Vasopressors for	3. Vasopressors, if
b. Normal saline	congestion is present	nonresponsiveness	necessary
c. Blood products	and venous pressure	4. Blood cultures	4. Atropine for
3. No vasopressors	is elevated. Close	5. IV antibiotics	symptomatic
4. Electrolyte	monitoring CVP and		bradycardia
replacement	PCWP		
	3. Vasopressors, if		
	necessary		
	4. Antiarrythmics		
	Sodium nitroprusside,		
	nitroglycerin/NTG;		
	(decrease preload and		
	decrease afterload)		
	Intropic drugs (e.g.,		
	dobutamine,		
	amrinone)		
	Sedatives		
	Diuretics		

Note: Examples of vasopressors are (1) levarterenol bitartrate/Levophed, (2) dopamine hydrochloride, (3) epinephrine infusion.

constricting blood vessels does not aid in the circulation of blood when the cause is most obvious—a lack of blood, causing hypovolemia. Replacing blood volume loss should correct this type of shock. Remember, removal of the cause is first and foremost in alleviating various types of shock.

Study Table 17-10 carefully and be able to explain the treatments for each type of shock.

77. a state of inadequate perfusion; low circulating blood volume or hypovolemia. This can be due to loss of blood from the body or "pooling" of blood in selected areas.

77.

What is shock? *_____

  What is a common feature of shock? *_____

_____

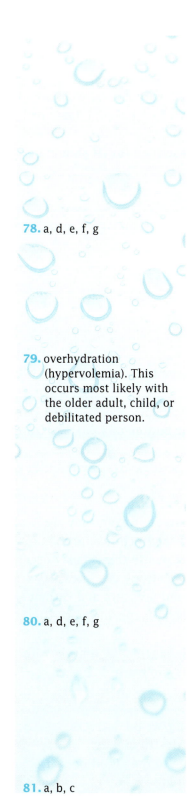

78.

The clinical management for *hypovolemic shock* may consist of which of the following:

( ) a. Blood products
( ) b. Digitalization
( ) c. Vasopressors
( ) d. Oxygen
( ) e. Lactated Ringer's solution
( ) f. Normal saline
( ) g. Electrolyte replacement
( ) h. Lidocaine

78. a, d, e, f, g

79.

When administering crystalloids, such as normal saline or lactated Ringer's solution, for hypovolemic shock, these IV solutions may be given rapidly at first to decrease the symptoms of shock and prevent fluid shift into the interstitial space at the injured site. Later, the flow rate should be slowed.

What type of fluid imbalance can occur if massive quantities of crystalloids are rapidly administered intravenously?

_____

79. overhydration (hypervolemia). This occurs most likely with the older adult, child, or debilitated person.

80.

Clinical management for *cardiogenic shock* may consist of which of the following:

( ) a. IV therapy
( ) b. No vasopressors
( ) c. Antibiotics
( ) d. Oxygen
( ) e. Intropic drugs
( ) f. Sedation
( ) g. Sodium nitroprusside

80. a, d, e, f, g

81.

Clinical management for *septic shock* may consist of which of the following:

( ) a. Blood culture
( ) b. Antibiotics in IV fluids
( ) c. Vasopressors
( ) d. Digitalization
( ) e. Massive IV therapy with whole blood

81. a, b, c

82. Not always. Please check with the health care provider. Frequently, regular doses are given diluted in 50–100 mL of IV solution. IV morphine is given slowly (approximately 5 minutes).

83. b, c

84. Vasopressors constrict blood vessels with the goal of improving circulation; levarterenol bitartrate/Levophed, dopamine HCl, and epinephrine

85. cardiac dysrhythmias

86. strong

82.

Antibiotics and pain medications should be given intravenously if the patient is in shock. Since circulation is poor, medications given intramuscularly (IM) are not fully absorbed. If given IM, after circulation is restored, the accumulated drug in the tissue spaces can be toxic.

Do you think the same dosage prescribed for IM should be given intravenously? *_____

83.

Clinical management for *neurogenic shock* may consist of which of the following:

( ) a. Blood culture
( ) b. Vasopressors
( ) c. IV therapy as needed
( ) d. Massive IV therapy

84.

Explain the action of vasopressors (see introduction to Table 17-10, if necessary). *_____
_____.

The three vasopressors listed at the bottom of Table 17-10 are
* _____
_____.

85.

Vasopressors should be used with care; however, they are helpful at the right time and with the right clinical problem. When vasopressors are used, cardiac dysrhythmias may occur.

Levophed (levarterenol bitartrate), a strong vasopressor, is norepinephrine, which increases blood pressure and cardiac output by constricting blood vessels. Epinephrine works in the same manner.

Maintaining the blood pressure higher than 90 mm Hg with Levophed and epinephrine infusions can cause *_____.

86.

Levophed and epinephrine are (strong/weak) _____ vasopressors and can cause cardiac dysrhythmias.

Vasopressors are titrated according to the blood pressure and should be continuously monitored.

87. dopamine HCl

87.

Dopamine HCl is a catecholamine precursor of norepinephrine. It increases blood pressure and cardiac output.

Levophed causes vasoconstriction, which affects the renal arteries and can decrease kidney function. The vasopressor that is a precursor of norepinephrine is *_____.

88.

Dopamine is helpful in the treatment of cardiogenic shock but is limited when severe hypotension exists.

What two vasopressors can be used in severe shock? *_____
_____

88. Levophed and epinephrine

89. Dobutamine has only a moderate effect on increasing blood pressure.

89.

Dobutamine is an adrenergic drug that increases blood pressure moderately by raising the heart rate and cardiac output. Dobutamine is effective in increasing myocardial contractility. It is frequently used with sodium nitroprusside.

Explain why dobutamine is not used to treat severe hypotension. *_____
_____

90.

Identify the treatments listed below that may be used in various types of shock by placing:

H for hypovolemic shock
C for cardiogenic shock
S for septic shock
N for neurogenic shock

Some treatments may be used for more than one type of shock.

_____ a. IV therapy: lactated Ringer's, normal saline
_____ b. Digitalis products
_____ c. Electrolyte replacement
_____ d. Sedatives
_____, _____, _____ e. Vasopressors
_____, _____, _____, _____ f. Oxygen
_____, _____ g. Limited IV therapy
_____ h. IV antibiotics

90. a. H; b. C; c. H; d. C; e. C, S, N; f. H, C, S, N; g. C, N; h. S

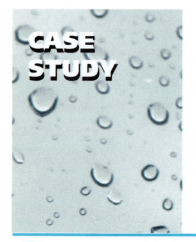

CASE STUDY

REVIEW

A 58-year-old male diagnosed with a ruptured diverticulum, causing peritonitis and systemic septicemia came to the ER. His vital signs are temperature 104°F (40°C), pulse 126 rapid and thready, respirations 32, and blood pressure 65/45. His urinary output is 25 mL/hr. His skin is warm and dry. He is markedly apprehensive and restless. He is diagnosed as being in septic shock.

 ANSWER COLUMN

1. circulation or blood volume

2. capillary permeability, permitting plasma to pass into the surrounding tissues

3. pulse 126, respiration 32, blood pressure 65/45 and low pulse pressure, and apprehension and restlessness

4. septicemia (bacterial infection)

5. shock

6. 30; kidney dysfunction or insufficiency

7. decreased renal function and output. It can lead to renal failure if prolonged.

1. Shock occurs when the hemostatic circulatory mechanism fails to maintain adequate *_____.

2. Septic shock is characterized by *_____
_____.

3. Identify four clinical signs and symptoms of shock.
*_____
_____
_____.

4. The patient's temperature was elevated due to _____.

5. His pulse pressure was 20 mm Hg (65 minus 45), which is indicative of _____.

6. His urine output is _____ mL/hr which is in the low "normal" range. If his urine output goes below 30 mL/hr, what may this indicate? *_____

7. Since his systolic blood pressure dropped below 70 mm Hg, what can occur to his renal function? *_____

8. pulse rate increases; heart beats faster to maintain circulating blood volume. Increased pulse rate is an early compensatory mechanism to overcome shock.

9. severe

10. oxygen, crystalloids, blood culture, IV antibiotics, vasopressors as needed

11. dopamine or Levophed

8. In shock, which frequently occurs first, does blood pressure decrease or does pulse rate increase? * _____
   _____
   Why? * _____

9. Based on his blood pressure, the state of shock is (mild/moderate/severe) _____.

10. Name the five methods for managing septic shock. * _____
    _____

11. If vasopressors were used for the patient, which two would be indicated? _____ or _____

CARE PLAN

PATIENT MANAGEMENT

Assessment Factors

● Check vital signs and report signs and symptoms that may indicate hypovolemia and shock: tachycardia, narrowing of the pulse pressure [difference between systolic and diastolic (less than 20 mm Hg is an indicator of shock)], tachypnea (rapid breathing), and skin cool and clammy.

● Obtain a drug history of the injured patient. Report if the patient is regularly taking insulin, potassium-wasting diuretics, digitalis, steroid preparations, beta blockers or calcium channel blockers.

● Relate acute clinical problem with the signs and symptoms of hypovolemia and shock.

● Assess the behavioral and neurologic status of the injured patient and/or the patient in shock. Irritability, apprehension, restlessness, and confusion are symptoms of deficient fluid volume. Apprehension and restlessness are early symptoms of shock.

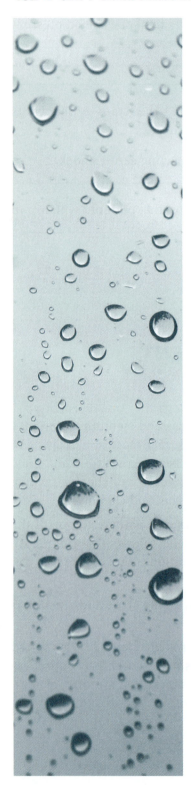

● Check urinary output. Less than 30 mL/hr or 200 mL/8 hr can indicate deficient fluid volume or renal insufficiency. In severe shock, severe oliguria or anuria might occur.

● Check laboratory results, especially ABGs, hemoglobin, hematocrit, serum electrolytes, BUN, and serum creatinine. Report abnormal laboratory results immediately.

Nursing Diagnosis 1

Deficient fluid volume related to traumatic injury and/or shock.

Interventions and Rationale

1. Monitor vital signs. Compare the vital signs with those taken on admission, and report abnormalities immediately. Significant vital sign changes that could be due to fluid loss or shock include rapid, thready pulse rate, drop in blood pressure, and narrowing of the pulse pressure (<20 mm Hg)

2. Check skin color and turgor. Note changes. Pallor, gray, cold, clammy skin, and poor skin turgor are symptoms of shock and deficient fluid volume.

3. Record amounts of vomitus, diarrhea, stools, secretions from nasogastric suction, and drains that contribute to fluid losses.

4. Check the mucous membranes for dryness. Observe for dry tenacious secretions.

5. Monitor IV therapy. Crystalloids are usually rapidly administered initially to hydrate the patient and to increase urine output. Normal saline solution and/or lactated Ringer's solution are the choice crystalloids for fluid replacement. Colloids may be used in combination with crystalloids for the older patient with a cardiac problem (excess fluid should be avoided).

6. Monitor central venous pressure (CVP) and pulmonary capillary (arterial) wedge pressure (PCWP) that is needed to adjust fluid balance. Norm for CVP is 5–12 cm/H_2O and for PCWP it is 4–12 mm Hg. Keeping PCWP between 12 and 15 mm Hg in shock conditions provides the filling

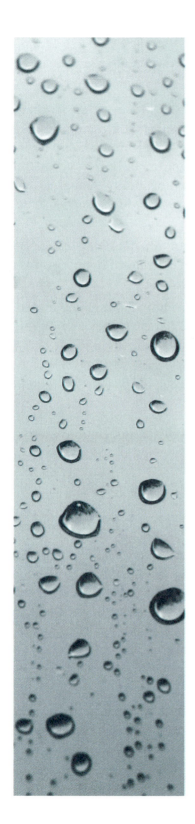

pressure required for adequate stroke volume and cardiac output. If PCWP drops below 8 mm Hg, administration of fluids is usually needed. If PCWP is greater than 15 mm Hg, fluid restriction may be necessary.

7. Draw blood chemistry, hematology, and arterial blood gases as ordered. Report abnormal findings immediately to the physician.

8. Monitor laboratory results, especially the serum electrolytes. The serum potassium (K) levels can vary after trauma. The low K serum level can be due to excess urine output. The serum K level may be normal even though there is a cellular potassium deficit. Hyperkalemia can occur due to excessive cellular breakdown and oliguria (decreased urine output). The serum potassium level should be known before administering potassium in IV fluids.

9. Monitor ECG readings and report arrhythmias, ST-T changes, potassium imbalance, or cardiac ischemia.

Nursing Diagnosis 2

Excess fluid volume related to massive infusions of crystalloids.

Interventions and Rationale

1. Monitor IV fluid therapy. Regulate flow rate to prevent overhydration (hypervolemia).

2. Auscultate the lungs for crackles. Overhydration from excess fluids and rapid administration of IV fluids can cause pulmonary edema and heart failure.

3. Instruct the patient to cough and breathe deeply and/or obtain an order for an incentive spirometer.

4. Check for neck vein engorgement when overhydration is suspected. Check jugular vein at a 45° angle.

5. Check for pitting edema in the feet and legs. Weigh patient daily to determine if there is fluid retention.

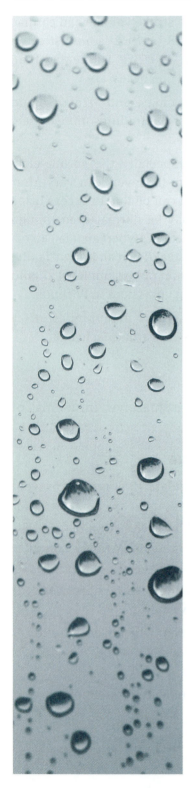

Nursing Diagnosis 3

Urinary retention related to deficient fluid volume and shock.

Interventions and Rationale

1. Monitor urine output. Hourly urine should be measured and, if less than 30 mL/hr, the IV fluid rate should be increased as ordered. Don't forget to check for overhydration when pushing fluids—IV or orally. Renal artery vasoconstriction occurs in shock, which causes a decrease in kidney perfusion.

2. Report systolic blood pressure of 80 mm Hg or *less* immediately. Kidney damage can occur due to hypotension if SBP is less than 70 mm Hg.

3. Check the BUN and creatinine. If both are highly elevated, it could be due to renal insufficiency. If they are slightly elevated and return to normal when the patient is hydrated, it could be due to deficient fluid volume.

Nursing Diagnosis 4

Ineffective tissue perfusion: renal, cardiopulmonary, cerebral, and peripheral, related to decreased blood volume.

Interventions and Rationale

1. Monitor blood pressure continuously when administering vasopressors. Monitor for cardiac dysrhythmias.

2. Monitor arterial blood gases (ABGs). Metabolic acidosis frequently results from cellular damage due to severe hypovolemia and shock. In acidosis, the pH is below 7.35, HCO_3 is below 24 mEq/L, and base excess (BE) is less than -2. Signs of Kussmaul breathing (rapid, vigorous breathing) may be present. Respiratory acidosis may also result due to the lungs' inability to excrete carbon dioxide. The ABGs that indicate respiratory acidosis include pH <7.35 and $PaCO_2$ >45 mm Hg. Dyspnea may be present.

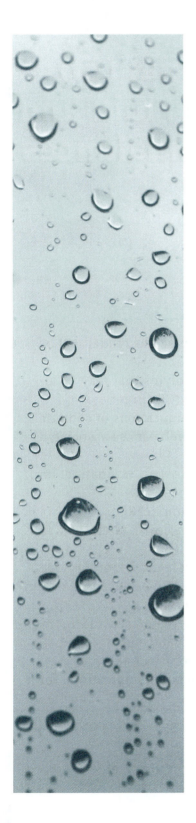

Evaluation/Outcomes

1. Skin warm and dry, mucous membranes moist, pulse and blood pressure within normal range, urine volume and specific gravity within normal range.

2. Weight stable, patient has no crackles, breathing pattern and rate are normal; peripheral pulses are present, no venous neck engorgement, CVP and PCWP are within patient's normal baseline.

3. BUN, creatinine, arterial blood gases, hemoglobin, and hematocrit stable and within normal limits.

4. Patient alert and oriented to person and place, not restless, and there is no peripheral edema.

5. Electrocardiogram ST segment and T wave are within normal limits.

6. Nail beds, oral mucous membranes, and conjunctiva show good oxygenation.

Gastrointestinal (GI) Surgery with Fluid and Electrolyte Imbalances

Erlinda Wheeler, DNS, RN

LEARNING OUTCOMES

Upon completion of this chapter, the reader will be able to:

- Identify five major electrolytes that may be affected by gastrointestinal (GI) surgery.
- Discuss the physiologic implications of sodium, potassium, and chloride imbalances associated with major GI surgery.
- Discuss the effects of gastric intubation on fluid and electrolyte balance.
- Describe the physiologic implications of hydrogen and bicarbonate balance with alterations in the GI system.
- Identify important assessment factors associated with fluid and electrolyte balance that may occur with major GI surgery.
- Identify selected nursing diagnoses and interventions related to fluid and electrolyte balance associated with major GI surgery.
- Identify possible significant complications for bariatric surgery patients.

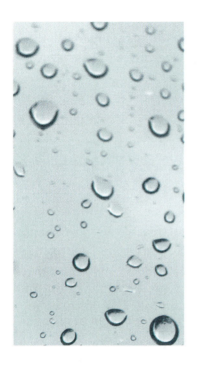

● INTRODUCTION

The main functions of the gastrointestinal (GI) tract are the ingestion, absorption, and transportation of fluids and nutrients. Diseases and illnesses that interrupt these daily functions place the patient at risk for developing fluid and electrolyte imbalances. Diagnostic testing and preparation for gastrointestinal surgery may further increase the patient's risk for fluid and electrolyte imbalance. Postoperatively, the patient may be NPO, have gastrointestinal drainage tubes, and delayed peristalsis. Pre-existing cardiopulmonary, endocrine, and renal conditions in conjunction with diuretics, glucocorticoids, mineralocorticoids, and insulin requirements place the patient undergoing major surgery at risk for fluid and electrolyte imbalances. Impairments in fluid volume status can occur rapidly; astute assessment skills and timely interventions may prevent or decrease potential complications.

● ANSWER COLUMN

1. ingestion, absorption, and transportation

1.
Three of the main functions of the GI tract are *_____ of fluids and electrolytes.

2.
Diseases and illnesses that interrupt the normal functions of the GI tract place the patient at risk for _____ and _____ imbalances.

2. fluid; electrolyte

3.
Postoperative treatment modalities that increase the patient's risk for fluid and electrolyte imbalance include _____, *_____, and *_____.

3. NPO; drainage tubes; decreased peristalsis

4. a. cardiopulmonary disorders (heart failure); b. endocrine disorders (diabetes mellitus), glucocorticoid disorders (Cushing's disease), mineralocorticoid disorders (Addison's disease); c. renal disease (renal impairment or kidney failure). You may have included other conditions as well as the ones mentioned.

4.

Name at least three pre-existing conditions that increase the surgical patient's risk for fluid and electrolyte imbalances.

a. *_____

b. *_____

c. *_____

FLUID AND ELECTROLYTE IMPAIRMENTS

5.

Many patients undergoing gastrointestinal surgery experience fluid and electrolyte imbalances prior to surgery. Treatment of these imbalances must be considered prior to surgery in conjunction with concurrent fluid losses. Replacement of fluid losses is necessary before, during, and following surgery.

Frequently, these patients have a fluid deficit and will need additional fluids to reestablish renal function. Which type of intravenous solution is indicated to reestablish renal function:

( ) a. Hydrating solutions

( ) b. Plasma expanders

( ) c. Replacement solutions with potassium replacement

5. a.

6.

Some patients undergoing gastrointestinal surgery may require fluid and electrolyte replacement therapy for which of the following:

( ) a. Before surgery

( ) b. During surgery

( ) c. After surgery

6. a, b, c

7.

Surgery causes aldosterone secretion, enhancing sodium reabsorption and water retention. When sodium is retained, potassium is excreted. Before administering potassium replacement, it is necessary to make certain that:

( ) a. The patient can tolerate food

( ) b. Renal function is adequate

7. b

8.

After major surgery, there is a tendency for sodium _____, water _____, and potassium _____.

9.

Gastric or intestinal intubation (tube passed into the stomach or intestines) for suctioning purposes may be inserted before surgery. This alleviates vomiting due to an obstruction in the gastrointestinal tract or decompresses the stomach or bowel, or both, before and after an operation.

For gastric intubation, a Levine tube or Salem sump is inserted via the nose into the stomach. For an intestinal intubation, a Miller-Abbott tube or Cantor tube is inserted via the nose and stomach into the intestines. The intestinal tubes are longer than the gastric tube and they contain a small balloon filled with air or mercury on the end which helps the tube pass into the lower intestines. A gastric or an intestinal tube is frequently used following abdominal surgery in order to remove secretions until peristalsis returns and to relieve abdominal distention.

Gastric or intestinal intubation before abdominal surgery is used to *_____

_____

Gastric or intestinal intubation after abdominal surgery is used to *_____ and to *_____.

Table 18-1 lists the electrolytes that are in the stomach and intestines. Note which electrolytes are more concentrated in gastric and intestinal fluids. The patient experiencing vomiting, diarrhea, or intubation (gastric or intestinal) loses fluid and electrolytes. Study Table 18-1 and be able to state which electrolytes are lost.

Table 18-1	Concentration of Electrolytes in the Stomach and Intestine (mEq/L)				
Area	**Body Fluid**	**Na$^+$**	**K$^+$**	**Cl$^-$**	**HCO$_3^-$**
Stomach	Gastric juice	60.4	9.2	100*	0–14	H^{+*}
Small intestine	Intestinal juice	111.3*	20*	104.2*	31*	

*Electrolytes that are highly concentrated in these areas.

10. potassium, chloride, and hydrogen; sodium and bicarbonate (chloride is in high concentration in the stomach and the intestines)

11. sodium, chloride, and bicarbonate; potassium

12. hypokalemia; intestines

13. metabolic acidosis

14. stomach; metabolic alkalosis

15. hypokalemia; metabolic alkalosis

10.
Identify three highly concentrated electrolytes that are lost with vomiting and gastric intubation. *_____
Name two other electrolytes that are lost from the stomach.
*_____

11.
What are the three major electrolytes lost by patients with diarrhea or intestinal intubation? *_____
Another electrolyte lost from the intestines is _____.

12.
Diarrhea can cause (hyperkalemia/hypokalemia) _____.
Potassium ions are more plentiful in the (stomach/intestines) _____.

13.
Intestinal fluids are relatively alkaline. Loss of intestinal fluids due to diarrhea can lead to (metabolic acidosis/alkalosis)
*_____.

14.
Hydrogen is more plentiful in the (stomach/intestines) _____.
What type of acid-base imbalance results when hydrogen is lost? *_____

15.
Name the electrolyte-acid-base imbalances that can occur if potassium, chloride, and hydrogen are lost from the stomach.
*_____

● CLINICAL APPLICATIONS

A retired 68-year-old man was admitted to the hospital for a probable bowel obstruction due to an incarcerated inguinal hernia. He complained of cramping abdominal pain that started 3 days ago and has gradually worsened, becoming severe and continuous pain. He felt bloated, nauseated, and weak. He has been unable to "keep anything down" for the past 3 days. On admission, he had a temperature of 100°F,

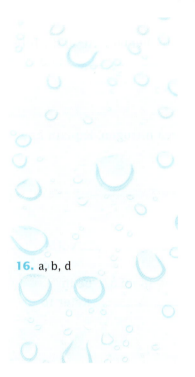

BP 100/70, pulse 90, and respiration 12. Examination of the abdomen revealed a mass in the left lower quadrant and diminished bowel sounds. He has had no bowel movement in the past 3 days. His skin was warm and dry with poor turgor.

16.

Which of the following signs and symptoms might indicate a deficient fluid volume:

( ) a. Vomiting—unable to retain food for 3 days

( ) b. Skin warm, dry, and lacking elasticity

( ) c. Not having a bowel movement for 3 days

( ) d. Weakness

( ) e. Hernia could be manually reduced

( ) f. Severe abdominal pain in left lower quadrant

16. a, b, d

Table 18-2 gives the laboratory studies for the patient and shows how his results changed from the norm at the time of his illness. Use the values throughout the chapter. Refer to Table 18-2 as needed.

Table 18-2   **Laboratory Studies**

Laboratory Tests	On Admission	First Day	Second Day	Third Day	Fourth Day
Hematology					
Hemoglobin (12.9–17.0 g)	21.2	18.4	13.1	13.2	
Hematocrit (40–54%)	58	54	38	39	
WBC (white blood count) (5000–10,000/mm³)	10,700				
Biochemistry					
BUN (blood urea nitrogen) (10–25 mg/dL)*	85	68	68	19	19
Plasma/serum† CO_2					
50–70 vol%	52	61	—	72	50
22–32 mEq/L	24	28	—	38	22
Plasma/serum chloride (98–108 mEq/L)	73	78	73	91	97
Plasma/serum sodium (135–146 mEq/L)	122	128	122	132	145
Plasma/serum potassium (3.5–5.3 mEq/L)	5.2	4.0	4.0	4.2	4.1

*mg/100 mL = mg/dL.

† *Plasma* and *serum* are used interchangeably.

17. 12.9–17.0 g; 40–54%;
5000–10,000/mm³

18. by-product of protein
metabolism; through the
kidney; 10–25 mg/dL

19. 50–70; 22–32; alkalosis

20. K, 3.5–5.3; Na, 135–146

21. a, b, e, f

22. deficient fluid volume (If
you answered
hemoconcentration or
dehydration, OK.)

17.
The "normal" ranges from hemoglobin, hematocrit, and white blood count are *_____, *_____, and *_____, respectively.

18.
BUN is the abbreviation for blood urea nitrogen. Explain how urea is formed. *_____
   How is it excreted? *_____
   What is the "normal" BUN range? _____

19.
The "normal" serum CO_2 range is _____ vol %, or _____ mEq/L.
   Would a patient with a serum CO_2 of 38 mEq/L be in metabolic (acidosis/alkalosis)? _____ Refer to Chapter 12 for further clarification.

20.
The "normal" range of the serum chloride is 98–108 mEq/L. Identify the "normal" range of the serum potassium and serum sodium: serum potassium: *_____ mEq/L; serum sodium: *_____ mEq/L. Refer to Chapters 6–7 for further clarification.

21.
Which of his admission laboratory results indicate a fluid and electrolyte imbalance:
   ( ) a. Hemoglobin 21.2 g
   ( ) b. Hematocrit 58%
   ( ) c. Serum CO_2 52%
   ( ) d. Serum CO_2 24 mEq/L
   ( ) e. Serum chloride 73 mEq/L
   ( ) f. Serum sodium 122 mEq/L
   ( ) g. Serum potassium 5.2 mEq/L

22.
His elevated hemoglobin and hematocrit on admission and the first day postoperatively indicate *_____.

23.

A high BUN is indicative of renal impairment or dehydration or both. His elevated BUN indicates which of the following:

( ) a. An increased urine output

( ) b. A retention of urea, the by-product of protein metabolism, in the circulating blood

( ) c. An abnormal excretion of urea, the by-product of protein metabolism

23. b

24.

The third day postoperatively, his plasma CO_2 increased. This indicates which of the following:

( ) a. An increased bicarbonate ion in the plasma

( ) b. A decreased bicarbonate ion in the plasma

( ) c. Metabolic acidosis

( ) d. Metabolic alkalosis

24. a, d

25.

Below are some of his laboratory results. Use the following symbols to label the imbalance that they might indicate:

D for dehydration

K for kidney dysfunction

E for electrolyte imbalance

M for metabolic alkalosis

O for normal range or for those that do not pertain to the above four

Some results may be associated with more than one imbalance.

_____ a. Hematocrit 40%

_____ b. Hemoglobin 21.2 g

_____ c. BUN 68 mEq/L

_____ d. BUN 19 mEq/L

_____ e. Serum potassium 4.0 mEq/L

_____ f. Serum sodium 122 mEq/L

_____ g. Serum CO_2 38 mEq/L

_____ h. Serum CO_2 28 mEq/L

_____ i. Serum chloride 73 mEq/L

25. a. O; b. D; c. K, D; d. O; e. O; f. E; g. M; h. O; i. E

● CLINICAL MANAGEMENT

Preoperative

The preoperative management for this patient should include:

1. Hydrate rapidly utilizing 4–5 liters over the next 6–8 hours.
2. Insert a Levine tube and connect to low intermittent suction.
3. Prepare for OR for a left inguinal herniorrhaphy and bowel resection to relieve obstruction as soon as he is hydrated.
4. Monitor renal function—urine output.

Solution for hydration: 4500 cc 5% D/$\frac{1}{2}$ NS (dextrose in $\frac{1}{2}$ normal saline or 0.45%)

26.

Which of the following conditions resulted from vomiting?

( ) a. Severe fluid volume deficit
( ) b. Water intoxication
( ) c. A loss of sodium and chloride
( ) d. A low serum bicarbonate level
( ) e. A low serum potassium level

26. a, c

27. before. On admission his potassium was high normal, probably because of the severe fluid volume deficit that caused hemoconcentration.; a, b, c

27.

He was hydrated (before/after) _____ the herniorrhaphy. A gastric tube was inserted to do which of the following:

( ) a. Relieve distention
( ) b. Remove secretions from the stomach
( ) c. Lessen vomiting
( ) d. Provide nutrition

Postoperative

28.

The postoperative fluid and electrolyte management should include the following:

1. Connect gastric tube to low suction and check drainage hourly.

2. Administer and monitor parenteral therapy to run at 125 mL/h.
   1000 cc 5% D/$\frac{1}{2}$ NS
   1000 cc 5% D/NS
   1000 cc 5% lactated Ringer's
3. Ranitidine (Zantac) 50 mg in 100 mL/D$_5$W; infuse 15–20 minutes every 6–8 hours.
4. Check urine output hourly and test for specific gravity and pH.
5. Assess serum electrolyte laboratory findings.
6. Administer antibiotic as prescribed for febrile condition.
7. Encourage patient to cough and deep breathe every 30 minutes for the first 4 hours.

Gastric intubation was initiated following surgery to
_____ and *_____.

28. relieve abdominal distention; remove gastric secretions

29.

Gastrointestinal secretions contain solid particles that may accumulate and obstruct the tube. Irrigating the tube will assure patency and proper drainage.

Frequent irrigations, using large amounts of water, should be avoided to prevent electrolyte washout. Normal saline (0.9% sodium chloride) should be used for irrigation.

Irrigation of the tube assures *_____.

Name the "major" electrolytes lost through frequent gastric irrigation with large quantities of water. _____,
_____, and _____

29. patency for proper drainage; potassium; hydrogen; chloride

30.

The gastric tube should be irrigated at specific intervals with small amounts of normal saline to keep it patent.

A change in the patient's position helps to alleviate tube obstruction.

The use of small amounts of air to check for patency and/or placement of the tube is no longer recommended. Research has determined that the auscultatory method (introducing air and listening with the stethoscope over the stomach for a "whoosh" sound when air is injected into the tube) is not an accurate way of determining patency or placement.

30. irrigate at specific intervals with small amounts of saline and change the patient's position

31. The electrolytes in the stomach would be diluted, and suction would remove them. H_2 receptor antagonists (cimetidine, famotidine, ranitidine) are commonly administered to patients with a gastric tube. These drugs suppress HCl production, thus minimizing the amount of HCl removed by suction.

32. is not; a feeling of fullness, vomiting, abdominal distention, and diminished bowel sounds

33. has not; a small amount of fluid return indicates peristalsis has returned

Two methods to maintain the patency of the gastric tube are

*_____

_____.

31.

Sips of water are allowed to alleviate the dryness of the mouth and lessen irritation in the throat.

Special attention should be taken to limit the amount of water by mouth, because water dilutes the electrolytes in the stomach and the suction then removes them.

What might happen to his electrolytes if he drinks too much of water during gastric intubation? *_____

_____

32.

After the gastric tube is removed, the nurse should observe for:
1. A feeling of fullness
2. Vomiting
3. Abdominal distention
4. Diminished bowel sounds

These symptoms indicate that the gastrointestinal tract (is/is not) _____ functioning.

The four signs and symptoms that indicate peristalsis has not returned to normal are *_____

_____.

33.

Frequently, the tube is clamped for a period of time and then unclamped. The amount of residual gastric fluid is measured. A large residual of gastric fluid released when the tube is unclamped indicates that peristalsis has not returned.

A feeling of fullness, vomiting, and abdominal distention are signs and symptoms that indicate that peristalsis (has/has not) _____ returned.

Using the clamping and unclamping method, how would one know if peristalsis has returned? *_____.

34.

Since suction removes fluids and electrolytes, oral fluid intake is restricted and parenteral therapy is initiated.

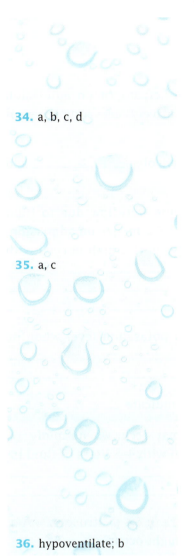

Intravenous fluids containing dextrose, saline, and lactated Ringer's are given to:

( ) a. Replace sodium and chloride loss
( ) b. Maintain nutritional needs
( ) c. Maintain electrolyte balance
( ) d. Replace and maintain the fluid volume

34. a, b, c, d

35.

The patient was given an ampule of sodium bicarbonate IV push. This was given to do which of the following:

( ) a. Increase the plasma CO_2 or bicarbonate
( ) b. Decrease the plasma CO_2 or bicarbonate
( ) c. Reduce his metabolic acidotic state
( ) d. Reduce his metabolic alkalotic state

35. a, c

36.

The patient should be encouraged to cough and deep breathe to help keep the lungs inflated and promote effective gas exchange. Inadequate ventilation due to pain, narcotics, and anesthesia causes alveolar collapse and eventually leads to CO_2 retention (respiratory acidosis).

In respiratory acidosis, the patient would (hypoventilate/hyperventilate) _____.

Indicate the type of breathing associated with alveolar collapse and CO_2 retention (respiratory acidosis). (Refer to Chapter 14 if needed.)

( ) a. Deep, rapid, vigorous breathing
( ) b. Dyspnea—difficult or labored breathing
( ) c. Overbreathing

36. hypoventilate; b

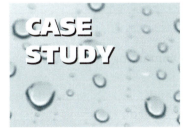

CASE STUDY

REVIEW

Preoperatively, the patient's fluid and electrolyte status and kidney function should be assessed. All laboratory findings should be checked to assess the fluid balance.

ANSWER COLUMN

1. dehydration or hypovolemia

2. dehydration; renal impairment

3. With dehydration, potassium is lost from cells and accumulates in ECF. If urine volume is low, the serum potassium level could increase.

4. serum potassium level decreased, with hydration

5. metabolic alkalosis

6. hypervolemia or overhydration

7. water intoxication. Dextrose is metabolized rapidly by the body, leaving water or hypo-osmolar fluid, which passes into cells.

8. a. sodium; chloride; b. nutritional; c. electrolyte; d. fluid volume

---

1. An elevated hemoglobin and hematocrit on admission and the first day postoperatively are indicative of _____.

2. An elevated BUN is also indicative of _____ and possibly of *_____.

3. The serum sodium and chloride were low due to fluid loss. His serum potassium was 5.2 mEq/L on admission. Explain why his serum potassium is a high normal with vomiting and dehydration. *_____
_____
_____

4. What happened to the serum potassium level when he was hydrated? *_____
_____

5. The increased serum CO_2 may indicate *_____.

6. What type of fluid imbalance may occur when rapidly hydrating a debilitated individual with 4–5 liters of fluid intravenously? *_____
_____

7. If he is hydrated with 4–5 liters of 5% dextrose in water, what type of fluid imbalance might occur?
*_____
Explain why. *_____
_____

8. He received intravenous fluids containing dextrose, saline, and lactated Ringer's for:
   a. Replacing _____ and _____ loss
   b. Maintaining _____ needs
   c. Maintaining _____ balance
   d. Replacing and maintaining *_____

9. depletion of electrolytes in the GI tract

10. irrigating with small amounts of saline and changing the patient's position

11. to determine kidney function. Also, it can be an indication of overhydration. When fluids—orally and parenterally—are being pushed and urine output is low, overhydration can occur.

12. to inflate the lungs and promote effective gas (O_2 and CO_2) exchange

9. Frequent irrigations of the gastric tube with a large quantity of water might have what effect?

_____

10. The two methods used to maintain the patency of his gastric tube are *_____

_____.

11. Why is it important to assess his urine output pre- and postoperatively? *_____

_____

_____

12. Why is it important for him to cough and deep breathe after surgery? _____

_____

● BARIATRIC SURGERY

Obesity is a national health problem that has increased significantly over the past decades. The National Center for Health Statistics shows an increasing proportion of the population to be obese. For the morbidly obese (BMI > 40), surgery is the only treatment that has been proven to have long-term impact on weight control and the comorbidity effects of obesity. With the increasing numbers of obese individuals, the need for bariatric surgery has also increased during the last 5 years. The two most common bariatric surgeries are Roux-en-Y gastric bypass (malabsorption and restrictive) and the adjustable gastric banding (restrictive). The Roux-en-Y gastric bypass creates a pouch by separating the stomach with staples just below the junction of the esophagus, and the jejunum is connected to the pouch. Adjustable gastric banding restricts the volume capacity of the stomach by placing an implantable, adjustable silicon band around the top of the stomach. Long term weight loss and resolution of comorbidities due to obesity can be accomplished through bariatric surgery.

The nursing care of patients after bariatric surgery is similar to most major GI surgery; however, there are some important fluid balance considerations to remember. Patients with gastric bypass surgery commonly experience vomiting and diarrhea, which can lead to dehydration. Early signs of possible dehydration are persistent tachycardia, decreased blood pressure, and decreased urine output. Careful monitoring of the patient's fluid and electrolyte status can prevent dehydration or overhydration. Changes in intake and output, BUN, creatinine, and potassium levels may indicate dehydration.

The use of a nasogastric tube (NG) is dependent on the surgeons' preference. Some surgeons do not insert NG tubes on bariatric patients in order to prevent inadvertent anastomotic complications. If the patient has an NG tube, do not insert air or manipulate the tube for any reason. If the tube accidentally falls out, do not re-insert it.

Bariatric surgery patients remain NPO until a GI series is performed and anastomotic complications ruled out. Unexplained tachycardia, fever, restlessness, and abdominal pain may indicate an anastomotic leak. Patients are maintained on a liquid diet starting with water and advancing to full liquids 30 mL at a time.

Dumping syndrome is a common complication of bariatric surgery occurring in 70% to 75% of bypass surgeries. Signs and symptoms of dumping syndrome include nausea, vomiting, abdominal cramping, diarrhea, diaphoreses, tachycardia, and palpitations. These symptoms are due to fluid shifts from the intravascular space into the lumen of the intestine. The fluid shifts result in rapid gastric emptying, allowing hyperosmolar chyme into the large intestines. Symptoms may appear 30 minutes to hours after eating food with 10 grams of sugar or more.

37.

37. Roux-en-Y and adjustable gastric banding (LAP-BAND)

Bariatric surgery for the morbidly obese has been proven to have long term weight loss effects with a resolution of comorbidities. What are the two most common types of bariatric surgery? * _____

38.

38. vomiting; diarrhea

The two most common side effects of bariatric surgery that can lead to dehydration are _____ and _____.

39. tachycardia, decreased blood pressure, and decreased urine output.

40. increase

41. Fluid shifts from the intravascular space into the intestinal lumen, resulting in a rapid gastric emptying of hyperosmolar chyme into the large intestines.

42. food containing more than 10 grams of sugar

39.
Name the 3 most common signs of dehydration after bariatric surgery. *_____

40.
Dehydration causes the BUN, creatinine, and potassium levels to (increase/decrease).

41.
Dumping syndrome is another common complication in bariatric surgery patients. Explain the physiologic cause of dumping syndrome. *_____

42.
The syndrome occurs within 30 minutes to hours of ingesting: *_____.

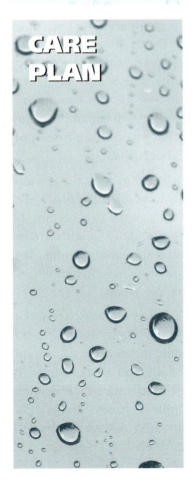

CARE PLAN

PATIENT MANAGEMENT

Assessment Factors

● Patients undergoing gastrointestinal surgery are at an increased risk for fluid and electrolyte disturbances. Preexisting health status and medications further increase the potential risk for fluid and electrolyte disturbances. Patients with pre-existing cardiac, pulmonary, endocrine, and renal disease who have gastrointestinal surgery add further challenges. Uncorrected preoperative hypovolemia and anemia may increase the risk of fluid and electrolyte disturbances postoperatively.

● Astute assessments and early interventions improve the patient's recovery rate and decrease postoperative complications. Fluid and electrolyte imbalances may have deleterious effects on cardiac conductivity, contractility, and rhythm. Pulmonary gas exchange and renal tissue perfusion are also affected by fluid and electrolyte imbalances. Gastrointestinal intubation tubes are used postoperatively to decompress the stomach and intestines to prevent abdominal distension and

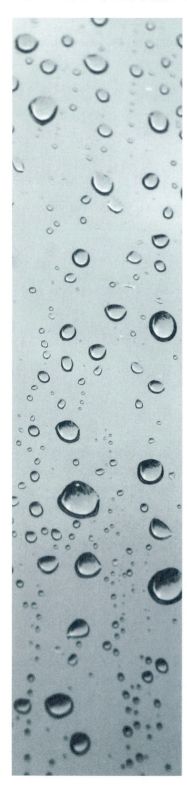

prevent or relieve nausea and vomiting. The amount of GI drainage must be considered when assessing fluid and electrolyte balance.

● To reduce the patient's risk for postoperative complications, assess vital signs with close attention to blood pressure and pulse rate, rhythm, and volume. Decreased fluid volume causes hypotension, orthostatic hypotension, decreased pulse pressure, and reflex tachycardia. Potassium disturbances may cause cardiac conduction and rhythm disturbances. Assess peripheral pulses for presence and quality. Hypovolemic states may decrease peripheral pulse quality and may ultimately lead to peripheral thrombosis in extreme states.

● Auscultate cardiac sounds for presence or worsening of an S_4, which may indicate an overstretched myocardium from a fluid volume excess. Check respirations every 2 hours or more frequently if indicated. Hypoventilation may occur as a result of the decreased rate and depth of respirations due to pain from the abdominal incision and the side effects of anesthesia and pain medications. Ausculate lungs for crackles, which indicate retention of fluid in the alveoli. Frequent coughing and deep breathing will expand the lung alveoli, help prevent the occurrence and buildup of pulmonary secretions, and prevent atelectasis.

● Measure intake and output hourly in the acute stage and every 8 hours for patient's who have stabilized. Careful monitoring of intake and output is essential to ascertain the patient's ongoing fluid volume status. Daily weights are essential for monitoring the overall fluid volume status. Urinary output relative to specific gravity also helps determine the adequacy of the patient's renal perfusion.

● Assess skin turgor at least every 8 hours: Hot, dry, scaly skin with poor turgor indicates a fluid volume deficit. Sacral and/or peripheral edema may indicate an excess fluid volume. Assess serum electrolytes daily and more frequently according to the patient's overall health status. Low potassium (hypokalemia) levels may indicate excess diuresis, inadequate replacement, or postoperative excess antidiuretic hormone release. High potassium levels (hyperkalemia) may

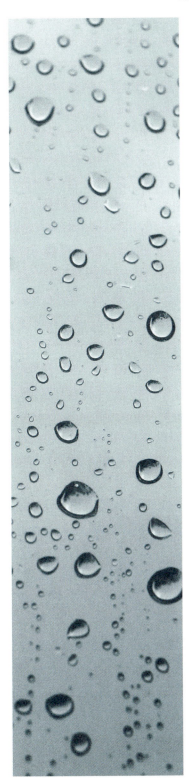

indicate excess potassium administration or impaired renal tubule function even when the total output is adequate in volume. Monitor creatinine/BUN and hemoglobin-hematocrit ratios as an indicator of fluid volume status as well as impaired renal functioning. Creatinine/BUN ratios greater than 1:20 indicate a fluid volume deficit. Hemoglobin-hematocrit ratios greater than 1:3 also indicate a fluid volume deficit.

● Ascertain current and preoperative medication regimes. Potassium-wasting diuretics such as HydroDiuril may further aggravate low potassium levels. Potassium-sparing diuretics such as aldactone may precipitate or further aggravate high potassium levels. Patients receiving steroids also need close monitoring of potassium. Steroids may cause or aggravate hypokalemia and hypernatremia as well as increase fluid retention.

● Assess patient's bowel sounds. Oral fluids and foods are not introduced postoperatively until bowel sounds have returned. Be sure to turn off the suction to GI intubation tubes before auscultation of the abdomen.

● Maintain patency of GI tubes to ensure proper functioning. Irrigating GI tubes with normal saline or air every 2 hours will help ensure their patency. For post–bariatric surgery patients, do not irrigate NG tube with air or manipulate tube. Changing the patient's position frequently helps to prevent the tube lumen from lodging against the gastric mucosa.

● Assess the patient's mental status pre- and postoperatively. Changes in mental status reflecting irritability and confusion may be a primary indicator of excess or deficient fluid volume. Left untreated, the patient's condition may deteriorate to the point of seizures or coma.

● Assess blood glucose for patients with pre-existing hyperadrenal secretions and diabetes mellitus. Uncontrolled hyperglycemia will cause osmotic diuresis and fluid volume deficit.

● Special consideration for post–bariatric surgery patients include possible anastomotic leak manifested by increasing pain to back, shoulder, and abdomen; tachycardia; and restlessness.

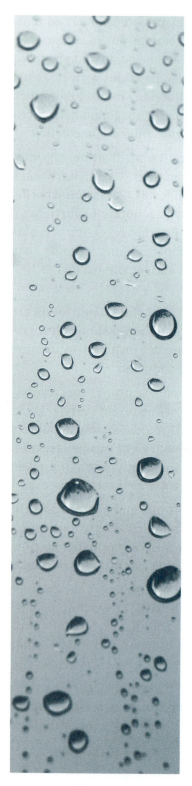

Nursing Diagnosis 1

Ineffective airway clearance related to pain, ineffective coughing, deep breathing, and viscous mucous secretions.

Interventions and Rationale

1. Elevate head of bed 45°–90° and change every 2 hours to promote lung expansion and take advantage of gravity decreasing diaphragmatic pressure.

2. Encourage coughing and deep breathing hourly while awake, and wake every 2–4 hours during sleeping hours, to improve alveolar expansion, mobilize secretions, and prevent atelectasis.

3. Splint abdominal incision to decrease pain and maximize effects of coughing and deep breathing exercises. (Administer pain medication as often as needed.)

4. Suction orally and/or nasotracheally to clear airway.

5. Auscultate lung fields for crackles and respiratory movement.

6. Observe for signs of respiratory distress—tachypnea, restlessness, anxiety, moistness of mucous membranes, and use of accessory muscles of breathing.

7. Maintain adequate hydration to liquify and mobilize pulmonary secretions.

8. Provide opportunities for rest to prevent fatigue and facilitate coughing and deep breathing.

Nursing Diagnosis 2

Deficient fluid volume related to GI loss, decreased fluid intake, and fluid volume shift.

Interventions and Rationale

1. Monitor intake and output at least every 8 hours and weigh daily to determine changes in fluid volume. In normovolemic patients, intake should be approximately 500 mL more than output in a 24-hour period. For hypovolemic patients intake should be greater than 500 mL for the total

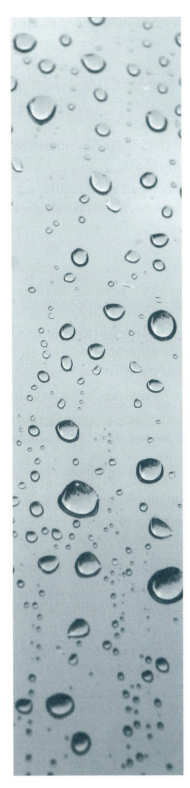

output in 24 hours. Hypervolemic patients should have an output equal to or greater than their intake.

2. Take blood pressure and pulse (include orthostatics) every 4 hours or more frequently if patient is unstable. Hypovolemic patients will have reflex tachycardia and hypotension. A blood pressure decrease of more than 20 mm Hg systolic or a pulse increase of more than 10 beats per minute with position changes indicates hypovolemia.

3. Check mucous membranes and skin turgor. Poor skin turgor with dry, scaly skin and dry mucous membranes indicates a fluid volume deficit.

4. Check temperature every 4 hours. Body water acts as a coolant and temperature increases as body water decreases.

5. Monitor for peripheral and sacral edema to determine fluid shifts from ECF to ICF volume.

6. Palpate peripheral pulses every 4 hours for presence and volume. Hypovolemia decreases the volume of peripheral pulses.

7. Assess creatinine/BUN and Hgb-Hct ratios for hemoconcentration, which indicates hypovolemia versus renal failure.

8. Assess serum potassium and sodium to determine changes. Hyperkalemia and hypernatremia may be early indicators of decreased body waters.

9. Measure urine specific gravity every 8 hours as the fluid volume decreases, unless there is renal failure.

10. Note medications that can alter fluid status and electrolyte alterations such as diuretics, insulin, and steroids.

Nursing Diagnosis 3

Acute pain related to trauma of abdominal surgery, decreased or absent bowel sounds, and decreased GI motility.

Interventions and Rationale

1. Ascertain cause of pain and treat accordingly. Medicate for surgical wound pain. Ascertain and maintain the correct

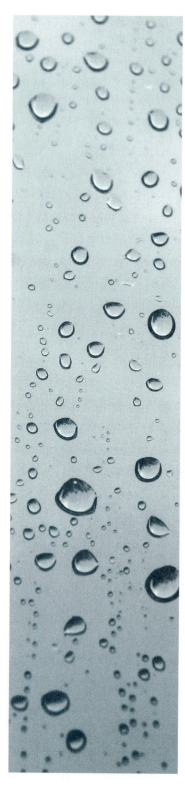

functioning of GI tubes to decrease distention, nausea, and vomiting.

2. Evaluate patient's response and tolerance of pain. Determine pain characteristics and degree of pain; use a 0–10 scale. Observe verbal and nonverbal cues. Explore cultural aspects of pain and methods of control.

3. Medicate for pain to enhance effectiveness of ambulation, coughing, and deep breathing exercises.

4. Use diversional activities to increase pain threshold, e.g., visitors, television, calm environment, relaxation exercises, and reading.

Evaluation/Outcomes

1. Confirm that the source of the ECFV problem has been eliminated or controlled.

2. Evaluate the effectiveness of interventions (fluid replacement therapy, medications, pain control measures, etc.) in balancing fluid needs and promoting comfort.

3. Monitor intake and output for effective regulation of fluid and electrolyte replacement.

4. Monitor vital signs (particularly BP and pulse) for stability or indications of a fluid imbalance.

5. Evaluate mucous membranes and skin turgor for appropriate oxygenation and return to normal pink status.

6. Monitor creatinine/BUN and Hgb-Hct ratios for return to normal range.

7. Monitor electrolyte (Na, Cl, K, Ca) and blood gas levels to confirm fluid and electrolyte balance.

8. Monitor urine specific gravity to detect potential renal problems.

9. Evaluate effectiveness of medications (diuretics, insulin, steroids, etc.) in maintaining fluid balance.

Renal Failure: Hemodialysis, Peritoneal Dialysis, and Continuous Renal Replacement Therapy

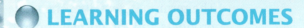

LEARNING OUTCOMES

Upon completion of this chapter, the reader will be able to:

- Discuss the physiologic changes related to acute and chronic renal failure.
- Identify the etiologic factors associated with acute renal failure and chronic kidney disease.
- Discuss common fluid, electrolyte, and acid-base imbalances in renal failure.
- Define the three types of clinical management for renal failure.
- Discuss the purposes for continuous renal replacement therapy (CRRT), hemodialysis, and peritoneal dialysis.
- Discuss the important assessment factors associated with the clinical management of renal failure.
- Describe selected complications associated with the clinical management of renal failure.
- List selected nursing diagnoses and interventions with rationales for patients with renal failure.

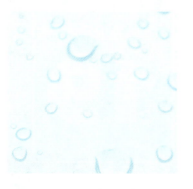

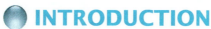

● INTRODUCTION

Renal failure is the inability of the kidneys to excrete the waste of cell metabolism and normal amounts of body water. Renal failure is classified as acute or chronic. *Acute renal failure (ARF)* results from an acute insult, primarily ischemia, toxicity, or obstruction. *Chronic kidney disease (CKD)* frequently results from a disease process that affects the renal parenchyma and eventually causes cessation of renal function.

● ANSWER COLUMN

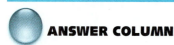

1. renal failure

1.

The term that describes the kidneys' inability to excrete waste products and the normal amounts of body water is *_____.

● PATHOPHYSIOLOGY

Acute renal failure (ARF) may progress through four phases: (1) initiating, (2) oliguric, (3) diuretic, and (4) recovery. The characteristics of these four phases are described in Table 19-1.

2.

When the urinary volume is less than 400 mL/day and azotemia is present, the patient is in the _____ phase.

Table 19-1   Phases of ARF

Phases	Characteristics
Initiating	This phase begins when the insult occurs and continues until signs of azotemia and/or oliguria appear. This can last hours to days.
Oliguric	Urine output is less than 400 mL/day. BUN and creatinine are markedly elevated. Dialysis is initiated in this phase. This phase can last from 10–14 days.
Diuretic	It starts with a gradual increase in urine output, 1–3 liters (1000 mL to 3000 mL) or more per day up to 5–6 L (5000 mL to 6000 mL) per day. Nephrons do not concentrate urine sufficiently to conserve electrolytes and water. Risk of dehydration and death are high. This phase can continue for days to weeks.
Recovery	This phase is noted by a decrease in azotemia with kidneys showing an ability to concentrate urine. It may last from weeks to months.

2. oliguric; diuretic; dehydration (if you answered electrolyte loss, true, but the greatest risk is ECFV deficit or dehydration)

3. recovery phase

If a sudden increase in urine output occurs (1.5 liters or more per day), the patient is in the _____ phase. In the diuretic phase the greatest risk is _____.

3.

The phase of ARF in which the kidneys can concentrate urine and azotemia is less apparent is called the *_____.

Chronic kidney disease (CKD) is defined as an insidious progressive loss of renal function that is irreversible. The five stages are characterized by the presence or absence or kidney damage and the level of kidney function. The level of functioning is measured by the GFR (glomerular filtration rate). This is a measurement of kidney function obtained by estimating the kidneys' capacity to filter. The higher the number, the better the kidneys are able to filter. Individuals with higher CKD stages have lower GFR levels. Table 19-2 lists the five stages and the characteristics associated with these stages.

4. end-stage renal disease (ESRD)

4.

Stage 5 of chronic kidney disease is also known as *_____.

5. slightly damaged with normal of increased filtration; mildly decreased; moderately decreased; severely decreased; failed

5.

In stage 1, kidney function is *_____.
In stage 2, kidney function is *_____.
In stage 3, kidney function is *_____.
In stage 4, kidney function is *_____.
In stage 5, kidney function has *_____.

Table 19-2	**Stages of CKD**	
Stage	**Characteristics**	**GFR mL/min/1.73m²**
1	Slight kidney damage with normal or increased filtration	More than 90
2	Mild decrease in kidney function	60–89
3	Moderate decrease in kidney function	30–59
4	Severe decrease in kidney function	15–29
5	Kidney failure requiring dialysis or transplantation (also known as end-stage renal disease, or ESRD)	Less than 15

Adapted from "Clinical practice guidelines for chronic kidney disease: evaluation, classification, and stratification," by National Kidney Foundation K/DOQI, 2002, *American Journal of Kidney Diseases*, 39 (Suppl. 1), p. S1.

6. filter

6.

Glomular filtration rate (GFR) measures the kidneys' capacity to _____.

7. lower

7.

Individuals with higher stages of CKD have (higher/lower) _____ GFR levels.

● ETIOLOGY

The causes of ARF are listed in three categories: ischemia, toxicity, and obstruction. Table 19-3 lists examples of the causes, with contributing problems.

8. ischemia, toxicity, and obstruction

8.

Acute renal failure usually results from insult to the kidney causing a rapid deterioration of renal function. The three major categories of the causes of ARF are *_____.

9. shock; antibiotics such as aminoglycosides; arterial emboli (prerenal) or ureteral obstruction (postrenal)

9.

Give examples of the following major causes of ARF:

Ischemia: _____

Toxicity: _____

Obstruction: *_____

Table 19-3	**Causes of ARF**	
Ischemia	**Toxicity**	**Obstruction**
Dehydration	Antibiotics:	Prerenal:
Shock:	Aminoglycosides	Arterial emboli
Distributive/sepsis	Penicillins	Aneurysm
Hypovolemic/hemorrhagic	Cephalosporins	Postrenal:
Cardiogenic	Nonsteroidal anti-inflammatory drugs	Ureteral obstruction
Type I and Type II diabetes	Organic compounds or solvents	Bladder obstruction
	Carbon tetrachloride	Catheter obstruction
	Methyl alcohol	
	Miscellaneous:	
	Myoglobin, transfusion reactions	
	Contrast media	

Table 19-4	Causes of CKD
Etiology	**Examples**
Congenital/developmental disorders	Bilateral renal hypoplasia
	Fused kidney
	Ectopic or displaced kidney
	Bilateral renal dysplasia
Cystic disorders	Polycystic kidney disease
	Medullary cystic kidney disease
Tubular disorders	Renal tubular acidosis (RTA)
	Fanconi's syndrome
Glomerular disorder	Glomerulonephritis (major cause of ESRD)
Neoplasms	Benign tumor
	Malignant tumor
	Wilms' tumor
Infectious diseases	Pyelonephritis
	Renal tuberculosis
Obstructive disorders	Nephrolithiasis
	Retroperitoneal fibrosis
Systemic diseases	Diabetes mellitus (DM): approximately 25% of ESRD patients with DM. Approximately 50% of Type I DM (juvenile onset) develop ESRD within 20 years of onset of DM.
	Diabetes insipidus
	Systemic lupus erythematosus (SLE)
	Hepatorenal syndrome
	Hypertensive nephropathy
	Amyloidosis
	Scleroderma
	Primary hyperparathyroidism
	Goodpasture's syndrome
	Henoch-Schöenlein purpura

10. pyelonephritis; glomerulonephritis

10.

An example of an infectious disease causing (CKD) is _____. A major cause of end-stage renal disease (ESRD) is _____.

11. diabetes mellitus

11.

Approximately 25% of the patients with ESRD have the systemic chronic disease *_____.

12. diabetes mellitus, diabetes insipidus, hepatorenal syndrome, hypertensive nephropathy, and systemic lupus erythematosus (others: scleroderma, amyloidosis)

12.

Name five systemic diseases that can lead to ESRD. *_____

_____

13.

Urine output in renal failure varies. No urine output is labeled *anuria*. In ARF the cause of anuria may be prerenal or postrenal obstruction. In CKD anuria indicates total loss of parenchymal function.

ARF means *_____.

CKD means *_____.

   Anuria, which is *_____, differs in ARF and CKD.

In ARF anuria may be the result of *_____, and in CKD anuria may cause _____

*_____.

13. acute renal failure; chronic kidney disease; no urine output; prerenal or postrenal obstruction; total loss of parenchymal function

14.

Normal urine output exceeds 30 mL. Urine output of less than 400–500 mL per 24 hours is *oliguria*. No urine output is called

_____.

   In ARF ischemia and nephrotoxicity are the causes of oliguria, whereas in CKD oliguria indicates a decline in parenchymal function.

14. anuria

15.

Symptoms of ARF and CKD appear when renal function decreases to at least 20%. When renal function decreases to less than 10%, death results if dialysis treatment is not initiated.

   Indicate which of the following problems contribute to acute and chronic renal failure by using ARF for acute renal failure and CKD for chronic kidney disease.

_____ a. Severe dehydration (hypovolemia)
_____ b. Diabetes mellitus
_____ c. Bladder obstruction
_____ d. Glomerulonephritis
_____ e. Hypertension nephropathy
_____ f. Severe fluid volume deficit
_____ g. Systemic lupus erythematosus
_____ h. Aminoglycoside therapy
_____ i. Pyelonephritis

15. a. ARF; b. CKD; c. ARF;
d. CKD; e. CKD; f. ARF;
g. CKD; h. ARF; i. CKD;
j. CKD; k. ARF; l. ARF

_____ j. Nephrosclerosis

_____ k. Carbon tetrachloride

_____ l. Sepsis

● CLINICAL MANIFESTATIONS

16.

Two measurements of nitrogenous waste products, by-products of protein metabolism, are BUN and creatinine. A rise in the level of BUN and creatinine is known as azotemia.

The two by-products of protein metabolism or nitrogenous waste products are *_____. Azotemia occurs when *_____.

16. BUN and creatinine; BUN and creatinine levels rise

17.

In ARF, the earliest sign after the insult is a rise in the BUN and serum creatinine accompanied by oliguria or nonoliguria.

The two renal laboratory results that can indicate an early sign of ARF are *_____.

The earliest manifestations of the disease that may lead to CKD are hematuria and proteinuria. At least 50% or more loss of renal tissue is required before signs are evident. If undetected, renal disease progresses, renal function degenerates, and azotemia ensues. No symptoms are evident until loss of renal tissue is at least 80%.

17. increased BUN and increased serum creatinine

18.

In ARF oliguria is usually caused by _____ and _____. In CKD oliguria indicates *_____.
In CKD two early manifestations of renal disease are _____.

18. ischemia and nephrotoxicity; a decline in parenchymal function; hematuria and proteinuria

Fluid, Electrolyte, and Acid-Base Imbalances

Table 19-5 outlines the fluid, electrolyte, and acid-base changes that occur in renal failure and lists the rationale for the signs and symptoms. Study Table 19-5 carefully, noting the changes that occur.

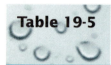

Table 19-5	Fluid, Electrolyte, and Acid-Base Imbalances in Renal Failure	
Imbalances	**Rationale**	**Signs and Symptoms**
Fluid Overload Decreased urine output	Inability of the kidneys to concentrate, dilute, and excrete urine with normal or excessive intake of fluid. When creatinine clearance is less than 4–5 mL/min, volume overload is usually the major problem.	Noninvasive: elevated jugular venous pressure Pitting edema: preorbital, hands, feet, sacral, anasarca
Sodium retention	Increased tubular reabsorption of sodium due to reduced renal perfusion and/or increased renin-angiotensin-aldosterone secretion. Occurs in ischemia and malignant hypertension.	Increased blood pressure Weight gain Moist crackles Dyspnea Pulmonary edema
Reduced oncotic pressure	Loss of intravascular protein through damaged glomeruli leads to decreased intravascular volume. ADH secretion increases water retention to maintain intravascular volume. Continued protein loss decreases oncotic pressure in capillaries and causes water to move into the interstitial space. Seen in nephrotic syndrome, glomerular diseases, and liver ascites.	Invasive: increased central venous pressure Elevated pulmonary artery and wedge pressure
Potassium Excess Potassium retention	*Hyperkalemia* Inability of the kidneys to excrete potassium in severe oliguric and anuric states.	Noninvasive: weakness, parathesia Nausea, vomiting ECG: elevated T wave Ventricular tachycardia Cardiac arrest
Cellular injury	Massive tissue injury, acidosis, and protein catabolism cause potassium to leave cells.	Invasive: serum K>5.3mEq/L Decreased pH (arterial blood) Decreased serum CO_2 and arterial HCO_3
Potassium Deficit Potassium loss	*Hypokalemia* Excessive loss of GI secretions or excessive loss in dialysis.	Noninvasive: muscle weakness Abdominal distention Arrhythmia
Diuretic phase of ARF	Excessive loss of electrolytes and water due to the kidneys' inability to concentrate urine.	Anorexia, N/V ECG: flat or inverted T wave, prominent U wave, and AV block
Renal tubular acidosis	Nonoliguric azotemia causes excretion of K^+. Present in Fanconi's syndrome, nephrotic syndrome, multiple myeloma, cirrhosis, and some drug toxicities.	Invasive: serum K<3.5 mEq/L
Sodium Excess Increased tubular sodium absorption	*Hypernatremia* With decreased intravascular volume, aldosterone secretion increases sodium retention to improve intravascular volume. May be seen in nephrotic syndrome and liver ascites.	Noninvasive: edema Dry tongue Tachycardia Thirst Weight gain Increased BP

(continues)

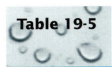

Table 19-5

Fluid, Electrolyte, and Acid-Base Imbalances in Renal Failure—*continued*

Imbalances	Rationale	Signs and Symptoms
Dietary sodium ingestion	Increased dietary ingestion of sodium, especially in anuric states.	Invasive: serum Na >145 mEq/L
Sodium Deficit	*Hyponatremia*	
Sodium loss	Excessive loss of gastrointestinal secretions through suction, vomiting, and diarrhea.	Noninvasive: decreased skin turgor Decreased BP
Diuretic phase of ARF	Excessive loss of electrolytes and water because of the kidneys' inability to concentrate urine.	Rapid pulse Dry mucous membrane Muscle weakness Invasive: serum Na <130 mEq/L
Excessive fluid intake	Increased fluid intake with oliguria or anuria dilutes the serum sodium level.	
Metabolic acidosis	Sodium shifts into cells as potassium shifts to plasma during acidosis.	
Phosphorus Excess	*Hyperphosphatemia*	
Phosphorus (phosphate) retention	Occurs because of decreased renal phosphate excretion, which increases metabolic acidosis. Phosphorus affects serum calcium level by altering the balance of their reciprocal relationships. Parathyroid hormone (PTH) (parathormone) enhances phosphorus or phosphate excretion in the urine.	Noninvasive: nausea and diarrhea Tachycardia Tetany with low Ca Hyperreflexia Muscle weakness Flaccid paralysis Invasive: serum P >4.5 mg/dL or >2.6 mEq/L
Calcium Deficit	*Hypocalcemia*	
Increased phosphorus retention	Decreases the balance between calcium and phosphorus. PTH demineralizes the bone to increase serum calcium. Untreated hypocalcemia and hyperphosphatemia lead to renal osteodystrophy and metastatic calcification (deposits of calcium phosphate crystals in soft tissues). The goal is to maintain serum Ca-P product of approximately 40 mg/mL.	Noninvasive: tetany Muscle twitching Tingling Carpopedal spasm Laryngeal spasm Abdominal cramps Muscle cramps Decreased clotting Cardiac dysrhythmias Positive Chvostek sign Positive Trousseau sign
Decreased absorption of calcium from intestines	Impaired vitamin D activity from renal impairment causes reduced calcium absorption.	Invasive: serum Ca <9 mg/dL or <4.5 mEq/L PTH >375 mEq/mL Ca-P product >70 mg/dL
Metabolic Acidosis		
Hydrogen ion retention	Inability of kidneys to excrete daily hydrogen ion load.	Noninvasive: weakness Lassitude; Increased respiration (rate and depth)
Reduced buffering mechanisms in tubules	Refer to Chapter 11, on renal regulatory mechanisms.	Restlessness Flushed skin
Ammonia	Reduced nephron function inhibits conversion of ammonia and HCl to NH_4Cl for excretion.	Invasive pH <7.35 HCO_3 <24 mEq/L Anion gap >16 mEq/L

(continues)

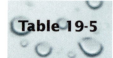

Table 19-5	Fluid, Electrolyte, and Acid-Base Imbalances in Renal Failure—*continued*	
Imbalances	**Rationale**	**Signs and Symptoms**
Phosphate salts	Reduced nephron function inhibits the combination of hydrogen ions with $NaHPO_4$ to form NaH_2PO_4 for excretion.	
Bicarbonate (HCO_3)	With damaged nephrons, less HCO_3 is regenerated and reabsorbed in the tubules.	
Retention of metabolic acids	Inability of the kidneys to excrete uric, sulfuric, phosphate, and other acids of metabolism.	
Lactic acid formation	Occurs from tissue hypoxemia from an ischemic insult.	
Increased fat breakdown	Malnutrition from decreased nutritional intake causes accumulation of ketone acids.	
Urine Sodium and Osmolality		
Urine sodium	Ischemic state increases ADH and aldosterone secretions. Renal efforts to conserve sodium show fewer Na ions in urine, <20 mEq. However, damaged nephrons cannot filter sufficiently; therefore it is possible that urine sodium level >20 mEq.	
Urine osmolality	Ischemic state increases renal filtration; thus urine osmolality >500 mOsm/kg/H_2O. Injured nephrons with impaired filtration have urine osmolality similar to plasma, 290 mOsm/kg/H_2O.	

19. a. decreased urine output; b. sodium retention; c. reduced oncotic pressure

20. elevated jugular venous pressure, pitting edema, weight gain, increased blood pressure, dyspnea, and increased central venous pressure (others: moist crackles, pulmonary edema, elevated pulmonary artery, and wedge pressures)

21. severe oligura and anuria; ventricular tachycardia and cardiac arrest

19.

In renal failure fluid overload can occur from the following pathologic responses:

a. *_____

b. *_____

c. *_____

20.

Name six symptoms of fluid overload (noninvasive and invasive).

*_____

_____

21.

A potassium excess occurs primarily with which urinary symptoms? *_____.

A potassium excess can cause cardiac muscle to exhibit which two symptoms? *_____.

22. a. loss of GI secretions or dialysis; b. diuretic phase of ARF; c. renal tubular acidosis

22.
Name the conditions that may cause potassium deficits.

a. *_____

b. *_____

c. *_____

23. a. increased tubular absorption; b. dietary ingestion

23.
Name the conditions that may cause sodium excess.

a. *_____

b. *_____

24. a. loss of GI secretions; b. diuretic phase of ARF; c. excessive fluid intake; d. metabolic acidosis

24.
Name the conditions that may cause sodium deficits.

a. *_____

b. *_____

c. *_____

d. *_____

25.
An excess serum phosphorus/phosphate level in renal failure is caused by *_____. The retention of phosphorus/phosphate alters the balance between calcium and phosphorus. The result of the calcium imbalance is

_____.

25. decreased excretion of phosphate; hypocalcemia or calcium loss (deficit)

26. muscle twitching, tingling, and laryngeal spasms (also carpopedal spasm and positive Chvostek's and Trousseau's signs); metabolic acidosis

26.
Calcium deficit results in symptoms of tetany, three of which are

*_____

In which acid-base imbalance are the symptoms of tetany decreased? *_____.

27.
Calcium deficits enhance the toxic effect of a high serum potassium by increasing cardiac muscle irritability.

When a low serum calcium exists, the serum potassium must be monitored to prevent *_____.

27. cardiac muscle irritability

28.
Name the metabolic changes associated with renal failure that cause metabolic acidosis.

a. *_____

b. *_____

28. a. hydrogen ion
retention; b. reduction of
buffering mechanisms;
c. retention of metabolic
acids; d. lactic acid
formation; e. increased
breakdown of fats

29. an increased respiratory
rate and depth or
Kussmaul breathing

30. urine sodium and urine
osmolality

31. increased

32. diluted

33. a, b, d, e, f, g, h, i

c. *_____

d. *_____

e. *_____

29.

What respiratory symptom occurs in metabolic acidosis?

*_____

30.

Two urinary tests for assessing damaged nephrons are

*_____.

31.

A low urine sodium indicates increased ADH and aldosterone
secretions. Nephrons damaged by ischemia or toxins cannot
filter sufficiently and the urine sodium can be _____.

32.

The urine osmolality measures the kidneys' ability to dilute
and concentrate urine. Damaged nephrons impair filtration
and decrease the kidneys' ability to concentrate urine. As a
result of damaged nephrons, the urine is (diluted/
concentrated) _____.

　　Table 19-6 explains the effects of renal failure on body
systems. Refer to Table 19-6 as needed to answer the following frames.

33.

Which of the following body systems are affected by renal
failure?

　　( ) a. Cardiovascular
　　( ) b. Respiratory
　　( ) c. Eye
　　( ) d. Neurologic
　　( ) e. Gastrointestinal
　　( ) f. Integumentary
　　( ) g. Musculoskeletal
　　( ) h. Endocrine
　　( ) i. Hematologic

Table 19-6	Systemic Effects of Renal Failure
Body Systems	**Rationale**
Neurologic	Uremic waste products cause slow neural conduction. Changes in personality, thought processes, levels of consciousness, and seizures can occur.
Cardiovascular	Fluid retention causes fluid overload, hypertension, and cardiac hypertrophy. Electrolyte imbalance causes arrhythmias. Uremic waste products can irritate the pericardium and lead to pericarditis and cardiac tamponade.
Respiratory	Fluid retention causes pulmonary edema. Thick bronchial secretions and impaired immune response increase susceptibility to bacterial infections.
Gastrointestinal	Ulcerations can develop anywhere in the mucosa of the GI tract from the breakdown of urea to ammonia. Metallic taste in mouth, hiccups, indigestion, nausea, and urine smell to breath from buildup of uremic waste products are added effects.
Hematologic	Failure of the kidneys to secrete erythropoietin results in decreased red cell production and anemia. Platelet survival is diminished and bleeding tendencies are increased. Immune deficiency develops from uremic waste products.
Musculoskeletal	Brittle bones and metastatic calcification result from bone demineralization in response to phosphorus and calcium imbalance.
Endocrine	Secondary hyperparathyroidism can develop from phosphorus and calcium imbalances. Sexual and menstrual dysfunctions are the result. Growth and mental retardation occur in children and carbohydrate and lipoprotein metabolism are altered.
Integumentary	Uremic waste products cause pruritis and dryness. Retained pigments and anemia give the skin a bronze cast.

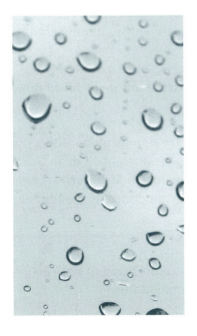

⬤ CLINICAL MANAGEMENT: DIALYSIS

Dialysis is the process of filtrating uremic waste products and excess body fluid through a semipermeable membrane to restore body homeostasis.

Diffusion is the movement of molecules/solutes in a solution. In diffusion the rate of movement across the permeable membrane is greater from the areas of higher concentration to the areas of lower concentration.

Osmosis is the movement of water molecules across a semipermeable membrane from an area of higher water concentration to an area of lower water concentration.

Ultrafiltration is the pressure gradient that enhances the movement of water molecules across the semipermeable membrane.

34.

The movement of molecules across a semipermeable membrane from an area of higher concentration to an area of lower concentration is _____.

The pressure gradient that enhances the movement of water molecules is called _____.

The movement of water molecules across a semipermeable membrane from an area of higher water concentration to one of lower water concentration is called _____.

34. diffusion; ultrafiltration; osmosis

35.

Types of dialysis therapy are continuous renal replacement therapy (CRRT), hemodialysis, and peritoneal dialysis.

The objectives for all types are to restore electrolyte balance, to remove uremic waste products, and to restore the patient's dry weight. *Dry weight* is normal body weight without excess fluid.

Name two goals of dialysis. *_____

35. to restore electrolyte balance and to remove uremic waste products (also to restore patient's dry weight)

Continuous Renal Replacement Therapy

36.

The type of dialysis most effective in the treatment of ARF is continuous renal replacement therapy (CRRT). In CRRT, an extracorporeal circuit is created with arterial to venous blood flow using the patient's mean arterial pressure (MAP) as the primary driving force. This acute treatment is administered in the ICU setting.

For CRRT, the patient's *_____ is used as the primary driving force for creating the arterial to venous blood flow.

36. mean arterial pressure (MAP)

37.

CRRT uses a hemofilter which is a very porous blood filter with a semipermeable membrane that is positioned in an extracorporeal circuit with arterial outflow to venous return access.

A very porous blood filter with a semipermeable membrane used in CRRT is called a _____.

37. hemofilter

38.

Unlike hemodialysis, CRRT requires cannulation of both an artery and a vein for extracorporeal blood flow.

Types of CRRT are (1) slow continuous ultrafiltration (SCUF), (2) continuous arteriovenous hemofiltration (CAVH), and (3) continuous arteriovenous hemodialysis (CAVHD).

CRRT requires cannulation in both an _____ and a _____.

38. artery; vein

39. slow continuous ultra-filtration, continuous arteriovenous hemofil-tration, and continuous arteriovenous hemodialysis

39.

The three types of CRRT are *_____

_____.

Indications for CRRT in the ICU setting include:

1. Patients with CKD with a preexisting vascular access who are clinically unable to tolerate routine hemodialysis procedures, such as with acute pulmonary edema, HF, recent gastrointestinal bleeding, and/or cardiogenic shock.

2. Patients with ARF who are too hemodynamically unstable for aggressive hemodialysis and for whom peritoneal dialysis is contraindicated. Examples include postoperative cardiac bypass surgery, recent myocardial infarction, sepsis, ARDS, and postoperative vascular bypass surgery.

3. Patients with ARF who are very catabolic and require daily clearance of uremic toxins and electrolyte and bicarbonate replacements.

4. Patients with oliguria who require large quantities of IV fluids either as medication or hyperalimentation.

40.

Indicate which patients with the following clinical health problems might be candidates for CRRT:

( ) a. Has CKD and cardiogenic shock occurs

( ) b. Has ARF and has an acute myocardial infarction

( ) c. Has an early stage pyelonephritis

( ) d. Has ARF and blood uremic toxins

( ) e. Has oliguria and requires large amounts IV therapy

( ) f. Has polyuria and does not receive sufficient fluids

40. a, b, d, e

41.

Hemodialysis and peritoneal dialysis are similar in the following ways: Both use dialysate, which is a solution that contains electrolytes approximating normal plasma, and both use a semipermeable membrane.

41. They both use dialysate similar in composition to normal plasma, and they both use a semipermeable membrane.

List two ways in which hemodialysis and peritoneal dialysis are similar. *_____

Hemodialysis

42.

In hemodialysis the artificial kidney (AK) is a semipermeable membrane made of a cellophanelike material through which only molecules of a particular size can diffuse.

The semipermeable membrane of the artificial kidney is a membrane through which only molecules of a *_____

_____.

42. particular size can diffuse

43.

The dialysate solution is prepared in the delivery system, where it is mixed to the correct concentration, heated, and pumped into the artificial kidney.

List the functions of the delivery system:

a. *_____

b. *_____

c. *_____

43. a. mixes dialysate in the correct concentration;
b. heats dialysate;
c. pumps dialysate

44.

Dialysate for hemodialysis contains five basic components: calcium chloride, magnesium chloride, potassium chloride, sodium chloride, and sodium acetate or bicarbonate. The concentration of these iso-osmolar/isotonic components resembles low plasma concentrations, but it can be prepared to correct an electrolyte or acid-base imbalance.

If a patient has a potassium excess, the dialysate can be prepared with low potassium. If a patient has metabolic acidosis, acetate or bicarbonate in dialysate can be used.

Dialysate can be individualized for correcting imbalances of _____ and _____.

44. electrolytes or potassium; acid-base or acidosis

45.

There are no uremic waste products in the dialysate. Therefore urea, creatinine, and other metabolic waste products diffuse rapidly from the blood across the membrane into the dialysate.

Uremic waste products rapidly diffuse from the _____ into the _____.

45. blood; dialysate

46.

Vascular access to the patient's bloodstream must be obtained to initiate hemodialysis. This access is surgically created or obtained by catheterizing a large vein.

46. bloodstream

To initiate hemodialysis, vascular access to the _____ must be obtained.

47.

During hemodialysis blood is pumped through tubing to the membranes of the AK. Two common types of AK design are the flat plate and hollow fiber. The flat plate is a stack of plastic plates with two membranes between each plate. Blood flows between these membranes. The hollow fiber has thousands of tiny hairlike fibers through which blood flows.

47. between the membranes; through the tiny hairlike fibers

By using the flat-plate AK blood flows *_____.
With the hollow-fiber AK blood flows *_____.

48.

A complication of hemodialysis is blood clotting in the blood lines and AK. This can be prevented by administering heparin, an anticoagulant, during the procedure.

48. clotting

Heparin administered during hemodialysis prevents _____.

49.

The delivery system pumps dialysate through the AK and around membranes. A negative pressure gradient, created by the delivery system, pulls excess water from the blood across the semipermeable membrane. A positive pressure gradient that pushes excess water across the membrane can occur. Ultrafiltration results and excess fluid is removed from the patient's bloodstream.

49. the pull of water across the semipermeable membrane; ultrafiltration

A negative pressure gradient results from *_____
_____.

Excess fluid is removed from the patient by _____.

50.

The goal of ultrafiltration is to obtain the patient's dry weight and prevent cardiovascular complications such as hypertension, pulmonary edema, and ventricular hypertrophy.

50. the normal body weight without excess fluid; cardiovascular

Dry weight is *_____.
Maintaining the patient's dry weight prevents _____ complications.

51. uremic waste products; electrolyte balance; excess fluid

51.

Hemodialysis treatment takes 3-4 hours to complete. The results should be the removal of *_____, restoration of *_____, and removal of *_____.

   Hemodialysis is done on a constant basis for patients with CKD and intermittently for those in ARF until renal function improves.

Peritoneal Dialysis

52.

In peritoneal dialysis the peritoneum that surrounds the abdominal cavity is used as the semipermeable membrane.

   The semipermeable membrane used in peritoneal dialysis is the _____.

52. peritoneum

53.

The dialysate for peritoneal dialysis is a sterile solution that contains similar levels of sodium, magnesium, calcium, and chloride as the plasma.

   The dialysate electrolyte levels of sodium, magnesium, calcium, and chloride are similar to _____.

   The dialysate solution is _____.

53. plasma; sterile

54.

Potassium is not included in peritoneal dialysate solutions. The health care provider prescribes the amount of potassium that can be added to the dialysate according to the patient's serum potassium level.

   Why do you think potassium is not added to the solution? *_____.

54. The patient's potassium level may be high. Adding too much potassium to the solution could increase the hyperkalemic state OR similar answer.

55.

Acid-base balance is corrected in peritoneal dialysis by adding acetate, a bicarbonate precursor, to the dialysate solution. This buffers metabolic acids.

   Acetate can be added to peritoneal dialysate to correct what acid-base disorder? *_____

55. metabolic acidosis

56.

Ultrafiltration is accomplished in peritoneal dialysis by creating an osmotic pressure gradient with glucose. The glucose concentration in the dialysate creates a hyperosmolar solution that pulls water across the peritoneal membrane.

Glucose in peritoneal dialysate creates an *_____ gradient. The dialysate solution in peritoneal dialysate is

_____.

56. osmotic pressure; hyperosmolar

57.

Peritoneal dialysate has four concentrations of glucose: 1.5, 2.5, 3.5, and 4.5%. The health care provider prescribes the concentration needed on the basis of the patient's state of fluid overload. The higher the glucose concentration, the more hyperosmolar the solution. The result is more ultrafiltration.

More ultrafiltration occurs in peritoneal dialysis when the dialysate has a *_____.

57. high glucose concentration

58.

Peritoneal dialysis begins by inserting a catheter into the peritoneal cavity. Capillary beds within the layers of peritoneum provide an indirect access to the bloodstream for the dialysate.

Access for peritoneal dialysis is obtained by a _____.

58. catheter

59.

A serious complication of peritoneal dialysis is peritonitis, the result of an infection caused by the peritoneal catheter, e.g., contamination.

Peritonitis is a serious complication of *_____. It is caused by an *_____.

59. peritoneal dialysis; infection associated with the catheter

60.

Two liters of dialysate are usually infused by gravity into the peritoneal cavity where it remains (dwells) for a prescribed time. Infusion of fluid by gravity takes approximately 10 minutes for a 2-liter volume. The dwell or equilibration period provides time for diffusion and osmosis to occur. A typical dwell or equilibration time for peritoneal dialysis is 20–30 minutes. The excess fluid, electrolytes, and uremic waste products (ultrafiltrate) move through the peritoneal membrane into the dialysate. The solution is then drained from the abdomen by gravity. The drainage of 2 liters of dialysate and ultrafiltrate takes approximately 15–30 minutes providing that the catheter is patent.

Dialysate solution is infused by gravity into the *_____.

How is the dialysate removed from the abdomen? *_____

60. peritoneal cavity; by gravity

61.

The approximate time for infusion or inflow of solution by gravity is _____ minutes.

The time for the dialysate to dwell (equilibrate) in the peritoneal cavity is _____ minutes.

The approximate time for the return of dialysate and ultrafiltrate (excess fluid, electrolytes, and uremic waste products) is _____ minutes.

61. 10; 20–30; 15–30

62.

Each infusion of fresh dialysate is referred to as an exchange. The treatment plan prescribed by the nephrologist includes the dialysis regimen, combined with the method of peritoneal dialysis, dialysis solution concentration, the frequency of exchanges, and the infusion volume and prescribed dwell time.

When ordering peritoneal dialysis, four of the treatment plans that the nephrologist must prescribe are *_____
_____.

62. dialysis regimen, method of peritoneal dialysis, dialysis solution concentration, and frequency of exchanges (others: infusion volume and dwell or equilibration time)

63.

When a peritoneal catheter is first inserted, heparin is added to the dialysate to maintain catheter patency by preventing obstruction of the peritoneal catheter with fibrin and/or blood.

The purpose of heparin in the dialysate is to *_____.

63. maintain catheter patency (prevent fibrin and clot formation)

64.

The amount of dialysate returned by gravity determines the amount of fluid loss from the body. The return must be accurately measured to maintain fluid balance. If the dialysate return is more than the amount of the infusion fluid being removed, there is a fluid imbalance.

The process by which this exchange occurs is called _____.

When the amount of dialysate returned is less than the amount infused, fluid is being (retained/excreted)

64. ultrafiltration; retained

_____. An accurate record of these differences must be maintained.

65.

If 2000 mL of dialysate is infused and 2500 mL is returned, an excess of 500 mL is being _____.

If 2000 mL of dialysate is infused and 1500 mL is returned, 500 mL is being _____.

65. ultrafiltrated or excreted; retained

66.

Retained dialysate can be reabsorbed and can lead to a fluid overload. Symptoms of fluid overload or overhydration are increased blood pressure, dyspnea, constant irritating cough, neck vein engorgement, chest crackles, and edema.

One cause of fluid overload during peritoneal dialysis is the * _____.

Name four symptoms associated with fluid overload. * _____
_____

66. retention of dialysate fluid; increased blood pressure, dyspnea, neck vein engorgement, and chest crackles (also edema and irritated cough)

67.

Excessive ultrafiltration can result in dehydration. Solutions such as 2.5% (398 mOsm/L) and 4.5% glucose dialysate (486 mOsm) or excessive exchanges can result in dehydration if not properly monitored. Symptoms of dehydration are decreased blood pressure, poor tissue turgor, tachycardia, dry mucous membranes, and hypernatremia.

Dehydration can result from * _____ or * _____.

Name three symptoms of dehydration and fluid loss. * _____
_____

67. 4.5% glucose dialysate; excessive exchanges; decreased blood pressure, poor tissue turgor, and tachycardia (also dry mucous membranes)

Table 19-7 compares the three types of dialysis treatment for renal failure. Unlike hemodialysis, CRRT is a continuous form of therapy that achieves a more stable maintenance of the volume and composition of body fluids. Rapid inter-compartmental fluid shifts observed in hemodialysis are avoided and blood pressure instability is prevented. The solute concentration changes observed in intermittent therapy are often avoided; thus the health care provider is able to remove or add electrolytes independent of changes in total body water. CRRT is used only as an acute therapy. This

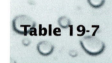

Table 19-7	Comparison of Hemodialysis, Peritoneal Dialysis, and CRRT	
Hemodialysis	**Peritoneal**	**CRRT**
Rapid removal of fluid	Fluid removed slowly	Rapid removal of fluid
Potassium lowered quickly	Potassium lowered slowly	Allows for removal or addition of electrolytes independent of changes in total body water
Waste products removed quickly	Waste products removed at a slower rate	
Rapid removal of poisonous drugs	Inefficient for removal of poisonous drugs	
Treatment time 3–4 hrs	Usual treatment process includes three to four exchanges per day	A continuous treatment process
Requires complex equipment and specialized training	Uses less complex equipment and less specialized personnel	Requires the use of a simple filter and ICU personnel
Requires vascular access	Requires no direct access to the bloodstream; causes no blood loss; used for patients with poor vascular access, i.e., children and the elderly	Requires vascular access
Requires large doses of heparin	Requires none or very small amounts of heparin	Requires the use of heparin and close monitoring for clotting in both the filter and tubing
Poorly tolerated by patients with cardiovascular disease	Minimal stress to patients with cardiovascular disease	Minimal stress for patients with cardiovascular disease
Contraindicated for patients in shock or hypotension	Can be used for patients with unstable cardiovascular status	Can be used for patients with unstable cardiovascular status
Can be used for patients with abdominal trauma	Contraindicated for patients with a colostomy, abdominal adhesions, ruptured diaphragm, or recent surgery	Can be used for patients with abdominal trauma or who are hemodynamically unstable
Cost is high	Cost effective	Cost effective
Risk of clotting increased with vascular access	Risk for peritonitis increased	Risk of access device clotting increased; Risk of dehydration from inappropriate fluid replacement increased
Treatment prescribed for chronic or acute conditions	Treatment prescribed for chronic or acute conditions	Treatment is prescribed only for acute conditions and is provided only in ICU setting

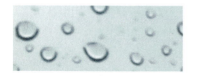

treatment takes place in an ICU (intensive care unit) for a limited period of time until there is a recovery in the patient's kidney function or either peritoneal dialysis or hemodialysis is instituted.

68.

Enter HD for hemodialysis, PD for peritoneal dialysis, and CRRT for continuous renal replacement therapy for the effect of the appropriate dialysis procedure:

_____ a. Removes fluid rapidly

_____ b. Removes excess potassium slowly

_____ c. Removes waste products quickly

_____ d. Needs no direct access to the bloodstream

_____ e. Is used in the ICU setting as an acute treatment

_____ f. Requires complex equipment and specialized training

_____ g. Can be used for hemodynamically unstable patients

_____ h. Is poorly tolerated by patients with cardiovascular disease

_____ i. Has high cost

_____ j. Risk of peritonitis

_____ k. Requires small amounts of heparin

68. a. HD and CRRT; b. PD; c. HD; d. PD; e. CRRT; f. HD; g. CRRT; h. HD; i. HD; j. PD; k. PD

● **CLINICAL APPLICATIONS**

A 36-year-old male sustained critical injuries in a motor vehicle accident. Assessment in the emergency department indicated that he suffered from blunt trauma to the chest and abdomen and two fractured femurs. He was also in shock. He went to surgery immediately for an exploratory laparotomy in which a splenectomy, aspiration of a large retroperitoneal hematoma, and repair of a ruptured diaphragm were performed. It was noted that he had bilateral contusion of both kidneys. An open reduction of his fractures was done and he was placed in balanced traction.

His urine after surgery was grossly bloody and the output ranged from 10 to 20 mL/hr. He experienced hypotension after his injury and surgery. He was transfused with eight units of whole blood. Postoperatively, he was sent to the SICU on ventilatory support with a subclavian line for fluids, nutritional support, and hemodynamic monitoring. Laboratory studies were done daily.

69.

Because the patient was hemodynamically acutely unstable due to an abdominal injury, the choice of treatment can be either _____ or _____.

69. hemodialysis; CRRT

70.

The intravascular fluid volume lost from his injuries can cause increased ADH and aldosterone secretion.

Two days after his accident the serum sodium increased. Which hormone prevents excretion of sodium?

_____

70. aldosterone

Table 19-8 lists the lab results, urine output, weight, and urinary sodium on admission, surgery, and the first four days of hospitalization. Refer to Table 19-8 as you respond to the questions.

71.

Which factors in the patient's history contributed to the development of the initial phase of ARF? _____ and * _____

71. hypotension; hemorrhagic shock

72.

A rise in serum potassium is noted the day after surgery. An increase in potassium in this situation is caused by * _____ .

72. massive tissue damage

Table 19-8	**Laboratory Studies 1**					
Tests	**Admission**	**Surgery**	**Day 1**	**Day 2**	**Day 3**	**Day 4**
Potassium (serum) (3.5–5.3 mEq/L)	3.6	4.2	6.5	5.1	5.9	6.8
Sodium (serum) (135–145 mEq/L)	138	142	144	143	144	143
Chloride (serum) (95–105 mEq/L)	110	110	110	108	103	104
CO_2 (serum) (22–30 mEq/L)	17	24	27	29	25	21
BUN (5–25 mg/dL)			30	34	57	84
Creatinine (serum) (0.5–1.5 mg/dL)			1.6	4.7	7.2	10.2
Urine output (mL/24 hr)			580	440	320	290
Weight (lb)		185	189	191	196	198
Urine sodium (mEq/L)						93

73. urine output less than 400 mL in 24 hours and elevated BUN and creatinine

73.

The patient shows signs of oliguric azotemia on the second and third days. What are the two clinical indicators of decreased renal function? *_____

_____

74. ischemia and toxicity

74.

The nephrologist who cared for him diagnosed his renal problem as acute kidney failure secondary to shock and myoglobinuria. Shock and myoglobinuria are listed under which two causes of kidney failure? *_____

75. hyperkalemia

75.

On the fourth day the patient's serum potassium measures 6.8 mEq/L. His ECG showed peaked T waves and signs of cardiac irritability. These are symptoms of (hypokalemia/hyperkalemia) _____.

76. a. Kayexalate and sorbitol; b. IV sodium bicarbonate; c. 10% calcium gluconate; d. insulin and glucose

76.

Hyperkalemia can be treated temporarily by methods that decrease serum potassium. (Refer to Chapter 6 on potassium if needed.)

List four methods used in the treatment of hyperkalemia:

a. *_____

b. *_____

c. *_____

d. *_____

77. sodium bicarbonate and glucose and insulin

77.

ECG changes indicate a need to rapidly lower the patient's serum potassium level. Name two methods that can be used to shift potassium back into the cells. *_____

78. Kayexalate

78.

Another treatment prescribed for the patient was a Kayexalate retention enema. Kayexalate, a cation exchange resin, is mixed with sorbitol and given orally or rectally to induce an "osmotic diarrhea." The sodium in Kayexalate is exchanged with potassium in the intestines to lower the serum potassium level.

The resin used in excreting potassium from the intestine is _____.

79. fluid overload OR overhydration

80. acidosis. If you answered metabolic acidosis—OK.

81. they are damaged

82. He is hemodynamically unstable and has abdominal trauma. Peritoneal dialysis is contraindicated after abdominal surgery. CRRT prevents the rapid intercompartmental fluid shifts that occur in hemodialysis and are poorly tolerated in a CRRT patient.

83. vascular access

84. ultrafiltration; the use of a low-potassium dialysate

79.

It is noted that the patient had a 13-pound weight increase since admission. Edema is evident in his hands, feet, and face. His blood pressure is 160/80 and his central venous pressure (CVP) and pulmonary artery wedge pressure (PAWP) are elevated. Auscultation of lung fields revealed coarse crackles bilaterally. These symptoms indicate what type of fluid imbalance? *_____

80.

His electrolytes for day 4 show a serum Na 143, Cl 104, and CO_2 21. He has an anion gap of 18. An anion gap greater than 16 mEq/L is indicative of what condition? _____ (Refer to Chapter 12 on anion gap if necessary.)

81.

Once the urine is clear of blood, a random urine sodium test is ordered. The result of 93 mEq/L means that the kidneys are unable to concentrate urine. What does this test indicate about the nephrons? *_____

82.

The decision is made to prescribe CRRT until the patient regains kidney function or becomes stable enough to tolerate hemodialysis. Explain why CRRT is selected over peritoneal dialysis or hemodialysis. *_____
_____
_____

83.

Several days later, a decision was made for the patient to have hemodialysis for 3 hours every day. What type of access is needed for hemodialysis? *_____

84.

During hemodialysis what method is used to remove excess fluid? _____

What can be done in hemodialysis to lower the serum potassium? *_____

85.

In hemodialysis the rapid shift of fluids and electrolytes can cause central nervous system disturbances such as agitation, twitching, and seizures. This is known as the *disequilibrium syndrome.*

This condition is caused by a _____.*

86.

Observe for signs of the disequilibrium syndrome that include _____, _____, and _____.

Table 19-9 lists the patient's test results on days 6, 14, 35, 37, 40, and 47. He is given hemodialysis until day 49. Refer to Table 19-9 as needed.

85. rapid shift of fluids and electrolytes during hemodialysis

86. agitation; twitching; seizures

Table 19-9	**Laboratory Studies II**					
Tests	**Day 6**	**Day 14**	**Day 35**	**Day 37**	**Day 40**	**Day 47**
WBCs (4500–10,000 mm³)		38,000				
Potassium (serum) (3.5–5.3 mEq/L)	5.3	5.2	3.8	3.9	3.8	4.8
Sodium (serum) (135–145 mEq/L)	142	135	134	128	133	147
Calcium (serum) (9–11 mg/dL)		8.5		8.6		
Chloride (serum) (95–105 mEq/L)	102	93	99	90	97	112
Phosphorus (serum) (2.5–4.5 mg/dL)		9.7		4.2		
CO_2 (serum) (22–30 mEq/L)	25	25	21	21	22	17
BUN (5–25 mg/dL)	71	110	86	89	86	140
Creatinine (serum) (0.5–1.5 mg/dL)	9.2	11.1	7.1	6.5	5.8	4.3
Weight (lb)	193	180	171	169	165	164
Intake (mL/24 hr)	600	600	600	600	3000	4955
Urine output (mL/24 hr)	170	0	250	550	3000	4650

87.

On day 14 the patient became anuric. He also developed a severe infection that caused catabolism and increased his BUN, creatinine, and WBC count. Hemodialysis time is increased to 5 hours per day. From Table 19-9 what three problems are controlled with dialysis on day 14? *_____

_____

87. acidosis, hyperkalemia, and fluid overload

88.

The serum phosphorus is very high (9.7 mg/dL). When the serum calcium and phosphate are multiplied, the Ca × P product is 82.4. This is an indication of *_____.

88. metastatic calcification

89.

The nephrologist ordered a phosphate binding agent to lower the serum phosphorus. This agent contains aluminum, which attracts and binds phosphorus compounds in the intestines for excretion in the stool.

    The drug/agent that lowers serum phosphate is *_____

_____.

89. a phosphate binding agent OR an agent that contains aluminum, such as Amphojel or Basaljel

90.

On day 35 the patient's urine output returned and hemodialysis was decreased to 4 hours per day. By day 37 his urine output increased further and dialysis times were reduced.

    Note: Electrolytes stabilize to low normal levels in daily dialysis therapy.

    His intake and output were about the _____. His serum phosphorus was within high normal limits because of the *_____ prescribed.

90. same; phosphate binding agent (phosphate binders)

91.

On day 40 the patient's urinary output increased to 3000 mL/24 hr. This indicates that he is in the _____ phase of ARF. Identify a potential serious complication of this phase. _____

91. diuretic; dehydration

92.

By day 47 the patient's urine output continues to be high, but his serum sodium and BUN are also high. Skin turgor is poor, mucous membranes are dry, and he complains of thirst. His blood pressure is 120/60 and his pulse is 92. These symptoms are indicators of what type of fluid imbalance?

92. dehydration

_____

93.

By day 55 the patient is no longer azotemic and his urine output and electrolytes are in normal range. This phase of ARF is _____.

93. recovery

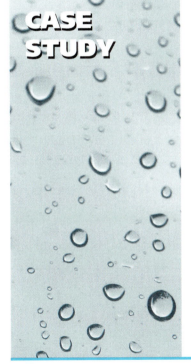

CASE STUDY

REVIEW

A 68-year-old female has a 3-year history of renal insufficiency from glomerulonephritis and a history of several myocardial infarctions. She is admitted to the hospital for shortness of breath with no dyspnea. Her laboratory results on admission are Hgb 6.1 g/dL, Hct 19%, BUN 78 mg/dL, creatinine 5.2 mg/dL, serum CO_2 13 mEq/L, serum potassium 5.6 mEq/L, serum sodium 124 mEq/L, serum calcium 8.4 mg/dL, and serum phosphorus 5.2 mg/dL. Physical assessment reveals edema of her face, hands, and lower legs. Lung sounds indicate bilateral coarse crackles but no frothy sputum. Blood pressure is 170/98 and her jugular venous pressure is elevated. She notes a weight gain of 5 pounds in the preceding 3 days and her urine output is approximately 500 mL per day. She complains of thirst.

ANSWER COLUMN

1. periods of time; nephrons

1. Chronic kidney disease usually develops over *_____. A progressive loss of _____ is the result.

2. What is the cause of her chronic kidney disease? _____

2. glomerulonephritis
3. Anemia; Kidneys are not producing erythropoietin to stimulate the bone marrow to build red blood cells.

3. The low hemoglobin and hematocrit indicate what clinical condition? _____. Explain why. *_____ _____

4. elevated; azotemia

5. decreased; acidosis

6. 3.5–5.3 mEq/L; potassium retention due to oliguria and massive tissue destruction

7. decreased; excessive fluid intake, and metabolic acidosis

8. It causes minimal stress to patients with cardiovascular disease; it is frequently used for patients with unstable cardiovascular disease.

9. weight gain, edema, increased blood pressure, and bilateral crackles (also elevated jugular venous pressure)

10. hyperosmolar; ultrafiltration; diffusion of potassium into the dialysate

11. respiratory distress

12. dehydration

13. strict measurement of dialysate from each exchange

14. fluid overload

---

4. Her BUN and serum creatinine are (elevated/decreased) _____, which is indicative of _____.

5. The patient's serum CO_2 is (elevated/decreased) _____, which is indicative of _____.

6. Her serum potassium is 5.6 mEq/L. The normal range of potassium is *_____. Identify two reasons why hyperkalemia occurs in kidney disease. _____ _____

7. Her serum sodium is (elevated/decreased) _____. Identify two reasons for her hyponatremia. *_____ _____

8. Peritoneal dialysis is chosen to treat her uremia. Why is peritoneal dialysis the best choice for her? *_____ _____

9. What four symptoms indicate signs of fluid overload? *_____ _____

10. After trocar insertion, the first exchange of peritoneal dialysate is a 4.25% dextrose dialysate with no potassium. The 4.25% dextrose dialysate is _____. It is used for _____. Dialysate without potassium increases *_____ _____.

11. When dialysate infuses into the peritoneum, it can push the diaphragm upward. One must assess the patient for signs of *_____ _____.

12. Excessive use of 4.25% dextrose dialysate can lead to _____.

13. An essential intervention during peritoneal dialysis to maintain fluid balance is *_____.

14. Retention of dialysate during exchanges can lead to *_____ _____.

15. hypokalemia; dialysate

16. phosphate binding agent such as Amphojel

17. dry weight

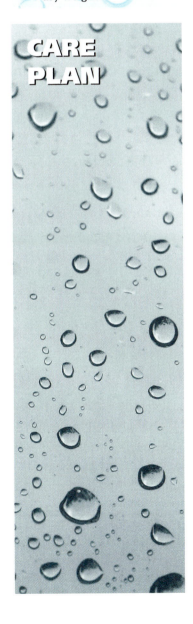

CARE PLAN

15. On the second day of peritoneal dialysis her potassium is 2.8 mEq/L, which indicates _____. Potassium must be added to the _____.

16. The patient's phosphorus is slightly elevated. The drug given to decrease her serum phosphorus is * _____.

17. To prevent fluid overload in the future, it is important to determine her * _____.

PATIENT MANAGEMENT

Assessment Factors

● Obtain a patient history concerning frequency and amounts of urination, fluid intake, and history of any past renal health problems.

● Obtain baseline vital signs for abnormal findings and for comparison with future vital signs. Obtain patient's weight.

● Record the amount of urine output for 8 hours. Report if the urine output amount is not within the desired range (>30 mL/hr).

● Check admitting laboratory results, especially the BUN, serum creatinine, serum electrolytes, and complete blood count (CBC).

● Assess for signs and symptoms that relate to the patient's abnormal laboratory values.

● Assess for edema in the extremities. A decrease in urine output in conjunction with edema in the lower extremities can indicate a renal disorder.

Nursing Diagnosis 1

Excess fluid volume related to decreased urine output, sodium retention, and inability of kidneys to regulate water balance.

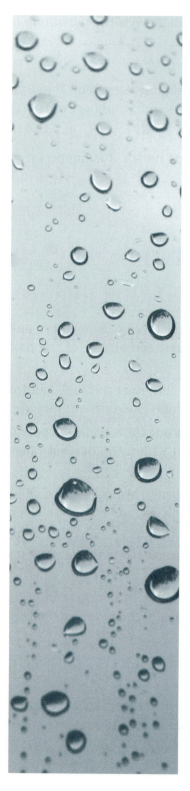

Interventions and Rationale

1. Monitor fluid intake and output. Report a decrease in urine output of less than 30 mL per hour.

2. Monitor vital signs. Report abnormal vital signs, such as an increase in pulse rate, an increase or decrease in blood pressure, and difficulty breathing.

3. Check for signs of hypervolemia, i.e., constant irritating cough, neck and hand vein engorgements, dyspnea, and chest crackles.

4. Check weights daily before breakfast. Weigh the patient with the same clothes and on the same scale. An increase in weight may indicate fluid retention. One liter of fluid weighs approximately 2.2 pounds.

5. Check for edema in the lower extremities early in the morning before the patient rises. The presence of feet, ankle, and/or leg edema in the morning frequently indicates a kidney or cardiac dysfunction.

6. Check abdominal girth. Monitor for fluid shifts by noting rigidity or girth changes in the abdomen.

7. Encourage patients to follow a restricted sodium diet and fluid limitation as ordered by the health care provider.

Nursing Diagnosis 2

Risk for deficient fluid volume related to excess ultrafiltration or diuresis.

Interventions and Rationale

1. Monitor vital signs, especially the pulse rate and blood pressure. An increased pulse rate with a decreased blood pressure may be indicative of a deficient fluid volume.

2. Monitor fluid balance associated with dialysis procedures. Excessive ultrafiltration during hemodialysis causes hypotension. If blood pressure postdialysis is low, it may cause decreased blood flow through the vascular access and result in clotting. Excessive ultrafiltration from peritoneal dialysis can produce hypovolemia and

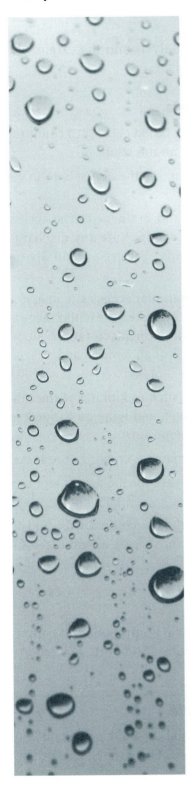

hypernatremia because of the rapid movement of water across the peritoneum.

3. Monitor urinary output in the diuretic phase of ARF. Excessive urine output can deplete the intravascular volume and cause severe dehydration.

4. Replace fluid loss rapidly as prescribed to increase blood pressure and perfusion to vital organs when hypovolemia is due to the dialysis procedure.

Nursing Diagnosis 3

Ineffective tissue perfusion: renal, cardiopulmonary, cerebral, related to hypovolemia and decrease in cardiac output secondary to dialysis.

Interventions and Rationale

1. Monitor vital signs and ECG. Report abnormal findings that may indicate poor tissue perfusion.

2. Check for signs of edema. Edema decreases tissue perfusion.

3. Monitor CVP and PAWP for early signs of decreased cardiac output and decreased perfusion.

4. Check specific gravity to detect changes in the concentration that result from decreased intravascular volume and may lead to decreased renal perfusion.

Nursing Diagnosis 4

Impaired urinary elimination related to inability of kidneys to regulate water excretion.

Interventions and Rationale

1. Check urine output daily at specified times.

2. Instruct patient with renal disorders to monitor their fluid intake and urine output. A decreased output may signify decreased function. Urinary output should be at a minimum of 30 mL/hr. The health care provider must be notified if theurine output drops.

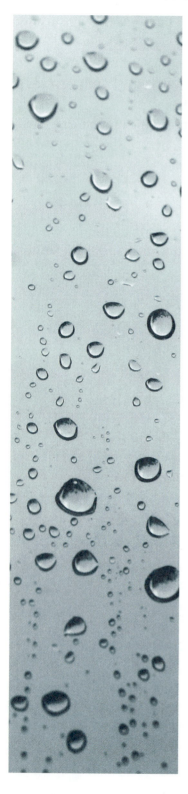

Nursing Diagnosis 5

Ineffective protection related to dialysis and the care of the vascular access site.

Interventions and Rationale

1. Monitor temperature and white blood cell (WBC) count for elevations, which can indicate an infection.

2. Use aseptic technique in caring for the access site to reduce risk of infection.

3. Check for swelling, redness, and drainage at the access site, which can indicate an infection. Note any discharge from the access sites or wounds. Culture potentially infected sites.

4. Check for the patency of the vascular access site used for hemodialysis. A surgically re-created vascular access should have bruits and pulsation on auscultation. Blood can be aspirated and infused through femoral and subclavian catheters.

5. Check for mechanical factors, such as kinking of the tubing, displacement of the catheter, and lying on the access site, which could cause poor blood flow.

6. Observe the peritoneal catheter site for crusting or redness.

7. Instruct the patient on how to care for the access site and maintain asepsis.

8. Teach the patient good hygiene, to avoid crowds, and to obtain yearly inoculation for flu viruses as indicated by the health care provider.

Nursing Diagnosis 6

Risk for injury related to mechanical equipment and central nervous system dysfunction from fluid and electrolyte imbalances.

Interventions and Rationale

1. Monitor new dialysis patients and catabolic patients in ARF for signs of central nervous system dysfunction that may

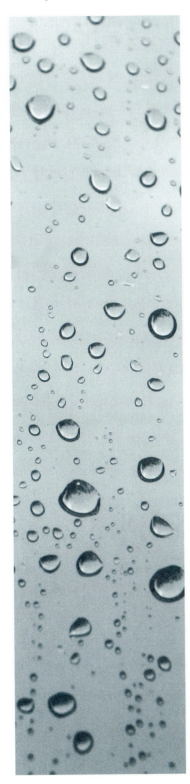

lead to disequilibrium syndrome. Observe for tremors, irritability, confusion, and seizures that indicate the disequilibrium syndrome.

2. Monitor serum electrolyte values associated with renal disorders and observe for symptoms of electrolyte imbalance. Report laboratory results that indicate hyperkalemia, hypocalcemia, and hyperphosphatemia immediately. These results can be life threatening.

3. Monitor the ECG for peaked T waves that can indicate hyperkalemia.

4. Administer phosphate binding agents as ordered to control the serum phosphorus level. A low serum calcium level can be caused by hyperphosphatemia, restricted calcium intake in the diet, and/or alterations in vitamin D metabolism needed for intestinal absorption of calcium. Overuse of aluminum-phosphate binding drugs can cause hypophosphatemia.

5. Check the symptoms of tetany when the serum calcium level is low and acidosis is corrected. Serum calcium deficits can indicate a need for vitamin D supplements.

Nursing Diagnosis 7

Ineffective breathing patterns related to peritoneal dialysate infusion.

Interventions and Rationale

1. Monitor respiratory rate. Report signs of dyspnea.

2. Check for dyspnea when administering solutions for peritoneal dialysis. Rapid infusion of dialysate can push the diaphragm upward, thus decreasing the area for lung expansion.

Evaluation/Outcomes

1. Confirm that the effects of hemodialysis or peritoneal dialysis for controlling fluid, electrolyte, and acid-base balance.

2. Monitor vital signs (particularly blood pressure and pulse rate) for stability or indications of a fluid imbalance.

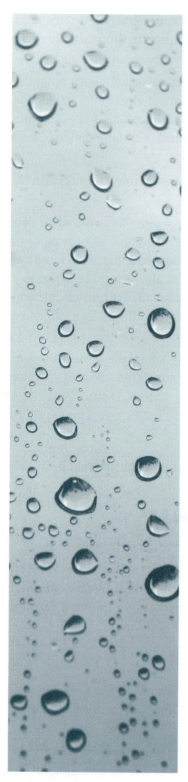

3. Monitor weight gain prior to and following dialysis to determine body fluid gains or losses.

4. Evaluate intake and output for fluid balance.

5. Evaluate that laboratory test results, i.e., electrolytes, creatinine, BUN, and CBC, prior to and following dialysis are in normal or in "near" normal ranges. Serum laboratory test results may be "alarmingly" elevated prior to dialysis.

6. Monitor for peripheral and pulmonary edema as a result of ECFVE.

7. Maintain a support system for the patient and family.

Chronic Diseases with Fluid and Electrolyte Imbalances

Erlinda Wheeler, DNS, RN
Judith Herrman, PhD, RN, ANP
Kathleen Schell, DNSc, RN

LEARNING OUTCOMES

Upon completion of this chapter, the reader will be able to:

- Identify the physiologic changes in fluid and electrolytes associated with chronic diseases such as heart failure, diabetes mellitus (DM), and chronic obstructive pulmonary disease (COPD).
- Explain the clinical manifestations related to HF, DM, and COPD.
- Identify abnormal laboratory results associated with HF, DM, and COPD.
- Discuss the major treatment modalities for correcting fluid and electrolyte imbalances associated with HF, DM, and COPD.
- Identify selected diagnoses and interventions with rationales for heart failure, DM, and COPD.

INTRODUCTION

A chronic disease, defined by the U.S. National Center for Health Statistics, is a chronic condition that has a duration of 3 months or longer. Chronic conditions usually progress slowly over a long period of time. Chronic illnesses frequently do not occur as a single health problem but are associated

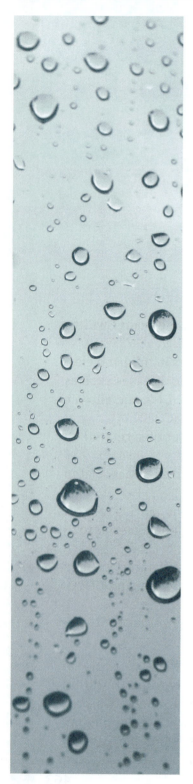

with multiple chronic health problems, e.g., a person with uncontrolled diabetes mellitus or chronic obstructive pulmonary disease (COPD) often develops heart failure. This chapter addresses three common chronic diseases: heart failure, diabetes mellitus, and COPD.

Heart failure is a condition in which the heart is unable to adequately supply blood to meet the metabolic needs of the body and a systemic response attempting to compensate for the inadequacy. Left ventricular failure (heart failure) is the result of systolic or diastolic ventricular dysfunction. Right ventricular failure can be secondary to left ventricular failure or can result from pulmonary disease (cor pulmonale).

Diabetes mellitus (DM) results from lack of insulin from the beta cells of the pancreas or an inability of the cells to use available insulin. Approximately 23.6 million people in the United States are affected by some form of DM. There are two common types of DM: Type 1, characterized by an absolute insulin deficiency, and Type 2, in which there is a relative deficiency in insulin compared to body needs. With noninsulin dependent diabetes mellitus (NIDDM) usually some insulin secretion occurs. The old term for Type 1 was juvenile-onset diabetes and for Type 2 was maturity-onset diabetes. These are misleading terms because either type of diabetes can occur in the very young or very old.

Diabetic ketoacidosis (DKA) is associated with insulin dependent diabetes mellitus (IDDM), Type I, and results from a severe or complete deficit of insulin secretion. DKA is characterized by a blood sugar exceeding 300 mg/dL, ketosis, a blood pH < 7.30, and a bicarbonate level < 14 mEq/L. *Hyperglycemic hyperosmolar state (HHS)* is characterized by a blood sugar > 500 mg/dL, dehydration, and a serum osmolality > 300 mOsm/kg and generally occurs in patients with Type 2 diabetes mellitus.

Chronic obstructive pulmonary disease (COPD) is a group of respiratory disorders characterized by airflow limitation that is not fully reversible. It is typically progressive and is considered an inflammatory pulmonary disease. Emphysema and chronic bronchitis have been considered the two types of COPD, but patients typically have elements of both types. Position papers from the American Thoracic Society (ATS), European Respiratory Society (ERS), and the

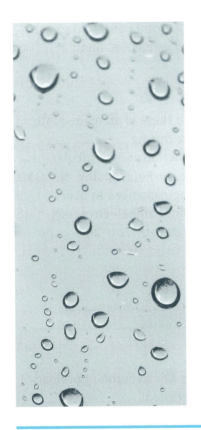

Global Initiative for Chronic Obstructive Lung Disease (GOLD) do not make this distinction. COPD leads to systemic effects such as skeletal muscle dysfunction, wasting, osteoporosis, sexual dysfunction, and cardiovascular diseases. It is the fourth leading cause of death in the United States and fifth in the world. The most common risk factor for COPD is cigarette smoking, and its prevalence in various countries is associated with time of introduction of tobacco smoking and total pack-years smoked. Other risk factors for COPD include alpha$_1$-antitrypsin (AAT) deficiency (genetic trait), occupational dusts and chemicals, indoor and outdoor air pollution, and severe recurring respiratory tract infections. Alpha$_1$-antitrypsin deficiency results in COPD because, without AAT, proteolytic enzymes (released in the lungs from bacteria or phagoctyic cells) damage lung tissue.

In this chapter, the three chronic diseases are presented in sections: Heart Failure, Diabetes Mellitus, and Chronic Obstructive Pulmonary Disease. The pathophysiology, clinical manifestations, clinical applications, and clinical management associated with specific diagnoses and clinical interventions are included in each section.

ANSWER COLUMN

HEART FAILURE

Pathophysiology

Heart failure is most commonly caused by dysfunction of the left ventricle (systolic or diastolic dysfunction, or both). Systolic dysfunction can result from inadequate pumping of blood from the ventricle (pump failure), leading to decreased cardiac output. Diastolic dysfunction happens when there is inadequate filling of the ventricle during diastole, causing decreased blood volume in the ventricle and therefore decreased cardiac output.

1.

Heart failure is a condition in which the heart is unable to deliver _____ to meet the needs of the body.

    Systolic dysfunction is referred to as _____.

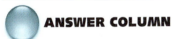

1. an adequate supply of blood; pump failure

Any condition that decreases myocardial contractility can cause systolic dysfunction (CAD, hypertension, dilated cardiomyopathy).

2.

Diastolic dysfunction happens when there is an inadequate amount of blood filling the ventricle during _____.

2. diastole

Conditions causing diastolic dysfunction are ventricular hypertrophy, myocarditis, restrictive cardiomyopathy, and CAD.

Table 20-1 lists the pathophysiologic changes in heart failure. These changes can lead to fluid and electrolyte imbalance. Study the changes and refer to Table 20-1 as necessary.

3.

3. preload; afterload; myocardial contractility; heart rate

Factors that affect cardiac output are _____, _____, * _____, and * _____.

4.

Increased preload initially increases CO. Eventually preload overstretches the myocardium also called * _____.

4. ventricular dilation

5.

Myocardial contractility is affected by what two factors?
* _____

5. preload and afterload

6.

Decreased cardiac output causes (increased/decreased) _____ renal perfusion.

6. decreased

7.

7. decreased; renin-angiotensin-aldosterone system

The effect of (increased/decreased) _____ renal perfusion causes the activation of the _____.

8.

What is the main vascular effect of these hormones?
_____

8. vasoconstriction

9.

9. sodium retention, fluid retention, and potassium excretion

Identify three effects of aldosterone on fluid and electrolytes.
* _____ _____ _____

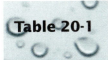

Table 20-1

Physiologic and Neurohormonal Changes Associated with Heart Failure

Physiologic Changes	Rationale
Cardiac output (CO) (decreased)	Factors that influence CO are preload, afterload, myocardial contractility, and heart rate. Diseases (hypertension, CAD, ventricular hypertrophy, etc.) that adversely affect these factors decrease CO. Decrease in CO causes the increase in preload, afterload, contractility, and heart rate to compensate for the failing heart.
Preload or left ventricular end-diastolic volume (LVEDV) (increased)	Increased volume in the ventricles after diastole increases CO initially, but it can eventually lead to overstretching of the myocardium (ventricular dilatation) and cause contractility to decrease.
Afterload (increased)	Increased systemic vascular resistance is due to activation of the sympathetic nervous system stimulated by decreased CO and peripheral vascular resistance (PVR). Increased PVR leads to increased work of the heart to eject blood to the systemic circulation, leading to hypertrophy of the myocardium.
Myocardial contractility (decreased)	Contractility is affected by diseases (MI, myocarditis, cardiomyopathy) that affect myocyte activity, causing inefficient contraction of the ventricles. Increased preload and afterload also affect contractility.
Heart rate (increased)	Tachycardia develops to compensate for decreased CO. Initially, cardiac output increases but eventually causes less ventricular filling time.
Renal perfusion (decreased)	Decreased CO causes decreased renal blood flow.
Renin-angiotensin-aldosterone system activated	Decreased renal blood flow activates this system, causing vasoconstriction and sodium and fluid to be retained, leading to increased preload and afterload. Excess fluid dilutes sodium and can cause hyponatremia. Aldosterone can also cause loss of potassium in the urine, leading to hypokalemia.
Sympathetic nervous system (SNS) stimulated	Stimulation of SNS due to decreased CO causes tachycardia, increased systemic vascular resistance (BP), and release of norepinephrine.
Left heart failure	Can be caused by either systolic or diastolic dysfunction or both. **Systolic dysfunction** is the inability of the left ventricle to pump enough blood to perfuse body tissues. **Diastolic dysfunction** is due to decreased compliance of the left ventricles, leading to increased left ventricular end-diastolic pressure (LVEDP). Diseases affecting myocardial contractility, preload, and afterload lead to heart failure.
Right heart failure	Can result from left heart failure as a result of increased pressure on the left side. Pulmonary disease is also a cause of right heart failure.

10. hyponatremia, hypokalemia, and hypervolemia (FVE)

10.

Activation of the renin-angiotensin-aldosterone system can cause which fluid and electrolyte imbalances? * _____,

_____, _____

11. left

11.
Systolic and diastolic ventricular dysfunction can lead to (right/left) _____ heart failure.

12. left heart failure and pulmonary disease

12.
The causes of right heart failure are *_____.

Clinical Manifestations

The heart compensates for inadequate blood flow by increasing the heart rate. Table 20-2 lists the common clinical manifestations and rationale associated with heart failure. Study Table 20-2 carefully, noting the reasons for the signs and symptoms related to heart failure.

13.
Vital sign changes associated with heart failure are:
  a. Pulse rate is _____.
  b. Respiratory rate is _____.
  c. Blood pressure may be _____.

13. a. increased;
b. increased; c. increased

14.
A rapid increase in respiration is known as _____.
The reason for an increased respiratory rate is to improve the
*_____. More (oxygen/carbon dioxide)
_____ intake occurs. Difficult or labored breathing is known as _____.

14. tachypnea; gas exchange; oxygen; dyspnea

15.
The two types of edema associated with heart failure are _____
_____.
  Initially, left heart failure causes _____ edema.
  Right heart failure is associated with _____ edema.

15. pulmonary and peripheral; pulmonary; peripheral

16.
Indicate which serum electrolyte results are most likely related to heart failure.
  ( ) a. Hypernatremia
  ( ) b. Hyperkalemia
  ( ) c. Hypermagnesemia

( ) d. Hyponatremia
( ) e. Normal serum sodium level
( ) f. Hypokalemia
( ) g. Hypomagnesemia

16. b, d, f

Table 20-2	Clinical Manifestations Associated with Heart Failure

Clinical Manifestations	Rationale
Increased pulse rate (tachycardia)	Increased heart rate is a compensatory mechanism to improve circulation of the blood.
Increased respiration (tachypnea)	Respirations increase to increase oxygen intake for tissue oxygenation.
Increased blood pressure (hypertension)	When hypertension occurs, it is usually because of atherosclerosis. Noncirculating vascular fluid can also increase blood pressure.
Dyspnea	Difficult or labored breathing due to inadequate cardiac output and oxygen to the tissues, leading to increased breathing difficulty.
Fatigue with exertion or at rest	Inadequate blood flow and oxygen to the tissues.
Blood-tinged sputum; cough	Increased pulmonary capillary pressure causes blood from capillaries to enter the alveoli, leading to pulmonary edema.
Abnormal lung sounds (crackles)	Caused by fluid in the lungs; pulmonary edema.
Decreased urinary output	Decreased renal perfusion.
Jugular venous distention	Hepatic congestion leading to venous distention.
Edema	
Pulmonary	Caused by left heart failure. (Because of pump failure, fluid "backs up" in the pulmonary system, causing fluid congestion in the lung tissues.) Fluid inhibits adequate gas exchange (O_2 and CO_2). Signs and symptoms of pulmonary edema are similar to the signs and symptoms of overhydration.
Peripheral	May result from right heart failure. Fluids accumulate in the extremities due to the fluid backup in the venous circulation.
Cyanosis	Cyanosis is a sign of hypoxia due to inadequate blood flow to body tissues.
Laboratory Results	
Plasma/serum sodium: increased (hypernatremia) or normal	Sodium retention in the extracellular fluid (ECF) usually occurs even when the serum sodium is within normal range or lower. Hemodilution can cause a normal or slightly lower serum sodium level.
Plasma/serum potassium: normal or decreased (hypokalemia)	The serum potassium level can be decreased with the use of potassium-wasting diuretics and due to hemodilution from fluid volume excess.
Plasma/serum magnesium: normal or decreased (hypomagnesemia)	Long-term use of potassium-wasting diuretics can cause both hypomagnesemia and hypokalemia.
Serum osmolality: < 280 mOsm/kg	Due to hemodilution. If the serum sodium level is increased, the serum osmolality increases.

Clinical Applications

A 68-year-old female was admitted to the hospital with a history of CAD and a diagnosis of heart failure. She has shortness of breath when walking up a flight of stairs. The health professional assessed her physiologic status and noted an irritating cough, dyspnea on exertion, crackles in the lungs, hand vein engorgement in upward position after 30 seconds, and swelling in the ankles and feet. Her blood pressure is 154/96 and pulse was 110. Her ECG showed ventricular hypertrophy.

17.
The patient presents two compensatory physiologic changes essential for maintaining cardiac function; these compensatory mechanisms are *_____.
Are these compensatory mechanisms effective? _____
Explain why. *_____
_____

17. tachycardia and ventricular hypertrophy; No; Most likely, ventricular dilatation is present and limiting the effectiveness of the increased heart rate and ventricular hypertrophy.

18.
According to the patient's symptoms, which type(s) of heart failure is (are) present?
( ) a. Left heart failure
( ) b. Right heart failure

18. a, b

19.
The assessment of the patient identifies four symptoms of pulmonary congestion, which are: *_____
_____

19. irritating cough, dyspnea, crackles, and hand vein engorgement

20.
Swelling in the feet and ankles is indicative of _____ heart failure.

20. right

Table 20-3 gives the laboratory results for the patient on the day of admission and the second and fourth days after admission. Identify laboratory results that are normal and abnormal. Explain the abnormal laboratory findings.

Table 20-3	Laboratory Studies		
Laboratory Tests	**On Admission**	**Day 1**	**Day 4**
Hematology			
Hemoglobin (12.9–17.0 g)	12.5		
Hematocrit (40–46%)	40		
WBC (white blood count)	8200		
Biochemistry			
BUN (blood urea nitrogen) (10–25 mg/dL)*	70	24	18
Plasma/serum CO_2† (22–32 mEq/L)	22	24	24
Plasma/serum chloride (95–108 mEq/L)	107	106	107
Plasma/serum sodium (135–146 mEq/L)	125	148	143
Plasma/serum potassium (3.5–5.3 mEq/L)	3.6	3.8	4.0

*mg/100 mL = mg/dL.
†*Plasma* and *serum* are used interchangeably.

21. decreased; rise; edema or ECFVE

22. increase; Potassium may be diluted due to the increase of ECF or hemodilution; A lack of adequate food intake containing potassium; If she were receiving diuretics, this might cause a low serum K.

21.

Her serum sodium is _____. Sodium retention can cause extracellular fluid volume to (rise/decrease) _____.

What type of fluid imbalance was present? _____

22.

Her low-average serum potassium may be due to a(n) (increase/decrease) _____ in ECF. Explain why. *_____
_____.

Another reason why her serum potassium may be low-average is *_____.

Clinical Management

The main goals in the management of heart failure patients are to decrease oxygen demand of the body (promote rest) and to increase cardiac output. Increasing cardiac output involves:
1. Decreasing preload
2. Decreasing afterload
3. Increasing myocardial contractility

Decrease Preload

23.

The patient was placed on a low-sodium diet and her fluid intake was limited to 1200 mL (300 mL below daily requirement).

Limiting sodium and water results in:
( ) a. increase preload
( ) b. decrease preload
( ) c. increase afterload
( ) d. decrease afterload

23. b

24.

Diuretics are used for the excretion of sodium and water. Many diuretics increase the excretion of sodium, water, and chloride, and the valuable electrolyte _____.

24. potassium

25.

Frequently, a potassium-sparing diuretic is prescribed with a potassium-wasting diuretic to prevent excessive loss of what ion? _____

25. potassium

26.

Identify diuretics that are potassium-wasting and potassium-sparing by placing K-W for potassium-wasting diuretics and K-S for potassium-sparing diuretics.
_____ a. Hydrochlorothiazide (HydroDIURIL)
_____ b. Triameterene (Dyrenium)
_____ c. Furosemide (Lasix)
_____ d. Mannitol
_____ e. Spironolactone (Aldactone)

26. a. K-W; b. K-S; c. K-W; d. K-W; e. K-S

27. muscular weakness, dizziness, arrhythmia, silent ileus (decrease peristalsis), and abdominal distention

27.

Identify at least five symptoms of hypokalemia (potassium deficit). (Refer to Chapter 6 if necessary.) * _____
_____

Decrease Afterload

The heart has to work harder to pump the blood against an increased vascular resistance (afterload). Diuretics and angiotensin-converting enzyme (ACE) inhibitors decrease afterload. Angiotensin-converting enzyme inhibitors (Vasotec, Zestril) prevent the conversion of angiotensin I to angiotensin II, decreasing vasoconstriction. Other drugs that are used to decrease afterload and preload are angiotensin II receptor blockers (losartan, valsartan), vasodilators (nitrates, Prazosin), beta-adrenergic blocking agents (Carvedilol), and phosphodiesterase inhibitors (Amrinone, Milrinone). BiDil is a new combination drug containing isosorbide and hydralazine. This drug has been recently approved for use in heart failure for African-Americans. Decreasing afterload and preload increases cardiac output.

Increase Myocardial Contractility

The most common drug used to increase myocardial contractility and decrease tachycardia is digoxin. Other drugs used to increase myocardial contractility (inotropes) are Dobutamine, Dopamine, Amrinone, and Milrinone.

Digitalization is the process of increasing the serum level of digoxin to achieve the desired physiologic effect. It is also referred to as a loading dose or doses.

Digitalis preparations are classified as cardiac glycosides (cardiotonic). The action of digitalis preparations is to slow the ventricular contractions and increase the forcefulness of the contractions. Examples of digitalis preparations are digoxin, digitoxin, gitaligin, deslanoside (Cedilanid), and digitalis leaf. Digoxin is the choice cardiac glycoside for prolonged use in the treatment of heart failure.

28.

28. cardiac glycoside; ventricular contractions (heart rate); more forcefully (stronger)

Digoxin is classified as a *_____.

   This drug slows the *_____ and makes the heart beat *_____.

29.

29. increases; improved or increased; increased

The patient was digitalized with digoxin and then placed on a daily maintenance dose of digoxin, 0.25 mg. This (increases/decreases) _____ cardiac output. Blood circulation is then _____. The urinary output is _____.

   It is important that you remember the toxic effects of digitalis preparations, which include pulse below 60, nausea, vomiting, and anorexia. Hypokalemia is one of the most common causes of digitalis toxicity.

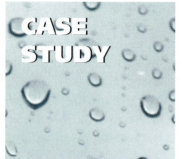

CASE STUDY

REVIEW

A 68-year-old female is diagnosed with heart failure on admission. The clinical assessment of her symptoms and findings are stated under clinical applications.

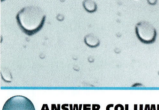

ANSWER COLUMN

1. decrease oxygen demand and increase cardiac output

2. decrease

3. decreased; increase

4. increase myocardial contractility and decrease heart rate

5. a. irritating cough;
b. dyspnea on exertion;
c. crackles; d. hand vein engorgement; e. pulse 110 (tachycardia);
f. ventricular hypertrophy

6. overhydration
7. swelling in the ankles and feet

1. Name the two main goals in the management of heart failure. *_____

2. The purpose of limiting the intake of salt and water in heart failure is to (increase/decrease) _____ preload.

3. ACE inhibitors and diuretics cause (increased/decreased) _____ afterload.
Decreasing preload and afterload (increases/decreases) _____ cardiac output.

4. The patient was given digoxin as part of her care management. Name two primary effects of digoxin on the heart.
*_____

The health professional assessed her physiologic status and identified symptoms of left and right heart failure.

5. Her signs and symptoms of left heart failure include:
a. *_____
b. *_____
c. *_____
d. *_____
e. *_____
f. *_____

6. The symptoms of left heart failure are similar to symptoms of _____.

7. Her symptom of right heart failure is *_____.

8. decrease preload, decrease afterload, and increase myocardial contractility

9. potassium-wasting; hypokalemia

10. Hypokalemia enhances the action of any digitalis preparation, making the digoxin stronger (cumulative action can occur).

11. a. bradycardia—pulse ↓ 60 or arrhythmia, or both; b. anorexia; c. nausea and vomiting

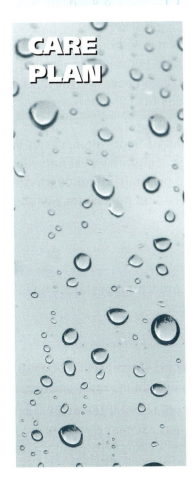

CARE PLAN

8. The main goals to increase her cardiac output are
   * _____.

9. The patient is receiving HydroDIURIL. Is this a (potassium-wasting/potassium-sparing) _____ diuretic? The potassium imbalance that can occur is (hypokalemia/hyperkalemia) _____.

10. If her serum potassium was below average, what effect does this have on digoxin. (Review Chapter 6 if necessary.)
    * _____
    _____

11. Give three symptoms of digitalis toxicity.
    a. * _____
    b. * _____
    c. * _____

PATIENT MANAGEMENT

Assessment Factors

● Obtain baseline vital signs to determine abnormal changes and for comparison with future vital signs.

● Assess for signs and symptoms of left heart failure (over-hydration (FVE) or pulmonary edema), i.e., constant, irritating cough, dyspnea, neck and/or hand vein engorgement, chest crackles.

● Assess for signs and symptoms of right heart failure, i.e., pitting peripheral edema, liver enlargement, fullness of abdomen.

● Check serum electrolyte levels, especially potassium and sodium. Report abnormal findings. Use baseline electrolyte results for comparison with future serum electrolytes.

Nursing Diagnosis 1

Excess fluid volume related to decreased output related to impaired excretion of sodium and water.

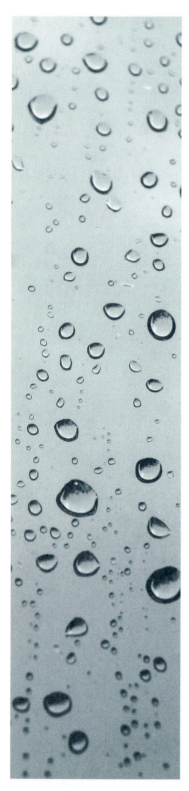

Interventions and Rationale

1. Auscultate lung areas to detect abnormal breath sounds, such as moist crackles due to lung congestion (pulmonary edema).

2. Monitor vein engorgement by checking hand veins for fluid overload. Lower the hand below the heart level until the hand veins are engorged; then raise the hand above the heart level. If the hand veins remain engorged above heart level after 15 seconds, excess fluid volume is most likely present.

3. Assess the feet and ankles daily in the early morning before patient rises. If edema is present, the reason is probably due to cardiac and/or renal dysfunction.

4. Instruct patient not to use table salt to season foods. Salt contains sodium, which can cause water retention. Suggest other ways to enhance flavor of foods.

5. Instruct the patient to eat foods rich in potassium (fruits, vegetables) if he or she is taking a potassium-wasting diuretic and digoxin. Hypokalemia can enhance the action of digoxin and can cause digitalis toxicity (slow, irregular pulse, nausea/vomiting).

6. Assess for signs and symptoms of hypokalemia (serum potassium deficit), i.e., dizziness, muscular weakness, abdominal distention, diminished peristalsis, and dysrhythmia, if patient has been receiving potassium-wasting diuretics for several months.

Nursing Diagnosis 2

Impaired gas exchange related to breathing pattern transudation of fluid into the lung tissues.

Interventions and Rationale

1. Monitor breathing patterns. Report the presence of dyspnea, shortness of breath, rapid breathing, and wheezing.

2. Elevate the head of the bed 30°–75° to lower the diaphragm and increase aveoli spaces for gas exchange. Patient may sit upright in a chair or in an orthopneic position to increase available air space.

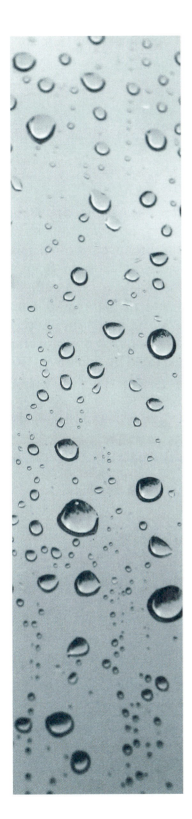

Nursing Diagnosis 3

Impaired tissue integrity related to fluid accumulation in the extremities and buttocks.

Interventions and Rationale

1. Encourage the patient to change positions frequently. Edematous tissue can break down due to hypoxia and constant pressure on skin surface.

2. Provide skin care, especially to edematous areas, at least twice daily.

Nursing Diagnosis 4

Self-care deficit: feeding, bathing, and hygiene, related to fatigue and breathlessness secondary to heart failure.

Interventions and Rationale

1. Assist patient with activities of daily living such as feeding and bathing. Heart failure increases body fatigue and the inability to perform small tasks without extreme exhaustion.

2. Encourage family member(s) to participate in meeting patient's needs as necessary.

3. Encourage the patient to be self-sufficient if he or she is able to perform basic tasks and meet his or her needs, such as dressing, bathing, and hygiene care (brushing teeth).

Other Nursing Diagnoses to Consider

Ineffective tissue perfusion related to cardiopulmonary insufficiency.

Evaluation/Outcomes

1. Confirm that the therapeutic effect of interventions to correct the underlying cause of heart failure.

2. Remain free of signs and symptoms of heart failure.

3. Evaluate the effectiveness of medications in reducing pulmonary and/or peripheral edema and cardiac symptoms.

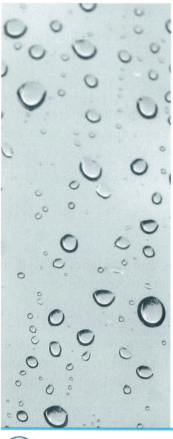

4. Evaluate the dietary intake and fluid intake and output.

5. Evaluate that a support system for the patient is available.

DIABETES MELLITUS (DM) AND DIABETIC KETOACIDOSIS (DKA)

Pathophysiology

Diabetes mellitus (DM) is a complex disease resulting from absolute or relative insulin deficiency. In Type 1 diabetes, the islet cells of the pancreas cannot produce insulin. Lacking insulin, the cells are unable to access glucose for energy needs. The body attempts to compensate for the cellular starvation in multiple ways. Fat and protein catabolism (breakdown) attempt to meet the body's needs for energy. Fatty acids released from the breakdown of fat produce acetone and ketones. The acetone is excreted by the lungs. The ketones cannot be oxidized in the liver and so they accumulate in the blood. This can lead to ketoacidosis. In Type 2 diabetes, insulin exists in insufficient quantities or the body is resistant to the action of insulin.

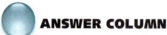

ANSWER COLUMN

30.
A cessation or deficit of insulin secretions (increases/decreases) _____ the body's utilization of glucose.

30. decreases

31.
Diabetic ketoacidosis (DKA) is more likely to occur with which type of diabetes mellitus? (Type 1 diabetes mellitus/Type 2 diabetes mellitus) *_____

31. Type 1 diabetes mellitus

32.
Failure to metabolize glucose leads to a(n) (increase/decrease) _____ in fat catabolism. Ketosis occurs, which results in a(n) (deficit/excess) _____ of ketone bodies (ketonic acids) in the blood.

32. increase; excess

33.

With an increase in bicarbonate ions excreted by the kidneys due to osmotic diuresis, more hydrogen ions are reabsorbed into the circulation. Cellular breakdown causes lactic acid to be released from the cells. The increase in ketone bodies, hydrogen ions, and lactic acid increases the (acidotic/alkalotic) _____ state of the body.

33. acidotic

34.

Failure of glucose metabolism can cause which of the following:

( ) a. Glucose utilization for energy

( ) b. Fat catabolism, which releases excessive amounts of ketone bodies

An excessive number of ketone bodies in the body is known as

_____.

Ketosis leads to diabetic _____.

34. b; ketosis; ketoacidosis

35.

An elevation of the blood sugar level, > 180 mg/dL, increases the glucose concentration in the glomeruli of the kidneys. When the concentration of glucose in the glomeruli exceeds the renal threshold for tubular reabsorption, glycosuria results. Increased glucose concentration acts as an osmotic diuretic, which causes diuresis.

What does *glycosuria* mean? *_____

What does *diuresis* mean? *_____

35. sugar in the urine; excess urine excretion

36.

An elevated blood sugar also increases the hyperosmolality of the extracellular fluid.

The hyperosmolality of the extracellular fluid leads to a withdrawal of fluid from the cells. Thus the ECF space is increased.

The fluid from the cells dilutes the extracellular sodium concentration, producing (hypernatremia/hyponatremia)

_____.

36. hyponatremia; a

The migration of intracellular fluid into the extracellular fluid results in which of the following:

( ) a. Cellular dehydration

( ) b. Cellular hydration

37.

In renal excretion, the ketones (strong acids) combine with the cation sodium, causing sodium depletion. Ketone bodies (ketones) are excreted as ketonuria. The additional solute load of ketones in the glomeruli results in which of the following:

( ) a. A decreased loss of water in the formation of ketonuria

( ) b. An increased loss of water in the formation of ketonuria

37. b

38.

Polyuria can result from which of the following:

( ) a. Glycosuria

( ) b. Anuria

( ) c. Ketonuria

With the loss of water, the solute concentration of the blood (increases/decreases) _____ and the blood volume (increases/decreases) _____.

38. a, c; increases; decreases

39.

In diabetic ketoacidosis (DKA), the body attempts to compensate for the acidosis through nausea and vomiting. By ridding the body of stomach acids, the system attempts to normalize the pH. This may lead to severe fluid and electrolyte imbalances.

There is an increase in water loss by way of the lungs due to Kussmaul breathing (rapid vigorous breathing).

Dehydration occurs from which of the following:

( ) a. Nausea and vomiting

( ) b. Kussmaul breathing

( ) c. Oliguria

( ) d. Polyuria

39. a, b, d

40.

The failure of cellular utilization of glucose causes potassium to leave the cells. The serum potassium level may therefore reflect normal or high serum values.

Potassium is lost as the result of vomiting and renal excretion. As a result of hemoconcentration, the serum potassium levels may appear *_____.

40. normal or high

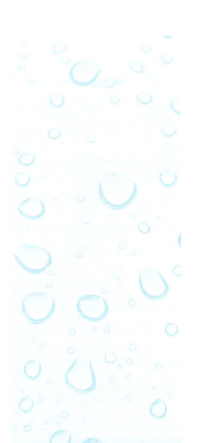

Table 20-4	Causes of DKA
Categories	**Causes**
Insulin deficiency	Undiagnosed DM, Type 1
	Omission of prescribed insulin
Acute incidence	Infection
	Trauma
	Pancreatitis
	Major surgical interventions
	Gastroenteritis
	Myocardial infarction
	Cerebrovascular accident
Miscellaneous	Hyperthyroidism
	Steroids and other drugs
	Adrenergic agonists
	Alcohol abuse

Etiology

Between 20% and 30% of DKA patients are those who are newly diagnosed with DM, Type I. Table 20-4 lists the causes of DKA.

41.

Two common causes of DKA due to insulin deficiency are
*_____.

41. undiagnosed DM and omission of a prescribed insulin dose

42.

Name three causes of an acute incidence of DKA. *_____
_____

42. infection, trauma, and pancreatitis (others: major surgery, gastroenteritis, myocardial infarction, and cerebrovascular accident)

Clinical Manifestations

The most common symptoms of DKA are extreme thirst, polyuria, weakness, and fatigue. Hyperglycemia induces osmotic diuresis. Table 20-5 describes the signs and symptoms and laboratory results related to DKA. Table 20-5 should be used as a guide for the assessment of patients with probable DKA.

Table 20-5	Clinical Manifestations of DKA

Signs and Symptoms	Rationale
Extreme Thirst	Elevated blood sugar and ketones increase the serum osmolality, causing thirst
Polyuria	and osmotic diuresis.
Weakness, Fatigue	Reduced cellular metabolism results in low energy levels.
Nausea, Vomiting	By ridding the body of stomach acids, the system attempts to normalize the pH.
	Continuous vomiting causes a loss of body fluids and electrolytes. Dehydration results.
Vital Signs	
Temperature elevated or N	Infection causes an elevated temperature; dehydration can cause a slightly
	elevated temperature.
Pulse rapid	With a loss of body fluid, the heart beats faster to compensate in order to maintain
	circulation. Tachycardia of greater than 140 bpm denotes a severe fluid loss.
Blood pressure slightly to	With early fluid loss from diuresis, the blood pressure decreases by 10–15 mm Hg.
severely decreased	
Respiration rapid,	Kussmaul breathing is a compensatory mechanism to decrease H_2CO_2 (acid) by
vigorous breathing	blowing off CO_2
Poor Skin Turgor; Dry,	Dehydration frequently results in these symptoms; poor skin turgor; dry, parched
Parched Lips;	lips; and confusion.
Disorientation, Confusion	
Abdominal Pain with	Abdominal pain usually indicates severe ketoacidosis.
Tenderness	
Laboratory Test Results	
Blood sugar 300–800 mg/dL	Blood sugar level is high; at times, it is not as high as HHS (hyperosmolar
	hyperglycemic state—more commonly occurring with Type 2 DM). Sugar is not
	metabolized and utilized by the cells.
Electrolytes	
Potassium N, ↓, ↑	Potassium in the cells is low, but the serum potassium level may be high due to a
	hemoconcentration. Normal or low levels can also occur.
Sodium N, ↓, ↑	Sodium is lost because of diuresis. Serum levels can be elevated due to dehydration.
Magnesium N, ↓, ↑	Magnesium and phosphorus react the same as potassium. Chloride is excreted with
Chloride N, ↓	sodium and water.
Phosphorus low N or ↓	
CO_2 ↓	The serum CO_2 is a bicarbonate determinant. With the loss of bicarbonate, the serum
	CO_2 is greatly decreased (<14 mEq/L).
Serum osmolality 300–350	Fluid loss (dehydration) increases the serum osmolality.
mOsm/kg	
Hematology	
Hemoglobin, hematocrit ↑	Because of fluid loss, hemoconcentration results, increasing the hemoglobin and
WBC ↑	hematocrit levels. Elevated white blood cells can indicate an infection.
Arterial Blood Gases (ABGs)	
pH ↓	The pH is low in the acidotic state. The $PaCO_2$ may be decreased as the lungs are
$PaCO_2$ ↓	expelling CO_2 (compensatory mechanism). The bicarbonate is lost through diuresis
HCO_3 ↓	with an increase in hydrogen and ketone (acid) levels.
Urine	
Glycosuria	Glucose and ketones spill into the urine.
Ketonuria	

Note: N = normal; ↑ = elevated; ↓ = decreased; bpm = beats per minute.

43. extreme thirst, polydipsia, polyuria, fatigue, and weakness

43.

The four early clinical manifestations related to DKA are

*_____.

44.

Indicate which of the following vital signs are related to DKA:

( ) a. Elevated temperature
( ) b. Tachycardia
( ) c. Bradycardia
( ) d. Decreased blood pressure of 10–15 mm Hg
( ) e. High blood pressure
( ) f. Vigorous, rapid breathing
( ) g. apnea

44. a, b, d, f

45.

Identify the changes that result in (a) the skin, (b) the lips, and (c) the sensorium from dehydration associated with fluid loss and diuresis:

a. *_____
b. *_____
c. *_____

45. a. poor skin turgor; b. dry and/or parched lips; c. disorientation or confusion

46.

The five electrolytes that frequently result in an imbalance due to DKA are *_____

_____

_____.

46. potassium, sodium, magnesium, phosphorus (phosphate), and bicarbonate or serum CO_2 (also chloride)

47.

With cellular breakdown, potassium is (lost/reabsorbed) _____ (from/into) _____ the cells.

When the acidotic state is corrected, potassium re-enters the cells and (hypokalemia/hyperkalemia) _____ may result.

47. lost; from; hypokalemia

48.

With early fluid loss, the sodium level may be elevated because of increased aldosterone secretion (sodium-retaining hormone) response.

With continuous diuresis, the serum sodium level is

_____.

48. decreased

49. hemoconcentration (due to deficient fluid volume); infection

49.

What causes the hemoglobin and hematocrit to be elevated?
*_____

An elevated white blood cell (WBC) count is often due to an

_____.

50. acidosis; it is a respiratory compensatory mechanism where the lungs blow off CO_2 to decrease the acidity in the blood

50.

A decrease in the pH and the arterial bicarbonate (HCO_3) indicates metabolic (acidosis/alkalosis) _____ resulting from DKA.

  Why is the $PaCO_2$ (arterial partial pressure carbon dioxide) decreased in DKA? *_____

_____

Clinical Applications

51.

Dehydration is one of the major symptoms and concerns for persons in DKA.

  When there is a marked intracellular and extracellular fluid depletion, the end result is which of the following:

( ) a. Decreased hemoconcentration
( ) b. Increased hemoconcentration
( ) c. Decreased blood volume
( ) d. Increased blood volume

51. b, c

52. If conscious, the patient can drink orange juice or milk, followed by a protein snack. If unconscious, cake icing in the buccal mucosa, IM glucagon, or IV dextrose may be given.

52.

While the patient is receiving IV fluids and insulin, observe for symptoms of hypoglycemia, also known as an insulin reaction, or a hypoglycemic reaction. These symptoms include cold, clammy skin; nervousness; weakness; dizziness; tachycardia; headache; irritability; visual changes; fatigue; diaphoresis; low blood pressure; and slurred speech. The blood sugar is frequently 50 mg/dL or lower.

  How can the insulin reaction be corrected quickly? *_____

_____

53.

When persons are treated for DKA with large doses of insulin, the health professional should observe for what type of reaction? *_____

53. insulin reaction; tachycardia, nervousness, and weakness (also low blood pressure, dizziness, headache, diaphoresis, irritability, visual changes, fatigue, and slurred speech)

Too much insulin causes symptoms similar to shock. Name three symptoms. _____

54.

Patients with diabetes who are ill are encouraged to rest to reduce their metabolic rate. This decreases fat and protein catabolism.

These patients should also be protected from overheating and chilling. If they are in a state of vascular collapse, extra heat should *not* be applied since it can increase vasodilatation and intensify the failure of the circulation.

Rest reduces metabolism in an ill diabetic patient; therefore, rest decreases the chance of _____ and _____ catabolism.

In the state of vascular collapse, extra heat may cause further (vasoconstriction/vasodilatation) _____.

54. fat; protein; vasodilatation

55.

The patient, a 22-year-old female, arrived in the emergency department in a semicomatose state. Prior to admission, she had been vomiting and complained of "feeling weak." The family stated she had a severe cold with a fever for a week. They felt the vomiting was due to a viral infection.

The mucosa in her mouth was dry. Vomiting and dry mucosa indicate _____.

Her respirations were rapid and deep, this can be an indication of which of the following:

( ) a. Kussmaul breathing

( ) b. Dyspnea

Her heart sinus rhythm was sinus tachycardia (pulse rate 120). Her breath had a very sweet smell. The family stated she did not have diabetes mellitus, but there was a familial history of it.

In the emergency room, a stat blood chemistry was done and a urethral catheter was inserted. The blood sugar was 476 mg/dL, the normal range being 70–110 mg/dL. This indicates a (hypoglycemic/hyperglycemic) _____ state. The serum CO_2 combining power was very low, which indicates an _____ state.

55. dehydration; a; hyperglycemic; acidotic

Table 20-6 identifies the laboratory studies, which show how her results deviated from the normal values at the time of her illness.

Table 20-6	Laboratory Studies				
Laboratory Tests	**On Admission**	**Day 1**		**Day 2**	**Day 3**
Hematology					
Hemoglobin					
(12.9–17.0 g)	17.8				
Hematocrit					
(40–46%)	52				
Biochemistry					
BUN (blood urea nitrogen)					
(10–25 mg/dL)*	15				
Sugar feasting—postprandial					
(under 150 mg/dL)	476	825	458	382	60	144
	+1	+1	Trace			
Acetone	1:10	1:10	1:8			
Plasma/serum CO_2†					
50–70 vol %	7	10	14	18	34	44
22–32 mEq/L	3	4	6	8	15	20
Plasma/serum chloride					
(95–108 mEq/L)	104		130	132	133	110
Plasma/serum sodium					
(135–146 mEq/L)	137		151	159	164	145
Plasma/serum potassium					
(3.5–5.3 mEq/L)	4.8		2.7	3.2	4.2	4.5

*mg/100 mL = mg/dL
†Plasma and serum are used interchangeably.

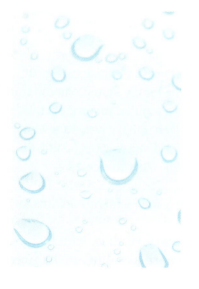

56.

Her urinalysis was as follows:

   Color, dark yellow

   Specific gravity, 1.024

   Reaction, acid

   Albumin, +3

   Sugar, +4

   WBC, many

Her specific gravity shows which of the following:

   ( ) a. A very high range

   ( ) b. A high average range

   ( ) c. A low range

   ( ) d. An indication of an increased amount of product in
      the urine

The +4 sugar in the urine indicates (hypoglycemia/hyperglycemia) _____.

The +3 albumin in the urine indicates which of the following:

( ) a. Normal range

( ) b. Pathologic involvement

56. b, d; hyperglycemia; b

57.

Her hemoglobin and hematocrit counts were which of the following:

( ) a. Normal

( ) b. Below normal

( ) c. Above normal

( ) d. An indication of mild edema

( ) e. An indication of mild dehydration

57. c, e

58.

The feasting blood sugars (blood drawn after eating) on admission and the first day were which of the following:

( ) a. Normal

( ) b. Below normal

( ) c. Above normal

( ) d. An indication of hyperglycemia

( ) e. An indication of hypoglycemia

The second day her blood sugar was 60 mg/dL, which indicates a _____ reaction.

58. c, d; hypoglycemic or insulin

59.

The patient's CO_2 combining power would indicate which of the following:

( ) a. Metabolic acidosis

( ) b. Metabolic alkalosis

( ) c. A bicarbonate loss

( ) d. A bicarbonate increase

59. a, c

60.

On admission, her serum chloride, sodium, and potassium were in the (high/low/normal) _____ range.

On the first day, the laboratory studies indicated which of the following:

( ) a. Hyperchloremia

( ) b. Hypochloremia

( ) c. Hypernatremia
( ) d. Hyponatremia
( ) e. Hyperkalemia
60. normal; a, c, f
( ) f. Hypokalemia

61.

In DKA there is frequently a serum sodium decrease before treatment due to which of the following:
( ) a. Fluid intake
( ) b. Vomiting
61. b, c
( ) c. Urine excretion

Clinical Management

Treatment modalities for DKA include (1) vigorous fluid replacement, (2) insulin replacement, and (3) electrolyte correction. Osmotic diuresis can cause a fluid volume deficit of 4–8 liters of body fluid. In such a case immediate restoration of fluid loss is essential.

Fluid Replacement

62.

In the first 24 hours, 80% of the total water and salt deficit should be replaced. There is less urgency for the other electrolytes since the rate of assimilation of the intracellular electrolytes is limited. Administration of potassium must be included, but *not in early treatment* (unless indicated) since an elevated serum potassium can be toxic. Potassium is not given until renal function is confirmed and the patient voids.

With DKA, 80% of (salt and water/potassium and magnesium) _____ should be replaced in the first 24 hours.

Cellular assimilation of electrolytes is (faster/slower)
62. salt and water; slower
_____ than extracellular assimilation of electrolytes.

63.

For the first hour, 1–2 liters of a crystalloid [normal saline solution (0.9% NaCl)] or lactated Ringer's solution may be rapidly infused to reestablish the fluid volume balance. This may be followed by 1 liter every hour for the next 2 hours as indicated.

Rapid fluid replacement decreases the hyperglycemic state by
63. hemodilution
causing a (hemoconcentration/hemodilution) _____.

64.

Alternating normal saline solution with lactated Ringer's solution may be the IV therapy of choice for improving fluid balance, renal perfusion, and blood pressure. ECF is restored directly from IV therapy. ICF replacement occurs in approximately 2 days.

When reestablishing fluid balance in the ECF space, the suggested amount of IV fluids for the first hour is

* _____. The purpose of rapid infusion of IV fluids is to improve * _____, * _____, and

* _____.

64. 1–2 liters; fluid balance; renal perfusion; blood pressure

65.

Restoration of ICF balance is somewhat (slower/faster) _____ than restoration of the ECF balance.

Indicate which solutions are used initially to correct the fluid imbalance:

( ) a. Dextrose in water (D₅W)

( ) b. Lactated Ringer's solution

( ) c. Normal saline solution (0.9% NaCl)

65. slower; b, c

66.

A fluid overload in the ECF space should be avoided. The healthcare provider should assess for signs of fluid overload. Overhydration or hypervolemia occurs from over-replacement of fluids and is noted by specific symptoms. What are four of the symptoms of overhydration or hypervolemia?

* _____

_____

Overhydration of the brain cells can result from over-replacement. This is known as _____.

66. constant, irritating cough, difficulty breathing (dyspnea), neck and hand vein engorgement, and chest crackles; cerebral edema

Insulin Replacement

Previously, massive doses of insulin were administered for the treatment of DKA. Today, less insulin is used when correcting DKA. The treatment of choice is administering regular insulin via intravenous infusion. The patient may receive a bolus of insulin prior to a continuous rate via the IV. Subcutaneous injection is an additional route, but should be avoided in patients with severe dehydration and poor perfusion.

67.

The preferred parenteral route for correction of DKA includes:

( ) a. Intravenous

( ) b. Subcutaneous

( ) c. Intramuscular

67. a

68.

A standard guideline for IV insulin replacement is an insulin bolus of 0.1 units/kg, followed by 0.1 units/kg per hour continuous IV infusion until blood sugar reaches 200 mg/dL. With children and adolescents, the infusion is begun without the insulin bolus, decreasing the incidence of cerebral edema. If the blood sugar does not fall, the infusion can be increased to 0.2 units/kg per hour. It is important to monitor the patient's hydration status throughout insulin infusion.

Sample Problem: A patient weighs 154 pounds or 70 kg. The order reads regular insulin bolus of 0.1 units/kg and 0.1 units/kg/hour in continuous normal saline solution. The amount of regular insulin to be administered as a bolus is _____ units. The amount of regular insulin to be administered per hour in continuous intravenous normal saline solution is _____ units. How much regular insulin is added to a 500-mL normal saline solution bag to run for 5 hours? _____ units

68. 10.5; 7; 35

69.

The blood sugar must be closely monitored during insulin replacement.

When the blood sugar level reaches _____ mg/dL, the IV fluids are usually switched to 5% dextrose in water. This prevents the possible occurrence of a (hypoglycemic/hyperglycemic) _____ reaction.

69. 250; hypoglycemic

70.

The longer the acidosis persists, the more resistant the person is likely to be to insulin.

If acidosis persists, the person may require (more/less) _____ insulin.

Which of the following types of insulin can be administered intravenously?

( ) a. NPH
( ) b. Regular
( ) c. Protamine zinc insulin (PZI)

70. more; b

Electrolyte Correction

71.

Potassium (K) replacement should start approximately 6–8 hours after the first dose of insulin has been administered (intravenously) and as the acidotic state is being corrected. Potassium replacement is dependent upon adequate renal function, and therefore, the patient must have voided in order to begin replacement. Serum potassium levels should be taken frequently. Potassium moves back into cells as fluid balance and the acidotic state are corrected.

If potassium is *not* given as acidosis is corrected, the serum potassium level may be (high/low) _____. State the rationale for the reaction. *_____

_____

71. low; Potassium moves back into the cells leaving a serum potassium (K) deficit.

72.

While fluid and insulin replacements are occurring, the serum potassium levels should be constantly monitored.

The serum potassium level (increases/decreases) _____ as fluids and insulin are being administered.

72. decreases

73.

When the pH returns to normal, the body is less resistant to insulin. The previously administered insulin becomes active leading to (hyperglycemia/hypoglycemia) _____.

73. hypoglycemia.

74.

Magnesium, phosphate, and bicarbonate serum levels should be closely monitored. If the serum magnesium level is low, correcting hypokalemia does not fully result until the magnesium level is corrected.

There is controversy related to phosphate replacement when treating DKA. Phosphates are needed for neuromuscular function; thus serum phosphorus should be monitored along with the other electrolytes.

Another controversial issue is the use of bicarbonate therapy in the treatment of DKA. Usually, fluids and insulin replacement correct the acidotic state. If the pH falls below 7.0, bicarbonate replacement is usually prescribed.

The three electrolytes other than potassium and sodium that should be closely monitored are *_____

_____.

74. magnesium, phosphate (phosphorus), and bicarbonate

75.

Indicate when a bicarbonate infusion may be ordered:
( ) a. pH 7.15
( ) b. pH 7.05
( ) c. pH 6.95
( ) d. pH 7.21

75. c

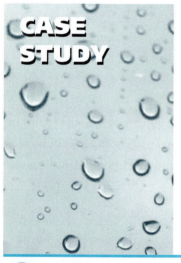

CASE STUDY

REVIEW

A 22-year-old female, unknown diabetic, was admitted to the emergency department in a semicomatose state. Her respirations were deep and rapid, and her breath had a sweet smell. She had been urinating frequently. She had been vomiting for several days. Her postprandial laboratory results were Hgb 17.8 g, Hct 52, sugar feasting or postprandial 476 mg/dL, serum CO_2 3 mEq/L, serum sodium 137 mEq/L, serum chloride 104 mEq/L, and serum potassium 4.8 mEq/L.

 ANSWER COLUMN

1. deep, rapid respirations (Kussmaul breathing), sweet smelling breath, and frequent urination

1. According to the patient's history, identify three clinical symptoms of hyperglsycemia. *_____

_____

2. frequent urination and prolonged vomiting; an elevated hemoglobin and hematocrit

2. Two clinical symptoms that indicated dehydration were
*_____

What two laboratory results also indicated dehydration?
*_____

3. 476; 70–110; 150 or
   lower

4. hyperosmolar

5. glycosuria

6. decreased; metabolic
   acidosis

7. ketone bodies or ketosis
   (strong acid); diabetic
   ketoacidosis

8. the 2 liters of normal
   saline solutions. One
   liter of normal saline
   (0.9% NaCl) supplies
   154 mEq/L of Na$^+$ and
   154 mEq/L of Cl$^-$.

9. Rehydration causing
   dilution of potassium.
   Also some of the
   potassium may be
   returning to the cells with
   the correction of DKA.

10. 6–8

3. Her feasting sugar or postprandial blood sugar was
   _____ mg/dL. The normal range for a fasting
   blood sugar is _____ mg/dL and for feasting
   sugar is _____ mg/dL.

4. Increased blood sugar causes the body fluids to be (hypo-
   osmolar/hyperosmolar) _____; thus, osmotic
   diuresis results.

5. Polyuria can occur from ketonuria and _____.

6. Her serum CO_2 was markedly _____. What type
   of acid-base imbalance is present? * _____
   _____

7. Her acidosis is the result of fat catabolism, producing
   * _____. This type of acidosis is referred to as
   * _____.

   In the emergency department, the patient received
   2 liters of normal saline (0.9% NaCl), NaHCO$_3$, and insulin.
   The health professional checked her laboratory results and
   noted that her blood sugar remained high and her serum
   CO_2 remained low. Her electrolytes were Na 151 mEq/L, Cl
   130 mEq/L, and K 2.7 mEq/L.

8. Her elevated serum sodium and chloride may be due to
   * _____
   * _____.

9. The low serum potassium level may be due to * _____
   _____.

10. Potassium should be administered * _____ hours
    after correction of acidosis.

    In the emergency department, the patient received 35
    units of regular insulin. The first day of admission she re-
    ceived a total of 175 units of regular insulin and 2 liters of
    normal saline solution (1 liter contained 5% dextrose).
    Also, the first day she received KCl—100 mEq/L in 2 liters
    of IV fluids.

    Her laboratory results the second day were blood sugar
    60 mg/dL, serum CO_2 15 mEq/L and 20 mEq/L, serum Na
    164 mEq/L, Cl 133 mEq/L, and K 4.2 mEq/L.

11. 200 mg/dL
12. nervousness, cold and clammy skin, tachycardia, and slurred speech (others: hunger, dizziness, low blood pressure, headache, irritability, visual changes, diaphoresis, and fatigue)
13. 2 liters of normal saline solutions administered the first day

11. Blood sugars need to be monitored frequently. When the blood sugar level drops to *_____, 5% dextrose in water should be given.

12. The health professional should observe for symptoms of hypoglycemia. Four of the symptoms are *_____ _____.

13. Her serum sodium and serum chloride levels were still elevated the second day. This may be due to *_____ _____.

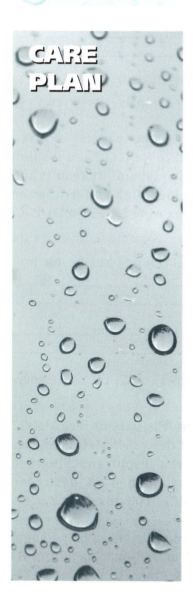

CARE PLAN

PATIENT MANAGEMENT

Assessment Factors

● Obtain a patient's history of signs and symptoms related to fluid loss and incidences leading to the health problem. Record the vital signs and note abnormal findings such as tachycardia, slightly decreased blood pressure, vigorous-rapid breathing, and slightly elevated or high temperature. These can indicate dehydration and a possible acidotic state.

● Check for abnormal laboratory results that indicate DKA, such as elevated blood sugar (>300 mg/dL); elevated hemoglobin and hematocrit; decreased serum CO_2, normal or low serum potassium, sodium, magnesium, chloride, and/or phosphorus levels; decreased pH; decreased arterial HCO_3; and decreased $PaCO_2$.

● Check urine for glycosuria and ketonuria. These are additional indicators of DKA.

● Assess urine output. Polyuria is an indicator of osmotic diuresis.

Nursing Diagnosis 1

Deficient fluid volume related to hyperglycemia and osmotic diuresis (polyuria).

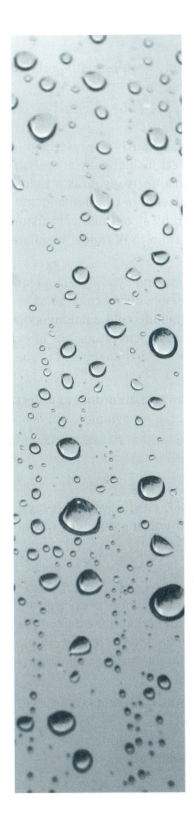

Interventions and Rationale

1. Monitor vital signs (VS). Vital signs that are indicative of fluid loss or dehydration include rapid, thready pulse rate; slightly decreased systolic blood pressure; rapid, vigorous breathing (Kussmaul breathing); and slightly elevated temperature. During the acute period of DKA management, monitor vital signs and other parameters hourly or as warranted by the patient's condition.

2. Check for other signs and symptoms of fluid loss such as poor skin turgor; dry, parched lips; dry, warm skin; and dry mucous membranes.

3. Check the serum osmolality from laboratory results or from assessment of physical changes. Normal serum osmolality is 280–295 mOsm/kg. The serum osmolality level may also be obtained by doubling the serum sodium level.

4. Monitor blood sugar level. Levels greater than 200 mg/dL indicate hyperglycemia. Increased blood sugar levels can cause osmotic diuresis.

5. Observe for signs and symptoms of hypokalemia and hyperkalemia. Symptoms of hypokalemia are malaise, dizziness, arrhythmias, hypotension, muscular weakness, abdominal distention, and diminished peristalsis. Hypokalemia can occur as the acidotic state is corrected. Symptoms of hyperkalemia are tachycardia and then bradycardia, abdominal cramps, oliguria, numbness, and tingling in extremities.

6. Instruct the patient to monitor blood sugar levels and/or urine to detect glycosuria. Patients can test their blood sugars with the use of a glucometer or some other approved testing device. Patients should also check their ketone levels when blood glucose levels exceed 300 mg/dL. This may be done via urine testing for ketones, or preferably, using a blood ketone meter.

7. Administer normal saline solution and/or lactated Ringer's solution as prescribed to re-establish ECF. IV fluids for the first hour are usually given rapidly.

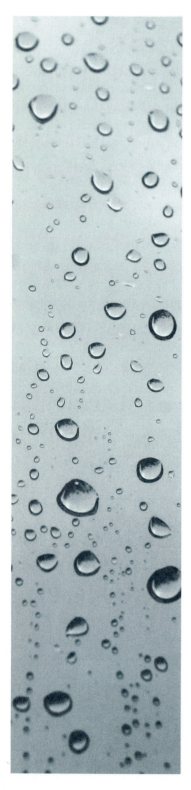

Nursing Diagnosis 2

Imbalanced nutrition: less than body requirements, related to insufficient utilization of glucose and nutrients.

Interventions and Rationale

1. Administer regular insulin intravenously as prescribed in a bolus and in IV fluids to correct insulin deficiency. Usually 0.1 units/kg of regular insulin is given as a bolus. (This bolus may not be administered in children and adolescents.) It is usually followed by a continuous infusion of 0.1 units/kg per hour of insulin in IV fluids. Regulate with an IV pump.

2. Observe for signs and symptoms of a hypoglycemic reaction (insulin reaction) from possible overcorrection of hyperglycemia. The symptoms include cold, clammy skin, nervousness, weakness, dizziness, tachycardia, low blood pressure, headache, irritability, visual changes, fatigue, and slurred speech.

3. Monitor IV fluids and adjust flow rate according to orders. If IV fluids are to run fast, observe for symptoms of overhydration.

Nursing Diagnosis 3

Ineffective tissue perfusion (renal, cardiopulmonary, peripheral) related to deficient fluid volume and lack of glucose utilization.

Interventions and Rationale

1. Monitor urine output, heart rate, blood pressure, and chest sounds for abnormalities. Fluid volume defect (dehydration) limits tissue perfusion and decreases circulatory volume and nutrients available to the vital organs. Report abnormal findings.

2. Monitor arterial blood gases (ABGs), particularly the pH, $PaCO_2$, PaO_2, and HCO_3. A decrease in pH and arterial HCO_3 determines the severity of the acidotic state. Tissue perfusion is decreased during acidosis.

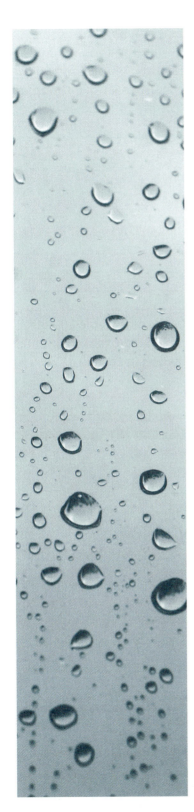

Other Nursing Diagnoses to Consider

Risk for injury: cells and tissues, related to glucose intolerance and infection secondary to DKA. Excess fluid volume (overhydration) related to excessive administration of IV fluids.

Risk for unstable glucose level, related to omission of insulin doses, infection, or excessive dosing of insulin.

Evaluation/Outcomes

1. Confirm that the therapeutic effect of interventions to correct the underlying cause of diabetic ketoacidosis.

2. Remain free of signs and symptoms of diabetic ketoacidosis.

3. Monitor the laboratory tests, serum electrolytes and glucose, and ABGs, that these tests remain within normal ranges.

4. Evaluate the dietary intake and fluid intake and output.

5. Evaluate that a support system for the patient is available.

Relevant Web Sites

American Diabetes Association
www.diabetes.org

Juvenile Diabetes Research Foundation
www.jdrf.org

Type 1 Diabetes Trial Net
www.diabetestrialnet.org

● CHRONIC OBSTRUCTIVE PULMONARY DISEASE (COPD)

Pathophysiology

In COPD, an abnormal inflammatory response is triggered by inhalation exposures, particularly tobacco smoking. Macrophages and lymphocytes increase, releasing cytokines and inflammatory mediators. There is an imbalance of proteinase and antiproteinase causing lung parenchymal destruction. Remodeling of the peripheral airways and pulmonary

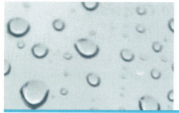

vascular changes also occur. These mechanisms produce several pathophysiologic changes including mucus hypersecretion and ciliary dysfunction, airflow limitation and hyperinflation. Gas exchange abnormalities and pulmonary hypertension develop later in the course of the disease.

ANSWER COLUMN

76. a. mucus hypersecretion
b. ciliary dysfunction
c. airflow limitation
d. hyperinflation

76.
List four pathophysiologic changes in COPD.
a. * _____
b. * _____
c. * _____
d. * _____

Bronchitis and emphysema generally coexist. Table 20-7 lists the pathophysiologic changes associated with COPD conditions. The rationale for pathophysiologic changes is included.

77. expiration; lung remodeling

77.
In COPD, airflow limitation is greatest on (inspiration/expiration) _____ due to *_____.

78. 35–45; hypercapnia; >45

78.
The normal value of PaCO$_2$ is _____ mm Hg.
The term for CO$_2$ retention is _____ when the PaCO$_2$ is _____ mm Hg.

79. respiratory acidosis; CO$_2$ combines with water to produce carbonic acid, thus causing acidosis; <7.35; >45 mm Hg

79.
An acid-base imbalance that occurs in advanced COPD is
* _____.

Explain how this acid-base imbalance occurs. *_____
_____

The pH is _____ and the PaCO$_2$ is _____.

80.
The name for reduced oxygen (O$_2$) concentration in the blood is _____.

| Table 20-7 | **Major Pathophysiologic Changes in COPD** |

Pathophysiologic Changes	Rationale
Mucus hypersecretion	Inflammation results in increased numbers and enlargement of goblet cells; inflammatory exudates form in airway lumens.
Ciliary dysfunction	Release of proteinases during inflammation causes epithelial damage and reduced ciliary beat frequency.
Airflow limitation particularly on expiration	Repeated cycles of injury & repair of peripheral airways cause lung remodeling; increased collagen and scar tissue in bronchial walls result in fibrosis; breakdown of intra-alveolar elastic fibers cause loss of elastic recoil; loss of alveolar attachments as a result of septal destruction.
Hyperinflation	Supporting structures of lung destroyed; lack of traction on bronchiole walls; bronchioles collapse on expiration trapping air in distal alveoli.
Gas exchange abnormalities:*	
Hypercapnia	Accumulation of carbon dioxide (CO_2) in the blood due to chronic alveolar hypoventilation; decreased surface area for gas diffusion as a result of alveolar wall and capillary loss; and inspiratory muscle weakness and airway obstruction (normal CO_2 35–45 mm Hg; hypercapnia > 45 mm Hg).
Respiratory acidosis	Retained CO_2 combines with water to produce carbonic acid (H_2O) + CO_2 = H_2CO_3); arterial blood gases reflect pH < 7.35 and $PaCO_2$ > 45 mmHg; may compensate with increased serum bicarbonate (HCO_3).
Hypoxemia	Reduced oxygen in the arterial blood (PaO_2 < 60 mm Hg, SaO_2 < 88%) caused by chronic alveolar hypoventilation, decreased surface area for gas diffusion and airway obstruction (normal PaO_2 is 80–100 mm Hg; normal SaO_2 is 94–100%).
Pulmonary hypertension*	Defined as elevated pulmonary pressures from increased pulmonary vascular resistance; due to inflammatory cells invading vessel smooth muscle, collagen deposited in vessels destroy capillary bed and decreased oxygen diffusion following alveolar wall loss.
Cor pulmonale*	Pulmonary hypertension causes right ventricular hypertrophy and may cause right-sided heart failure.
Secondary polycythemia*	Increased red blood cell count (RBC) occurs to compensate for chronic hypoxemia; hemoglobin concentration will also increase.

*late changes.

80. hypoxemia; increase; increased; More RBCs and hemoglobin are needed to carry oxygen.

Decreased arterial O_2 causes the number of red blood cells to (increase/decrease) _____.

The hemoglobin and red blood cells are (increased/decreased) _____.

Why? *_____

81. Yes. Antitrypsin deficiency permits the proteolytic enzymes in the lungs to damage lung tissue.

82. pulmonary hypertension; inflammatory cells invade vessel smooth muscles, collagen deposits destroy capillary beds, and alveolar wall loss decreases oxygen diffusion.

81.

Could a nonsmoker with an alpha$_1$-antitrypsin deficiency develop emphysema? _____.

Explain the rationale for your answer. * _____

_____

82.

Cor pulmonale is caused by * _____

_____.

Pulmonary hypertension can occur in COPD when
*
_____.

Fluid and Electrolyte Considerations

Respiratory acidosis with metabolic compensation may influence fluid and electrolyte balances by decreasing binding of calcium to albumin. An increase in serum ionized calcium results. On rare occasions, respiratory acidosis may cause an extracellular shift of potassium and subsequent hyperkalemia. Other disturbances in fluid and electrolyte balance relate to malnourishment associated with the dyspnea, sensation of fullness and distention common with air swallowing and hyperinflation, and increased caloric expenditure seen in COPD patients. Medications such as corticosteroids and theophylline also cause bloating and early satiety. Potassium-wasting diuretics used for patients experiencing heart failure from cor pulmonale may trigger hypovolemia, hypokalemia, and hyponatremia. Tachypnea and fever related to infections may also contribute to hypovolemia due to insensible losses.

Clinical Manifestations

One of the earliest symptoms of COPD is a chronic cough which is intermittent and occurs in the morning. COPD patients frequently produce small amounts of tenacious sputum with coughing. However, dyspnea, considered the hallmark of COPD, is often the reason why patients first seek medical attention. This progressive dyspnea typically interferes with activities of daily living and may be associated with an acute respiratory infection. These symptoms in addition to the history of exposure to risk

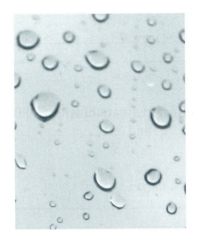

factors should prompt healthcare providers to consider a diagnosis of COPD.

Spirometry is the gold standard for diagnosing COPD and helps to classify the severity of the disease. Spirometry measures volume of air forcibly exhaled from the point of maximal inspiration (forced vital capacity or FVC) and the volume of air exhaled during the first second of this maneuver (forced expiratory volume in one second or FEV_1). The ratio of these two measures (FEV_1/FVC) is calculated and compared to reference values based on age, height, sex, and race. A ratio < 0.70 or 70% following bronchodilator use indicates airflow limitation.

Table 20-8	Major Clinical Manifestations of COPD
Signs and Symptoms	**Description/Explanation**
Dyspnea	Difficulty breathing due to airflow obstruction; patients report shortness of breath, gasping for air, heaviness, air hunger; prompted by exertion or infection but occurs at rest as disease progresses; ↑ respiratory rate (tachypnea).
Cough	Initially intermittent, typically earlier in the day; eventually occurs on a daily basis; may be nonproductive but often is productive as disease progresses.
Sputum	Clear or white, often tenacious; green or purulent with infection; amounts vary but increases with infection.
Prolonged expiration	Inspiration to exhalation ratio > 1:2 due to loss of lung elasticity.
Accessory muscle use	Use of muscles not typically used for breathing including the sternocleidomastoid, spinal, and neck muscles when patient is dyspneic/hypoxemic.
Intercostal retractions	Muscles between ribs draw in during inspiration when patient is dyspneic/hypoxemic.
Tripod position	While sitting, patient leans forward with hands resting on knees or with arms and elbows supported with table in order to relieve respiratory distress.
Barrel-shaped chest (A-P diameter = lateral diameter)	Distended alveoli trap air, flattening the diaphragm and increasing anterior-posterior diameter.
Abnormal breath sounds	Decreased sounds because of reduced airflow; wheezes due to air passing through narrow airways; crackles due to air passing through airway fluid. Also, heart sounds may be distant.
Cyanosis	Bluish color of skin, lips suggesting poor tissue perfusion, hypoxemia and/or hemoglobin < 5 g/dL.
Nail clubbing	Soft tissue thickening beneath the proximal nail plate that results in sponginess; cause poorly understood.

83. cough and dyspnea on exertion
84. a. use of accessory muscles
    b. intercostal retractions
    c. prolonged expiratory phase
85. loss of lung elasticity, chronic air trapping, and chest wall expansion with chest rigidity or dorsal kyphosis from a bent position and using accessory respiratory muscles

83.
Two early signs and symptoms of COPD are *_____
_____.

84.
Three qualities of the respiratory effort of a patient with COPD are: _____, _____, and _____.

85.
A common characteristic of COPD is a barrel-shaped chest. Explain. *_____
_____.

Table 20-9	Diagnostic and Laboratory Studies Used With COPD Patients
Test	**Explanation/Rationale**
Spirometry	Forced vital capacity (FVC) and forced expiratory volume in one second (FEV_1) − FEV_1/FVC < 70% following bronchodilator confirms COPD.
Arterial blood gases	Obtain baseline and for patients with FEV_1 < 40% or with COPD exacerbations; abnormalities usually develop late in the disease.
pH ↓ (< 7.35)	As a result of hypercapnia; retained CO_2 combines with water to produce carbonic acid.
$PaCO_2$ ↑ (> 45 mm Hg)	Decreased pH and increased $PaCO_2$ indicate respiratory acidosis.
HCO_3 ↑ (> 26 meq/l)	An increased bicarbonate level indicates metabolic compensation to neutralize or decrease acidosis. A normal HCO_3 (22–26 meq/L) indicates no compensation.
PaO_2 ↓ (< 70 mm Hg)	Hypoxemia develops as disease progresses.
SaO_2 ↓ (< 88%)	Decreased saturation of hemoglobin with oxygen; Often measured using pulse oximetry during evaluation of patient tolerance of activities.
Base Excess ↓ (< −2)	Indicates acidemia; Reflects body's attempt to neutralize metabolically-produced acids by using buffering compounds such as HCO_3, RBC proteins, phospates, etc. Normal base excess values are between −2 and +2 $mmoL^{-1}$.
Pulse oximetry	Reflects oxygen saturation through measurement of the proportion of light transmitted by oxygenated forms of hemoglobin using finger/earlobe/toe sensor; ABG analysis is recommended when SaO_2< 80%.
Chest X-ray	Used to rule out other etiology, to evaluate presence of cardiac disease; will reveal flattened diaphragm, hyperinflation; may detect blebs and bullae.
Red blood cells (RBCs) ↑ Hemoglobin (Hb) ↑ Hematocrit (Hct) ↑	Erythropoiesis stimulated by chronic hypoxemia; More Hb carries more oxygen.

86. bronchitis; Bacteria grows in retained mucous secretions and respiratory infection results.

87. b, d

88. Elevated HCO_3 level indicates metabolic compensation. Conservation of bicarbonate helps to decrease the acidotic state.

89. dyspnea, sensation of fullness common with hyperinflation, increased caloric expenditure, certain medications such as steroids and theophylline.

90. spirometry; a decrease in the FEV_1/FVC ratio to < 70% or 0.7

86.

A cough is more common with what COPD problem? —————
Respiratory infection is a complication of COPD. Explain why?
*————————————————————————————

————————————————————————————————

87.

Select the arterial blood gas parameters that often occur in patients with late stage COPD: (select all that apply)

( ) a. pH 7.51
( ) b. pH 7.33
( ) c. $PaCO_2$ 34 mm Hg
( ) d. $PaCO_2$ 49 mm Hg

88.

Explain the significance of an elevated bicarbonate (HCO_3) level in respiratory acidosis. *————————————

————————————————————————————————

89.

Malnourishment causing fluid and electrolyte disturbances in patients with late COPD is a result of *————————————,

————————————, ————————————, and ————————————.

90.

The gold standard for the diagnosis of COPD is ————————————, specifically *————————————————————————————.

Clinical Applications

A 54-year-old male who has smoked two packs of cigarettes per day for the last 35 years (70-pack years). He has repeatedly been admitted to the hospital over the last 7 years for COPD. The health professional assessed his physiologic status and noted dyspnea following exertion (breathlessness), barrel-shaped chest, and mild cyanosis. The patient complained of a chronic cough productive for thick white mucus. When checking his breath sounds, the health professional noted decreased breath sounds, and a prolonged expiration. Vital signs were BP 150/86, pulse rate 94, and respiration 26 and labored.

91.

Which of these clinical signs and symptoms taken on admission suggest COPD?

( ) a. Breathlessness
( ) b. Barrel-shaped chest
( ) c. Mild cyanosis
( ) d. Chronic cough
( ) e. Prolonged expiration

91. a, b, c, d, e

92.

A risk factor of COPD which can be linked to his problem is

92. smoking

_____.

The results of his laboratory studies are given in Table 20-10.

Table 20-10	Laboratory Studies		
Laboratory Tests	**On Admission**	**Day 1**	**Day 2**
Hematology			
Red blood cells (4.5–6 million)	6.6	6.5	6.2
Hemoglobin (Male: 13.5–18 g)	16.8	16.6	16.2
Hematocrit (Male: 40–54%)	57.8	57.2	55.6
White blood cells (5–10 mm³)	12.8	13.0	10.5
Biochemistry			
Potassium (K) (3.5–5.0 mEq/L)	3.5	3.6	3.7
Sodium (Na) (135–145 mEq/L)	140	138	139
Chloride (Cl) (100–106 mEq/L)	107	106	106
Carbon dioxide (CO_2) (24–30 mEq/L)	30	36	38
Arterial Blood Gases (ABGs)			
pH (7.35–7.45)	7.24	7.32	7.34
$PaCO_2$ (35–45 mmHg)	73	68	60
PaO_2 (70–100 mmHg)	45	70 (with O_2)	76 (with O_2)
HCO_3 (24–28 mEq/L)	28	34	37
BE (−2 to +2)	+2	+6	+9

93. poor oxygenation or hypoxemia
94. poor nutritional intake. He can be given a potassium-wasting diuretic for heart failure as a result of prolonged respiratory distress.

95. normal

96. metabolic (renal) compensation

97. respiratory acidosis; without; The pH is low, PaCO$_2$ is high, and HCO$_3$ and BE are normal values and thus there is no compensation.

98. respiratory acidosis; Yes; The HCO$_3$ and BE are elevated. This is a compensatory mechanism that brings the pH close to normal value.

99. low; hypoxemia or low oxygen content in the blood

93.

The patient's RBC, hemoglobin, and hematocrit were elevated because of * _____.

94.

His potassium is low average. This can be the result of * _____
_____.

95.

Sodium level may be normal or slightly elevated. His serum sodium value is in the (high/normal/low) _____ range.

96.

The serum CO$_2$ is a bicarbonate determinant. An increased value (alkalosis) may be due to base excess from bicarbonate intake or to metabolic (renal) compensation.

In this situation the cause is most likely * _____.

97.

On admission, his arterial blood gases (ABGs) indicate (respiratory alkalosis/respiratory acidosis) * _____ (with/without) _____ metabolic compensation.

Explain his ABGs in response to your previous answer.

* _____
_____

98.

On day 1 and day 2 his acid-base imbalance reflects * _____.
Is there metabolic compensation? _____. Explain.

* _____
_____

99.

His PaO$_2$ is (high/low) _____. His PaO$_2$ indicates

* _____
_____.

100.

The health professional rechecked his breath sounds and noted coarse crackles in the lower base of both lungs.

100. respiratory infection. This is the result of trapped mucous secretions and the presence of bacteria.

The patient's WBCs are elevated. Crackles and elevated WBCs could be indicative of *_____

_____.

Clinical Management

The patient received bronchodilators, and the health professional was considering the administration of oxygen. Breathing exercises were explained to him. Techniques for smoking cessation will be discussed with him prior to discharge. He is encouraged to eat five to six small, high-protein, high-calorie meals daily.

Table 20-11 lists methods of managing COPD.

Table 20-11

Clinical Management of COPD

Management Methods	Rationale
Smoking Cessation through counseling and pharmacotherapeutics	Smoking cessation slows the rate of decline in FEV_1 and decreases coughing and sputum production.
Oxygen (O_2) if PaO_2 55 mm Hg or less or evidence of tissue hypoxia, cor pulmonale, or altered mental status	Low-flow O_2: with a nasal cannula, transtracheal catheter, or other devices that focus on O_2 with delivery on inspiration. Noninvasive and invasive mechanical ventilation may be indicated during exacerbations of COPD. Provide enough oxygen to increase PaO_2 to at least 60 mm Hg and SaO_2 to at least 90%.
Hydration	Fluid intake should be increased to 2–3 L/day to thin secretions and ease expectoration unless cor pulmonale and/or heart failure is present.
*Bronchodilators** Beta$_2$ agonists (albuterol, salmeterol, terbutaline) Anticholinergics (ipratropium) Methylxanthines (theophylline)† Combivent (ipratropium with albuterol)	These agents dilate bronchioles, enhance mucociliary clearance, improve ventilation, and increase exercise tolerance. Depending on the agent, bronchodilators can be administered orally, intravenously, and through inhalers (with or without spacers) and nebulizers. Side effects may include tachycardia, cardiac dysrhythmias, changes in BP, tremor, agitation, insomnia, and nausea/vomiting. Combination therapy may improve efficacy and decrease risk of side effects. Choice of one or a combination of these medications depends on availability, cost, and individual patient response.
Glucocorticosteroids Prednisolone, Solu-Medrol } systemic Beclomethasone Triamcinolone } inhaled	These agents may improve airflow and gas exchange and may decrease dyspnea. Corticosteroids are typically reserved for acute COPD exacerbations. They may be given orally, intravenously, and through inhalation therapy. Long-term therapy is not recommended due to (1) inadequate evidence of its benefits and (2) side effects associated with use.

(continues)

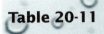

Table 20-11	**Clinical Management of COPD—*continued***
Management Methods	**Rationale**
Antibiotics	When a respiratory infection is present, narrow-spectrum antibiotics are usually given, orally or intravenously. *Streptococcus pneumoniae* and *Haemophilus influenzae* are common bacteria in this patient population.
Vaccinations	A one-time pneumococcal and an annual influenza vaccine decrease the incidence of serious illnesses and death.
Breathing Retraining	Pursed-lip breathing prevents airway collapse so that trapped air in the alveoli can be expelled.
Coughing Techniques	Huffing, a forced expiratory technique, is one to two forced expirations without glottis closure starting from mid-lung to low lung volume, followed by relaxed breathing.
Chest Physiotherapy	Routine chest percussion therapy (CPT), vibration, and postural drainage have not proven beneficial for COPD patients. These techniques may be used in patients who cannot clear excess bronchial secretions. Automatic CPT vests and hand-held devices are available.
Exercise	Exercises that are muscle group specific are used to strengthen respiratory muscle, arm, and leg strength. Improves respiratory status, endurance, and state of well-being.
Complementary and Alternative Therapies	Practicing relaxation techniques, biofeedback, and/or undergoing hypnosis helps to decrease anxiety, fear, and panic. Decreased dyspnea can result.
Nutritional Support with Attention to Electrolytes	Malnutrition is associated with wasting of respiratory muscles. Diaphragmatic functioning decreases with hypophosphatemia, hyperkalemia, hypocalcemia, and hypomagnesemia.
Pulmonary Rehabilitation Program	A multidisciplinary approach to exercise training, nutrition counseling, patient education, and psychosocial support. These programs improve survival and quality of life, reduce respiratory symptoms, increase exercise tolerance, decrease need for hospitalizations, and increase psychological functioning.

*May be given as needed for relief of persistent/worsening symptoms or on a regular basis to prevent/reduce symptoms.
†Not recommended during COPD exacerbations.

101. yes; provide enough oxygen to increase PaO_2 to at least 60 mm Hg and SaO_2 to at least 90%

101.

Based on the patient's admission arterial blood gases, does he need oxygen? Yes/no _____. If so, how much oxygen should be administered? * _____.

102. to liquify secretions and ease in expectoration; cor pulmonale; heart failure

103. a. to dilate the bronchial tubes/bronchioles; b. to enhance mucociliary clearance of mucus; c. to improve ventilation

104. b, c, d, e

105. to prevent airway collapse

106. smoking; smoking cessation

107. malnutrition and hypophosphatemia, hyperkalemia, hypocalcemia, and hypomagnesemia impair respiratory muscle functioning.

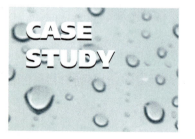

CASE STUDY

102.

Why is hydration important in the management of COPD?

*_____

_____

Increased fluid intake should be contraindicated when

_____ and/or _____ are present.

103.

Bronchodilators are used for the following purposes:

   a. *_____

   b. *_____

   c. *_____

104.

Indicate which of the following side effects may result from constant use or overuse of bronchodilators:

   ( ) a. Bradycardia

   ( ) b. Tachycardia

   ( ) c. Nausea, vomiting

   ( ) d. Cardiac dysrhythmias

   ( ) e. Insomnia

   ( ) f. Skin rash

105.

Identify the purpose of pursed-lip breathing.

106.

Because _____ is the major cause of COPD.

*_____ is one of the most important components of disease management.

107.

Adequate nutritional intake and electrolyte balance is vital for COPD patients because *_____.

REVIEW

  A 54-year-old male has had numerous admissions for severe dyspnea related to COPD. His clinical signs, symptoms, and findings are stated under clinical applications.

ANSWER COLUMN

1. airflow limitation that is not fully reversible and is typically progressive

1. Chronic obstructive lung disease is characterized by:
*_____

2.
a. inflammatory;
b. macrophages, lymphocytes;
c. cytokines, inflammatory mediators;
d. lung parenchymal;
e. peripheral airways

2. COPD is an abnormal _____ response during which _____ and _____ increase, releasing _____ and *_____. There is an imbalance of proteinase and antiproteinase causing *_____ destruction. Remodeling of the *_____ also occurs.

3. smoking

3. What is the major risk factor in COPD? _____

4. antitrypsin; damage to lung tissue; emphysema or COPD

4. Name the protein produced in the liver that inhibits proteolytic enzymes in the lung. _____ A deficit of this protein causes *_____ and the disease _____.

5. fatigue, dyspnea, barrel-shaped chest, and coughing (others: cyanosis, abnormal ABGs), any signs and symptoms listed in Table 20-8

5. Four signs and symptoms of COPD are *_____
_____

6. poor oxygenation or hypoxemia

6. The patient's RBC, hemoglobin, and hematocrit values are elevated. Identify the reason.
*_____

The patient's ABGs on admission are pH 7.24, PaCO$_2$ 73 mm Hg, and HCO$_3$ 28 mEq/L. On day 2 his ABGs were pH 7.34, PaCO$_2$ 600 mm Hg, HCO$_3$ 37 mEq/L, BE +9.

7. respiratory acidosis; No

7. His acid-base imbalance on admission is *_____
_____. Is there metabolic compensation? _____

8. respiratory acidosis; Yes; HCO$_3$ and BE are elevated to decrease acidotic state.

8. On day 2 his ABGs indicate *_____.
Is there metabolic compensation? _____ Explain. *_____

The patient received 3 liters per minute of oxygen and levofloxacin (Levaquin).

9. 90

9. A goal of oxygen therapy is to increase a COPD patient's oxygen saturation (SaO$_2$) to at least _____%.

10. His WBC is elevated, indicating a possible infection (respiratory).

11. huff coughing, teaching pursed-lip breathing, explaining relaxation technique, mild exercise, increase fluids (hydration)

12. exercise training; nutritional counseling; patient education; psychosocial support

---

10. Why was the patient given Levaquin? _____
   * _____

11. Name three actions to assist the COPD patient with his breathing and sputum expectoration.
   * _____
   * _____
   * _____.

Prior to discharge, the COPD patient is enrolled in a pulmonary rehabilitation program. A clinical nurse specialist from the program arrives to discuss the purposes, components, and scheduling of the program.

12. The major components of a pulmonary rehabilitation program are
   * _____
   * _____
   * _____
   * _____

CARE PLAN

PATIENT MANAGEMENT

Assessment Factors

● Obtain a patient history of respiratory-related problems such as dyspnea on exertion and at rest, cough with or without sputum production, wheezing, fatigue, and activity intolerance.

● Assess for history of risk factors such as exposure to tobacco smoke, occupational dusts, gases and fumes, and air pollution. Determine if patient has a history of numerous respiratory infections, or a family history of alpha$_1$-antitrypsin deficiency.

● Inspect for use of accessory muscles, barrel-shaped chest, clubbing, and cyanosis.

● Percuss and auscultate the lung areas noting decreased fremitus, hyperresonance, decreased lung expansion, diminished breath sounds, crackles, and wheezing.

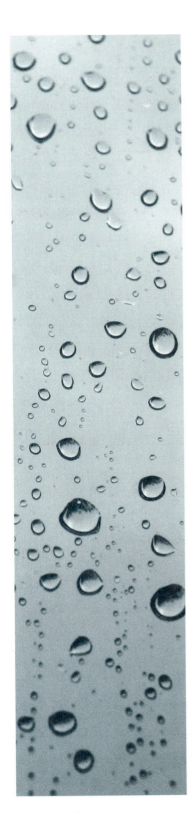

- Check vital signs (VS) for baseline reading to compare with future VS readings.
- Check the arterial blood gas (ABGs) report. Compare results with the norms: pH 7.35–7.45, $PaCO_2$ 35–45 mm Hg, HCO_3 22–26 mEq/L, BE −2 to +2. PaO_2 80–100 mm Hg. SaO_2 94–100%. Consider the COPD patient's norms.

Nursing Diagnosis 1

Impaired gas exchange related to alveoli damage and the collapse of the bronchial tubes (bronchioles), and excessive mucous production.

Interventions and Rationale

1. Monitor ABGs. Report abnormal changes as noted. A marked decrease in pH, a marked increase in $PaCO_2$ (respiratory acidosis), and $pO_2 < 55$ mm Hg (severe hypoxemia) should be reported immediately.

2. Assess the electrolytes and hematology findings when returned and report abnormal results. Low phosphorus, low calcium, low magnesium, and high potassium levels can cause weakened diaphragm functioning. Elevated hemoglobin and hematocrit suggest hypoxemia.

3. Perform a pulmonary physical assessment at frequent intervals.

4. Administer low-flow oxygen therapy to relieve symptoms of hypoxemia and hypoxia. Monitor effectiveness through ABG analysis and/or pulse oximetry.

5. Provide education to patient and family about the oxygen equipment and safe administration in the home setting.

6. Assist with the use of aerosol bronchodilators. Check breath sounds after use of aerosol treatments. If breath sounds are not clear or improved, the physician or nurse practitioner should be notified.

Nursing Diagnosis 2

Ineffective airway clearance related to excess mucous secretions and the collapse of the bronchial tubes, fatigue, and ineffective cough secondary to COPD.

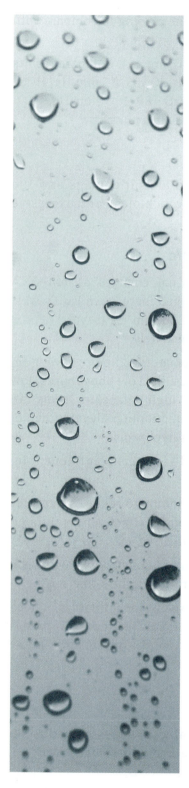

Interventions and Rationale

1. Assess breath sounds for coarse and fine crackles. Provide chest physiotherapy (chest clapping and postural drainage) for crackles and excessive secretions. Have patient deep breathe and cough to clear bronchial secretions.

2. Instruct patient on the huff coughing technique.

3. Nasotracheal suctioning may be necessary for patients with a weak cough and inability to expectorate effectively. Suctioning is only indicated when abnormal breath sounds are present.

4. Instruct the patient to use bronchodilators as directed. Overuse of pressurized bronchodilator aerosol can cause a rebound effect.

5. Promote hydration. Encouraging 2–3 L/day helps liquefy tenacious mucous secretions. Humidifiers may be helpful for patients living in dry climates or using dry heat. Humidifiers must be cleaned daily to prevent mold spore growth.

6. Assist patients to position themselves to mobilize secretions and allow diaphragm-free movement. Sitting in a chair and walking periodically are recommended.

7. Instruct the patient to recognize early signs of respiratory infections, i.e., change in sputum color, elevated temperature, and coughing.

Nursing Diagnosis 3

Ineffective breathing patterns related to airway obstruction, diaphragm flattening, and fatigue.

Interventions and Rationale

1. Instruct the patient how to do pursed-lip breathing (to prevent airway collapse).

2. Assist the patient to an upright position to alleviate dyspnea. Sitting on the edge of a bed with arms folded and resting on several pillows over a nightstand, as well as sitting in a chair with feet shoulder-width apart, leaning forward, and with elbows on knees are two helpful positions.

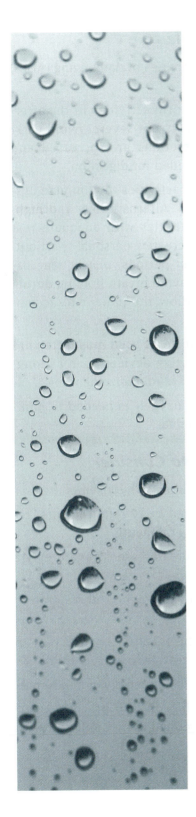

These positions increase chest expansion, relax chest muscles, and position the diaphragm for proper contraction. Another position that facilitates easier breathing when a chair is unavailable is standing with the back and hips against a wall and with feet about a foot from the wall. Shoulders are relaxed and bent slightly forward. This position supports the thorax to allow better use of accessory muscles.

3. Advise the patient not to get overfatigued, alternate rest with activity, and to avoid conditions that increase oxygen demand or irritate the airways such as exposure to stressful situations, temperature extremes, tobacco smoke, chemical irritants, heavy air pollution, and excess dust.

Nursing Diagnosis 4

Anxiety related to breathlessness, dependence on others, and the treatment regime.

Interventions and Rationale

1. Stay with the patient or have a significant other stay with the patient during periods of dyspnea. Provide care in a calm, supportive manner. Encourage the use of pursed-lip breathing.

2. Explore complementary and alternative approaches to dyspneic and anxiety attacks. Examples include relaxation techniques, biofeedback, and hypnosis therapy. Controlling anxiety will improve breathing patterns and decrease oxygen need by the tissues.

3. Explain the treatment and care to the patient and family members and answer questions or refer them to the health care provider.

4. Be supportive of patient and family members.

5. Refer to pulmonary rehabilitation programs, support groups, community agencies, and/or assistance programs.

Nursing Diagnosis 5

Activity intolerance related to breathlessness and fatigue.

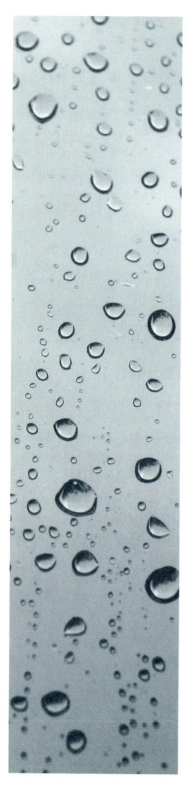

Interventions and Rationale

1. Assist the patient with the activities of daily living (ADLs) as needed.

2. Encourage the patient to perform activities in the afternoon or when breathlessness is not severe. Avoid early mornings when mucous secretions are increased and after meals when energy is needed for digestion.

3. Encourage the patient to pace activities to minimize dyspnea, fatigue, and hypoxemia. Alternate low- and high-energy tasks. Intersperse activities with adequate rest periods. Assist the patient to create a personal chart outlining daily activities and rest periods. Instruct the patient to minimize talking and avoid breath-holding during activities. These measures allow the patient to accomplish more, using less energy.

4. Organize living space so that items used most often are within easier reach. Use adaptive devices such as long-handled dustpans and brushes to minimize bending.

5. Use prescribed supplemental oxygen as needed to minimize exercise-induced hypoxemia.

Other Nursing Diagnoses to Consider

1. Ineffective tissue perfusion related to hypoxemia.

2. Imbalanced nutrition: less than body requirements, related to breathlessness and poor appetite.

3. Ineffective coping related to breathlessness and lifestyle changes.

4. Risk for injury: lungs, related to smoking and respiratory infections.

5. Self-care deficit related to the inability to take part in ADLs because of dyspnea or breathlessness.

6. Fatigue related to change in metabolic energy or hypoxemia.

7. Knowledge, deficient regarding disease process, treatment, and lifestyle changes related to unfamiliarity with information sources.

8. Sleep deprivation related to dyspnea.

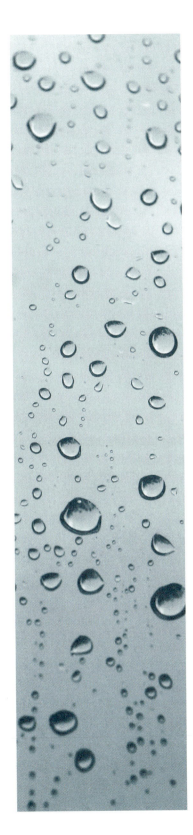

9. Altered thought processes related to hypoxemia, hypercarbia, or sleep deprivation.

10. Ineffective sexuality patterns related to extreme fatigue.

11. Risk for hopelessness.

12. Health-seeking behaviors related to desire to stop smoking.

13. Risk for infection, related to ineffective airway clearance, weak cough, and possible corticosteroid use.

Evaluation/Outcomes

1. Patient's arterial blood gases are within his or her chronic baseline range.

2. Patient is free of signs and symptoms of respiratory acidosis.

3. Patient's breath sounds are clear or improved.

4. Patient exhibits less tachypnea and dyspnea.

5. Patient is able to use breathing exercises, coughing, and positioning to improve gas exchange and mucous expectoration.

6. Patient demonstrates increased activity tolerance and decreased fatigue.

7. Patient minimizes exposures to emotional or physical conditions that precipitate ineffective breathing patterns and hypoxia.

8. Patient participates in smoking cessation activities.

9. Patient exhibits and/or verbalizes less anxiety and identifies appropriate personal and professional sources of support.

Relevant Web Sites

Some useful Web sites for students or health care professionals working with fluid balance issues and or patients with COPD:

National Heart, Lung and Blood Institute
www.nhlbi.nih.gov

American Lung Association
www.lungusa.org

National Lung Health Education Program
www.nlhep.org

Appendix A

Common Laboratory Tests and
Values for Adults and Children

Reference Values

Hematology	Color-Top Tube	Adult	Child
Bleeding time		Ivy's method: 3–7 minutes Average: 8 min	
Erythrocyte sedimentation rate (ESR)	Lavender	<50 years old (Westergren) Male: 0–15 mm/hr Female: 0–20 mm/hr >50 years old (Westergren) Male: 0–20 mm/hr Female: 0–30 mm/hr Wintrobe method: Male: 0–9 mm/hr Female: 0–15 mm/hr	Newborn: 0–2 mm/hr 4–14 years old: 0–10 mm/hr
Factor assay	Blue		
I Fibrinogen		200–400 mg/dL Minimum for clotting: 75–100 mg/dL	Same as adult
II Prothrombin		Minimum hemostatic level: 10%–15% concentration	
III Thromboplastin		Variety of substances	
IV Calcium		4.5–5.5 mEq/L or 9–11 mg/dL	
V Proaccelerin labile factor		Minimum hemostatic level: 50%–150% activity; 5%–10% concentration	Same as adult
VI		Not used	
VII Proconvertin stable factor		Minimum hemostatic level: 65%–135% activity; 5%–15% concentration	
VIII Antihemophilic factor (AHF)		Minimum hemostatic level: 55%–145% activity; 30%–35% concentration	
IX Plasma thromboplastin component (PTC Christmas factor)		Minimum hemostatic level: 60%–140% activity; 30% concentration	

(continues)

Hematology	Color-Top Tube	Reference Values	
		Adult	Child
X Stuart factor, Prower factor		Minimum hemostatic level: 45%–150% activity; 7%–10% concentration	
XI Plasma thromboplastin antecedent (PTA)		Minimum hemostatic level: 65%–135% activity; 20%–30% concentration	
XII Hageman factor		0% concentration	
XIII Fibrinase, fibrin stabilizing factor (FSF)		Minimum hemostatic level: 1% concentration	
Fibrinogen	Blue	200–400 mg/dL	Newborn: 150–300 mg/dL; Child: same as adult
Hematocrit (Hct)	Lavender	Male: 40%–54%; 0.40–0.54 SI units; Female: 36%–46%; 0.36–0.46 SI units	Newborn: 44%–65%; 1–3 years old: 29%–40%; 4–10 years old: 31%–43%
Hemoglobin (Hb or Hgb)	Lavender	Male: 13.5–17 g/dL; Female: 12–15 g/dL	Newborn: 14–24 g/dL; Infant: 10–17 g/dL; Child: 11–16 g/dL
Lymphocytes (T & B) assay	Lavender (2 tubes)	T cells: 60%–80%, 600–2400 cells/µL; B cells: 4%–16%, 50–250 cells/µL	
Partial thromboplastin time (PTT)	Blue	PPT: 60–70 seconds; APTT: 25–40 seconds	
Plasminogen	Blue	2.5–5.2 U/mL; 3.8–8.4 CTA	
Platelet aggregation and adhesion	Blue	Aggregation in 3–5 minutes	
Platelet count (thrombocytes)	Lavender	150,000–400,000 µL (mean, 250,000 µL); SI units: 0.15–0.4 $\times$ 10^{12}/L	Premature: 100,000–300,000 µL; Newborn: 150,000–300,000 µL

Test	Tube color	Adult value	Pediatric value
			Infant: 200,000–475,000 µL Same as adult
Prothrombin time (PT)	Blue or black	11–15 seconds or 70%–100% Anticoagulant therapy: 2–2.5 times the control in seconds or 20%–30%	
RBC indices (mil/µL)	Lavender	Male: 4.6–6.0 Female: 4.0–5.0	Newborn: 4.8–7.2 Child: 3.8–5.5
MCV (cuµ)		80–98	Newborn: 96–108 Child: 82–92
MCH (pg)		27–31	Newborn: 32–34 Child: 27–31
MCHC (%)		32–36	Newborn: 32–33 Child: 32–36
RDW (Coulter S)		11.5–14.5	
Reticulocyte count	Lavender	0.5%–1.5% of all RBCs 25,000–75,000 µL (absolute count)	Newborn: 2.5%–6.5% of all RBCs Infant: 0.5%–3.5% of all RBCs Child: 0.5%–2.0% of all RBCs
Sickle cell screening	Lavender	0	0
White blood cells (WBC)	Lavender	4,500–10,000 µL	Newborn: 9,000–30,000 µL 2 years old: 6,000–17,000 µL 10 years: 4,500–13,500 µL

(continues)

Chemistry	Color-Top Tube	Reference Values	
		Adult	**Child**
White blood cell differential	Lavender		
Neutrophils		50%–70% of total WBCs	29%–47%
Segments		50%–65%	
Bands		0%–5%	
Eosinophils		0%–3%	0%–3%
Basophils		1%–3%	1%–3%
Lymphocytes		25%–35%	38%–63%
Monocytes		2%–6%	4%–9%
Immunohematology (Blood Bank)			
Coombs direct	Lavender	Negative	Negative
Coombs indirect	Red	Negative	Negative
Cross matching	Red	Absence of agglutination (clumping)	Same as adult
Rh typing	Red	Rh+ and Rh−	Same as adult
Acetone (ketone bodies)	Red	Acetone: 0.3–2.0 mg/dL; 51.6–344 µmol/L (SI units)	Newborn: slightly higher than adult
		Ketones: 2–4 mg/dL	Infant and child: same as adult
Acid phosphatase (ACP)	Red	0.0–0.8 U/L at 37°C (SI units)	6.4–15.2 U/L
Adrenocorticotropic Hormone (ACTH)	Lavender	7–10 AM: 15–80 pg/mL; 4 PM: 5–30 pg/mL, 10 PM to Midnight: <10 pg/mL	
Alanine aminotransferase (ALT, SGPT)	Red	10–35 U/L	Same as adult
		4–36 U/L at 37°C (SI units)	Infant: could be twice as high

Test	Tube color	Values	Pediatric values
Albumin	Red	3.5–5 g/dL	
Aldosterone	Red or green	Fast: <16 mg/dL; 4–30 mg/dL (sitting position)	3–11 years: 5–70 mg/dL
Alkaline phosphatase (ALP)	Red	42–136 U/L	Infant: 40–300 U/L
Alpha-fetoprotein (AFP)	Red	(see table below)	
Ammonia	Green	Toxic level: >500 ng/mL; 15–45 µg/dL; 11–35 µmol/L (SI units)	Newborn: 64–107 µg/dL; Child: 21–50 µg/dL
Amylase		30–170 µ/L; Isoenzymes: S: 45–70%; P: 30–55%	
Angiotensin-converting enzyme (ACE)	Red or green	11–67 U/L	Not usually performed
Anion gap		10–17 mEq/L	
Antidiuretic hormone (ADH)	Lavender	1–5 pg/mL; 1–5 ng/L	
Arterial blood gases (See *Others.*)			
Aspartate aminotransferase	Red	0–35 U/L	
(AST, SGOT)		Average 8–38 U/L	
Bilirubin (indirect)	Red	0.1–1.0 mg/dL	Newborn: four times normal level; Child: same as adult

Weeks of Gestation	Serum (ng/ml)	Amniotic Fluid (µg/ml)
14	7–50	11.0–32.0
15	7–60	5.5–31.0
16	10–72	5.7–31.5
17	11–90	3.8–32.5
18	14–94	3.6–28.0
19	24–112	3.7–24.5
20	31–122	2.2–15.0

(continues)

Reference Values

Chemistry	Color-Top Tube	Adult	Child
Bilirubin (total and direct)	Red	1.7–17.1 μmol/L (SI units) Total: 0.1–1.2 mg/dL; 1.7–20.5 μmol/L (SI units) Direct (conjugated): 0.1–0.3 mg/dL; 1.7–5.1 μmol/L (SI units)	Newborn, total: 1–12 mg/dL; 17.1–205 μmol/L (SI units) Child, total: 0.2–0.8 mg/DL
Blood urea nitrogen (BUN)	Red	5–25 mg/dL	Infant: 5–15 mg/dL Child: 5–20 mg/dL
BUN/creatinine ratio	Red	10:1 to 20:1	
Calcitonin	Green or lavender	Male: <40 pg/mL	Newborn: usually higher
Calcium (Ca)	Red	Female: <25 pg/mL 4.5–5.5 mEq/L 9–11 mg/dL 2.3–2.8 mmol/L (SI units)	Child: <70 pg/mL Newborn: 3.7–7.0 mEq/L; 7.4–14 mg/dL Infant: 5.0–6.0 mEq/L; 10–12 mg/dL Child: 4.5–5.8 mEq/L; 9–11.5 mg/dL
Ionized calcium (iCa)		4.4–5.9 mg/dL 2.2–2.5 mEq/L 1.1–1.24 mmol/L	
Carbon dioxide combining power (CO_2)	Green	22–30 mEq/L 22–30 mmol/L (SI units)	20–28 mEq/L

Test	Tube Color	Value	Value (child)
Carbon monoxide (CO), Carboxyhemoglobin (may be done in hematology)	Lavender	< 2.5% saturation of Hb 2%–9% saturation of Hb (smokers)	Same as adult
Chloride (Cl)	Red	180–450 mg/L (SI units) 95–105 mEq/L 95–105 mmol/L (SI units)	Child: 30–65 mg/dL Newborn: 94–112 mEq/L Infant: 95–110 mEq/L Child: 98–105 mEq/L
Cholesterol	Red	Desirable level: < 200 mg/dL Moderate risk: 200–240 mg/dL High risk: > 240 mg/dL	Infant: 90–130 mg/dL 2–19 years: Desirable level: 130–170 mg/dL; Moderate risk: 171–84 mg/dL; High risk: > 185 mg/dL
Cortisol	Green	8 AM–10 AM: 5–23 µg/dL; 138–635 nmol/L (SI units) 4 PM–6 PM: 3–13 µg/dL; 83–359 nmol/L (SI units)	8 AM–10 AM: 15–25 µg/dL 4 PM–6 PM: 5–10 µg/dL
Creatinine phosphokinase (CPK)	Red	Male: 5–35 µg/mL; 30–180 IU/L, 55–170 U/L at 37°C (SI units) Female: 5–25 µg/mL; 25–150 IU/L; 30–135 U/L at 37°C (SI units)	Newborn: 65–580 IU/L at 30°C Child: Male: 0–70 IU/L at 30°C Female: 0–50 IU/L at 30°C
Creatinine	Red	0.5–1.5 mg/dL 45–132.3 µmol/L (SI units)	Newborn: 0.8–1.4 mg/dL Infant: 0.7–1.7 mg/dL 2–6 years: 0.3–0.6 mg/dL, 24–54 µmol/L (SI units) 7–18 years: 0.4–1.2 mg/dL, 36–106 µmol/L (SI units)

(continues)

		Reference Values	
Chemistry	**Color-Top Tube**	**Adult**	**Child**
Digoxin	Red	Therapeutic: 0.5–2 ng/mL; 0.5–2 nmol/L (SI units)	Therapeutic: Infant: 1–3 ng/mL; 1–3 nmol/L (SI units)
		Toxic: > 2 ng/mL; > 2.6 nmol/L (SI units)	Toxic: >3.5 ng/mL
D-xylose absorption	Red	25–40 mg/dL/2 hr	30 mg/dL/1 hr
		Older adult same as adult	
Estrogen	Red	Male: 10–50 pg/mL	1–6 years: 3–10 pg/mL
		Female:	8–12 years: <30 pg/mL
		Early menstrual cycle: 60–200 pg/mL	
		Midcycle: 120–440 pg/mL	
Fasting blood sugar (FBS)	Gray or red	Male: 40–155 pg/mL	Newborn: 30–80 mg/dL
		70–110 mg/dL (serum)	
Feasting blood sugar (See *Postprandial blood sugar, P. TK.*)		60–100 mg/dL (blood)	Child: 60–100 mg/dL
Ferritin	Red	Female:	Newborn: 20–200 ng/mL
		10–125 ng/mL	Infant: 30–200 ng/mL
		10–125 µg/L (SI units)	1–16 years: 8–140 ng/mL
		Male:	
		35–300 ng/mL	
		35–300 µg/L (SI units)	
Folate (folic acid) (may be done by nuclear medicine)	Red	3–16 ng/mL (bioassay)	Same as adult
		>2.5 ng/mL (RIA; serum)	
		200–700 ng/mL (RBC)	
Follicle-stimulating hormone (FSH)	Red	Pre/postovulation: 4–30 mU/mL	5–12 mU/mL
		Midcycle: 10–90 mU/mL	
		Postmenopausal: 40–170 mU/mL	
		Male: 4–25 mU/mL	
Gamma-glutamyl transferase (GGT)	Red	Male: 4–23 IU/l	
		Female: 3–13 IU/L; 4–33 U/L at 37°C (SI units)	

Glucose—fasting blood sugar (*See Fasting blood sugar, P. TK.*)

Glucose tolerance test (GTT) — Gray or red

Time	Serum (mg/dL)	Blood (mg/dL)	Child (6 years or older)
Fasting	70–110	60–100	Same as adult
0.5 hour	<160	<150	
1 hour	<170	<160	
2 hour	<125	<115	
3 hour	Fasting level	Fasting level	

Human chorionic gonadotropin (HCG) — Red

Nonpregnant female: <0.01 IU/mL

Pregnant (Weeks)	Values
1	0.01–0.04 IU/mL
2	0.03–0.10 IU/mL
4	0.10–1.0 IU/mL
5–12	10–100 IU/mL
13–25	10–30 IU/mL
26–40	5–15 IU/mL

Human immunosuppressive virus (HIV) — Red — Negative

Human leukocyte antigen (HLA) — Green — Histocompatibility match

Immunoglobulins (*See Serology, P. TK.*) — Red

Insulin — Red — 5–25 µU/mL

Iron — Red — 50–150 µg/dL; 10–27 µmol/L (SI units)

Infant (6 months–2 years): 40–100 µg/dL

Newborn: 100–270 µg/dL

(continues)

Reference Values

Chemistry	Color-Top Tube	Adult	Child
Iron-binding capacity (IBC, TIBC)	Red	250–450 μg/dL	Infant (6 months–2 years): 100–350 μg/dL Child: same as adult
Lactic acid	Green	Arterial blood: 0.5–2.0 mEq/L; <11.3 mg/dL Venous blood: 0.5–1.5 mEq/L; 8.1–15.3 mg/dL Critical: >5 mEq/L; >45 mg/dL	
Lactic dehydrogenase (LDH/LD)	Red	100–190 IU/L; 70–250 U/L	Newborn: 300–1500 IU/L Child: 50–150 IU/L
Lead	Lavender or green	10–20 μg/dL	10–20 mg/dL
Lipase	Red	20–40 μg/dL (acceptable) 20–180 IU/L 14–280 mU/mL 14–280 U/L (SI units)	20–30 μg/dL (acceptable) Infant: 9–105 IU/L at 37°C Child: 20–136 IU/L at 37°C
Lipoproteins (*See Cholesterol, P. TK; Phospholipids, P. TK; and Triglycerides, P. TK.*)			
Luteinizing hormone (LH)	Red or lavender	Pre/postovulation: 5–30 mIU/mL Midcycle: 50–150 mIU/mL Postmenopause: >35 mIU/mL Male: 5–25 mIU/mL	6–12 years: <10 mIU/mL 13–18 years: <20 mIU/mL
Magnesium (Mg)	Red	1.5–2.5 mEq/L; 1.8–3.0 mg/dL	Newborn: 1.4–2.9 mEq/L Child: 1.6–2.6 mEq/L
Osmolality	Red	280–300 mOsm/kg	270–290 mOsm/kg
Parathyroid hormone (PTH)	Red	PTH: 11–54 pg/mL C-Terminal PTH: 50–330 pg/mL; N-Terminal PTH: 8–24 pg/mL	
Phosphorus (P) (inorganic)	Red	1.7–2.6 mEq/L 2.5–4.5 mg/dL	Newborn: 3.5–8.6 mg/dL Infant: 4.5–6.7 mg/dL Child: 4.5–5.5 mg/dL

Test	Tube color	Adult values	Child values
Postprandial blood sugar (feasting: PPBS)	Gray Blood/ Plasma Serum Red	Adult: serum and plasma: <140 mg/dL/2 hr; <7.8 mmol/L (SI units) Whole blood: <120 mg/dL/2 hr; <6.7 mmol/L (SI units) Elderly: Serum: <160 mg/dL; <8.9 mmol/L (SI units) Whole blood: <140 mg/dL; <7.8 mmol/L (SI units) Serum: <140 mg/dL; <6.7 mmol/L (SI units)	Same as adult
Potassium (K)	Red	3.5–5.3 mEq/L 3.5–5.3 mmol/L (SI units)	Infant: 3.6–5.8 mEq/L Child: 3.5–5.5 mEq/L
Progesterone	Red	Female: Follicular phase: 0.1–1.5 ng/mL Luteal: 2–28 ng/mL Pregnancy: First trimester: 9–50 ng/mL Second trimester: 18–150 ng/mL Third trimester: 60–260 ng/mL Male: <1.0 ng/mL	
Prostate-specific antigen (PSA)	Red	Normal: 0–4 ng/mL BPH: 4–19 ng/mL Prostate cancer: 10–120 ng/mL	
Protein	Red	6.0–8.0 g/dL	Premature: 4.2–7.6 g/dL Newborn: 4.6–7.4 g/dL Infant: 6.0–6.7 g/dL Child: 6.2–8.0 g/dL

(continues)

Reference Values

Chemistry	Color-Top Tube	Adult	Child
Protein electrophoresis	Red	Albumin: 3.5–5.0 g/dL; 52%–68% of total protein	Premature: 3.0–4.2 g/dL; Newborn: 3.5–5.4 g/dL; Infant: 4.4–5.4 g/dL; Child: 4.0–5.8 g/dL
		Globulin: 1.5–3.5 g/dL; 32%–48% of total protein	
Renin	Lavender	Normal sodium diet: supine: 0.2–2.3 ng/mL; upright: 1.6–4.3 ng/mL. Restricted salt diet: upright: 4.1–10.8 ng/mL	3–5 years: 1.0–6.5 ng/mL; 5–10 years: 0.5–6.0 ng/mL
Serotonin	Lavender	50–175 ng/mL; 10–30 µg/dL; 0.29–1.15 µmol/L (SI units)	
Sodium (Na)	Red	135–145 mEq/L; 135–142 nmol/L (SI units)	Infant: 134–150 mEq/L; Child: 135–145 mEq/L
T_3	Red	80–200 ng/dL	Newborn: 90–170 ng/dL; Child, 6–12 years: 115–190 ng/dL
Thyroxine (T_2)	Red	4.5–11.5 µg/dL (T_4 by column); 5–12 µg/dL (T_4 RIA); 1.0–2.3 ng/dL (Thyroxine iodine)	Newborn: 11–23 µg/dL; 1–4 months: 7.5–16.5 µg/dL; 4–12 months: 5.5–14.5 µg/dL; 1–6 years: 5.5–13.5 µg/dL; 6–10 years: 5–12.5 µg/dL
Triglycerides	Red	10–150 mg/dL; 0.11–2.09 mmol/L (SI units)	Infant: 5–40 mg/dL; Child: 10–135 mg/dL
Uric acid	Red	Male: 3.5–8.0 mg/dL; Female: 2.8–6.8 mg/dL	2.5–5.5 mg/dL
Zinc	Navy-blue	60–150 µg/dL; 11–23 µmol/L (SI units)	

Reference Values

Urine Chemistry	Adult	Child
Aldosterone	6–25 µg/24 hr	Not usually done
Amylase	4–37 U/L/2 hr	Not usually done
Bilirubin and bile	Negative to 0.02 mg/dL	Same as adult
Calcium (Ca)	100–250 mg/24 hr (average calcium diet)	Same as adult
	2.50–6.25 mmol/24 hr	
Cortisol	24–105 µg/24 hr	Similar to adult
Creatinine clearance	85–135 mL/min	
Creatinine	Male: 20–26 mg/kg/24 hr;	
	0.18–0.23 mmol/kg/24 hr (SI units)	
	Female: 14–22 mg/kg/24 hr;	
	0.12–0.19 mmol/kg/24 hr (SI units)	
Follicle-stimulating hormone (FSH)	Follicular: 2–15 IU/24 hr	<10 mUU/24 hr (prepubertal)
	Luteal phase: 4–20 IU/24 hr	
	Menopause: >50 IU/24 hr	
Human chorionic gonadotropin (HCG)	Positive for pregnancy: no agglutination	Not usually performed
	Negative for pregnancy: agglutination	
Ketone bodies (acetone)	Negative	Negative
17-Ketosteroids (17-KS)	Male: 5–25 mg/24 hr	Infant: 1 mg/24 hr
	Female: 5–15 mg/24 hr	1–3 years: <2 mg/24 hr
	>65 years: 4–8 mg/24 hr	3–6 years: <3 mg/24 hr
		7–10 years: <4 mg/24 hr
		10–12 years:
		Male: <6 mg/24 hr
		Female: <5 mg/24 hr
		Adolescent:
		Male: <3–15 mg/24 hr
		Female: <3–12 mg/24 hr

(continues)

Reference Values

Urine Chemistry	Adult	Child
Myoglobin	None detected	
Osmolality	50–1200 mOsm/kg	Newborn: 100–600 mOsm/kg
	Average: 200–800 mOsm/kg	Child: same as adult
Phenylketonuria (PKU)	Not usually done	PKU: negative (positive when serum phenylalanine is 12–15 mg/dL)
		Guthrie: negative (positive when serum phenylalanine is 4 mg/dL)
Potassium (K)	25–120 mEq/24 hr	17–57 mEq/24 hr
	25–120 mmol/24 hr (SI units)	
Protein	0–5 μg/24 hr	
Sodium (Na)	40–220 mEq/24 hr	Same as adult
Uric acid	250–500 mg/24 hr (low-purine diet)	Same as adult
Urinalysis		
pH	4.5–8.0	Newborn: 5–7
		Child: 4.5–8
Specific gravity	1.005–1.030	Newborn: 1.001–1.020
		Child: Same as adult
Protein	Negative	Negative
Glucose	Negative	Negative
Ketones	Negative	Negative
RBC	1–2/low-power field	Rare
WBC	3–4	0–4
Casts	Occasional hyaline	Rare

Reference Values

Others	Adult	Child
Urobilinogen	Random: 0.3–3.5 mg/dL 0.05–2.5 mg/24 hr 0.5–4.0 Ehrlich units/24 hr 0.09–4.23 µmol/24 hr (SI units)	Same as adult
Arterial blood gases (ABGs)		
pH	7.35–7.45	7.36–7.44
$PaCO_2$	35–45 mm Hg	Same as adult
PaO_2	75–100 mm Hg	Same as adult
HCO_3	24–28 mEq/L	Same as adult
BE	+2 to −2 (∓2 mEq/L)	Same as adult
Cerebrospinal fluid (CSF)		
Pressure	75–175 mm H_2O	50–100 mm H_2O
Cell count	0–8 mm³	0–8 mm³
Protein	15–45 mg/dL	15–45 mg/dL
Chloride	118–132 mEq/L	120–128 mEq/L
Glucose	40–80 mg/dL	35–75 mg/dL
Culture	No organism	No organism

Adapted from *Laboratory and Diagnostic Tests with Nursing Implications* (7th ed.), by J. L. Kee, 2002, East Rutherford, NJ., Prentice Hall Health. Reprinted with permission.

Appendix B

Foods Rich in Potassium,
Sodium, Calcium, Magnesium,
Chloride, and Phosphorus

Classes	Potassium	Sodium	Calcium	Magnesium	Chloride	Phosphorus
Daily requirements	3–4 g	2–4 g	800 mg	300–350 mg	3–9 g	800–200 mg
Beverages	Cocoa, Coca-Cola, coffee, wines, orange juice, tomato juice	Pepsi-Cola, tea, decaffeinated coffee		Cocoa		
Fruit and fruit juices	Citrus fruits: oranges, grapefruit juices: grapefruit (canned), orange (canned), prune (canned), tomato (canned) Fruits: apricots (dry), bananas, cherries, cantaloupe, dates, figs, raisins (dry), strawberries watermelon, prunes, peaches		Fruit drink with added calcium figs	Bananas Average	High only in dates and banana	
Bread products and cereal	Average to low amount	White bread, soda crackers, and wheat flakes		Cereals with oats Whole grain cereal		Whole grain cereal
Dairy products	Average to low—milk, buttermilk	Butter, cheese, and margarine Low, except if salted	Milk, cheese	Milk (average)	Cheese, milk	Cheese, milk, eggs
Nuts	Almonds, Brazil nuts, cashews, and peanuts		Brazil nuts (moderate)	Almonds, Brazil nuts, peanuts, and walnuts		Peanuts

(continues)

Classes	Potassium	Sodium	Calcium	Magnesium	Chloride	Phosphorus
Vegetables	Baked beans, carrots (raw), celery (raw), dandelion greens, lima beans (canned), mustard greens, tomatoes, spinach *Note:* Nearly all vegetables are rich in potassium when raw; but K will be lost if water used in cooking is discarded	Average to low Celery (high average)	Baked beans, kale, mustard and turnip greens, broccoli, tofu	Leafy green's sag	Spinach, celery	Dry beans
Meat, fish, and poultry	Average—meats High average—sardines, codfish, scallops	Corned beef, bacon, ham, crab, tuna fish, sausage (pork) Low in poultry	Salmon, meats, chicken, egg yolks	Fish, shrimp Low in poultry Low in meats Egg, average	Eggs, crabs, fish (average), turkey	Beef, pork, fish, chicken, turkey
Miscellaneous	Catsup (average), spices, potato chips, and peanut butter	Catsup, mayonnaise, potato chips, pretzels, pickles, dill, olives, mustard, Worcestershire sauce, celery salt, salad dressing—French and Italian	Molasses	Chocolate and chocolate bars, chocolate syrup Molasses Table salt		

Appendix C

The Joint Commission's (TJC) List of Accepted Abbreviations

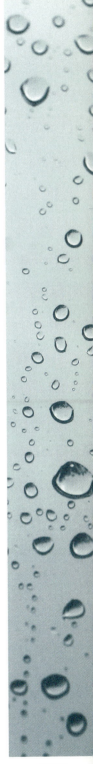

ABBREVIATIONS: DRUG MEASUREMENTS AND DRUG FORMS RECOMMENDED BY TJC

In 2005, The Joint Commission (TJC) (formerly known as the Joint Commission on Accreditation of Healthcare Organizations [JCAHO]) issued a new list of abbreviations that should not be used, but rather written out to avoid misinterpretation.

Below is the "Do Not Use" abbreviation list, followed by a list of abbreviations that could possibly be included in future "Do Not Use" lists.

Abbreviation	Preferred
q.d., Q.D.	Write "daily" or "every day."
q.o.d., Q.O.D.	Write "every other day."
U	Write "unit."
IU	Write "international unit."
MS, MSO$_4$	Write "morphine sulfate."
MgSO$_4$	Write "magnesium sulfate."
.5 mg	Use zero before a decimal point when the dose is less than a whole.
1.0 mg	Do not use a decimal point or zero after a whole number.

The following abbreviations could possibly be included in future Joint Commissions "Do Not Use" lists.

Abbreviation	Preferred
c.c.	Use "mL" (milliliter).
µg	Use "mcg."
>	Write "greater than."
<	Write "less than."
drug name abbreviations	Write out the full name of the drug.
apothecary units	Use metric units instead.
@	Write "at."

TJC lists of acceptable abbreviations follow in three categories:

- Drug measurements and drug forms
- Routes of drug administration
- Times of administration.

Selected abbreviations are listed below. These are frequently used in drug therapy and must be known by the nurse.

Drug Measurements and Drug Forms

Abbreviation	Meaning
cap	capsule
dr	dram
elix	elixir
g, gm, G, GM	gram
gr	grain
gtt	drops
kg	kilogram
l, L	liter
m^2	square meter
mcg	microgram
mEq	milliequivalent
mg	milligram
mL, ml	milliliter
m, min	minimum
oz	ounce
pt	pint
qt	quart
SR	sustained release
ss	one half
supp	suppository
susp	suspension
T.O.	telephone order
T, tbsp	tablespoon
t, tsp	teaspoon
V.O.	verbal order

Routes of Drug Administration

Abbreviations	Meaning
A.D., ad	right ear
A.S., as	left ear
A.U., au	both ears
ID	intradermal
IM	intramuscular
IV	intravenous
IVPB	intravenous piggyback
KVO	keep vein open
L	left

(continues)

Routes of Drug Administration—*continued*

Abbreviations	Meaning
NGT	nasogastric tube
O.D., od	right eye
O.S., os	left eye
O.U., ou	both eyes
PO, po, os	by mouth
®	right
SC, subc, sc, SQ, subQ	subcutaneous
SL, sl, subl	sublingual
TKO	to keep open
Vag	vaginal

Times of Administration

Abbreviations	Meaning
AC, ac	before meals
ad lib	as desired
B.i.d., b.i.d.	twice a day
c	with
hs	hour of sleep
NPO	nothing by mouth
PC, pc	after meals
PRN, p.r.n.	whenever necessary, as needed
q	every
qAM	every morning
qh	every hour
q2h	every 2 hours
q4h	every 4 hours
q6h	every 6 hours
q8h	every 8 hours
s	without
SOS	once if necessary: if there is a need
Stat	immediately
T.I.D., t.i.d.	three times a day

Please refer to the Joint Commission Web site at www.jointcommission.org and that of the Institute for Safe Medication practices at www.ismp.org for more detailed safety information.

Glossary

abdomen the portion of the body lying between the chest and the pelvis.

accessory muscles respiratory muscles of inspiration and expiration that are activated when the diaphragm becomes depressed as in chronic obstructive pulmonary disease.

acid any substance that is sour in taste and that neutralizes a basic substance.

acid metabolites see metabolites.

ascites an accumulation of serous fluid in the peritoneal cavity.

ACTH abbreviation for adrenocorticotropic hormone. A hormone secreted by the hypophysis or pituitary gland. It stimulates the adrenal cortex to secrete cortisone.

ADH abbreviation for antidiuretic hormone. A hormone to lessen urine secretion. Also known as vasopressin.

afterload arterial blood pressure which the ventricle must overcome when ejecting blood during systole; due largely to blood vessel resistance.

albumin the main protein in blood plasma. Its major function is to maintain the osmotic pressure of blood.

alimentary pertaining to nutrition; the alimentary tract is a digestive tube from the mouth to the anus.

alkaline any substance that can neutralize an acid and that, when combined with an acid, forms a salt. Having the properties of a base.

alveolus air sac or cell of the lung.

amphoteric ability to bind or release excess H^+.

anasacra generalized body edema.

anastomosis a procedure that reconnects healthy sections of body tissue after surgical removal of a piece of body tissue (as in bariatric surgery).

anesthetic an agent causing an insensibility to pain or touch.

anion a negatively charged ion.

anorexia a loss of appetite.

anoxia oxygen deficiency.

antipyretic a medication that reduces body core temperature.

anuria a complete urinary suppression.

aortic arch the arch of the aorta soon after it leaves the heart.

aphasia a loss of the power of speech.

arrhythmia irregular heart rhythm.

arterioles minute arteries leading into a capillary.

arteriosclerosis pertaining to thickening, hardening, and loss of elasticity of the walls of the blood vessels.

artery a vessel carrying blood from the heart to the tissue.

ascites an accumulation of serous fluid in the peritoneal cavity.

atrium the upper chamber of each half of the heart.

atrophy decrease in size of structure.

autoregulation control of blood flow to tissue by a change in the tissue.

azotemia an excessive quantity of nitrogenous waste products in the blood, increased BUN and creatinine.

bariatrics the practice of medicine that deals with the causes, prevention, and treatment of obesity. The term *bariatrics* comes from the Greek root *baro* ("weight") and *iatrics* ("treatment").

baroreceptor sensory nerve ending in a blood vessel (e.g., aorta, carotid sinus)

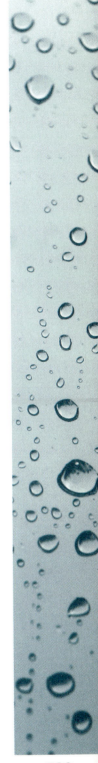

539

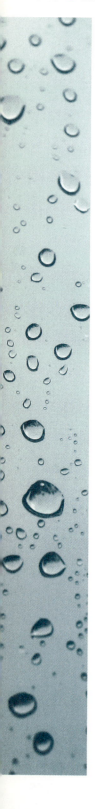

which is stimulated by blood vessel stretch (increase in blood pressure).

base any substance that can neutralize an acid and that, when combined with an acid, forms a salt.

base excess the amount of protons (H⁺ ions) required to return the pH of blood to 7.35 if the partial pressure of carbon dioxide is adjusted to normal.

BE abbreviation for base excess.

biliary pertaining to or conveying bile.

body mass index (BMI) medical standard for measuring degree of obesity. Determined by dividing a person's weight in kilograms by height in meters squared (kg/m²).

blood intravascular fluid composed of red and white blood cells and platelets.

bradycardia pulse rate less than 50 beats per minute.

brain interstitium spaces between the brain tissues.

brain parenchyma functional tissue of the brain.

brain stem herniation protrusion of the medulla, pons, and midbrain into the spinal canal.

bronchiectasis dilatation of a bronchus.

BUN abbreviation for blood urea nitrogen. Urea is a by-product of protein metabolism.

butterfly (winged tip) an infusion device designed for short-term parenteral therapy.

capillary a minute blood vessel connecting the smallest arteries (arterioles) with the smallest veins (venules).

capillary permeability diffusion of substances from capillary walls into tissue spaces.

carbonic anhydrase inhibitor an agent used as a diuretic that inhibits the enzyme carbonic anhydrase.

cardiac dysrhythmia an abnormal heart rhythm.

cardiac output amount of blood ejected by the heart each minute.

cardiac reserve capacity of the heart to respond to increased burden.

carotid sinus a dilated area at the bifurcation of the carotid artery that is richly supplied with sensory nerve endings of the sinus branch of the vagus nerve.

cation a positively charged ion.

cerebral hemorrhage bleeding into brain tissue from rupture in a blood vessel.

cerebral spinal fluid fluid contained within the ventricles of the brain and spinal cord.

cerebrospinal fluid fluid found and circulating through the brain and spinal cord.

cirrhosis a chronic disease of the liver characterized by degenerative changes in the liver cells.

colloid gelatin like substance, e.g., protein.

colloid osmotic pressure pressure exerted by nondiffusible substances.

contraindication nonindicated form of therapy.

conversion table:
  1 kilogram (kg) = 2.2 pounds (lb)
  1 gram = 1000 milligrams (mg) or 15 grains (gr)
  1 liter (L) = 1 quart or 1000 milliliters (ml)
  1 cubic centimeter (cc) = 1 milliliter (ml); 100 ml = 1dl
  1 deciliter (dl) = 100 ml
  1 drop (gtt) = 1 minim (m)
  qh = every hour
  x = times

COPD exacerbation an acute event in the disease, characterized by worsening symptoms, beyond the patient's baseline dyspnea, cough, and/or sputum, that may require alterations in medications and other treatment strategies.

cortisone a hormone secreted by the adrenal cortex.

crackle the sound heard in the chest due to the passage of air through the bronchi, which contain secretions of fluid.

creatinine end product of creatine (amino acid).

crystalloids diffusible substances dissolved in solution that pass through a selectively permeable membrane.

CVP abbreviation for central venous pressure. It is the venous pressure in the vena cava or the heart's right atrium.

cyanosis a bluish or grayish discoloration of the skin due to a lack of oxygen in the hemoglobin of the blood.

cytogenic originating within the cell.

decerebrate condition wherein the brain cells are affected, causing the extremities to be in rigid extension.

decompensation failure to compensate.

decorticate condition wherein the cortex of the brain is affected, causing the extremities to be in rigid flexion.

deficit lack of.

dehydration a state of extracellular fluid volume deficit commonly seen in infants and small children where sodium may be low, normal, or elevated.

dependent edema see edema.

dermis the true skin layer.

dextran colloid hyperosmolar solution.

dextrose a simple sugar, also known as glucose.

diabetes mellitus a disorder of carbohydrate metabolism due to an inadequate production or utilization of insulin.

diabetic acidosis an excessive production of ketone bodies (acid) due to a lack of insulin and inability to utilize carbohydrates, also called diabetic ketoacidosis.

dialysate an isotonic solution used in dialysis that has similar electrolyte content to plasma or Ringer's solution, with the exception of potassium.

diaphoresis excessive perspiration.

diaphragm a major inspiratory muscle that separates the abdominal and thoracic cavities.

diarrhea increased water in the stool, which results in increased stool frequency or loose consistency, yielding a stool output of greater than 10 g/kg/day in children and 200 g/day in adults.

diastolic dysfunction decreased comp-liance of the left ventricles leading to increased left ventricular end-diastolic pressure.

diffusion the movement of each molecule along its own pathway irrespective of all other molecules; going in various directions, mostly from greater to lesser concentration.

diplopia double vision.

disequilibrium syndrome rapid shift of fluids and electrolytes during hemodialysis which causes CNS disturbances.

dissociation a separation.

diuresis an abnormal increase in urine excretion.

diuretic a drug used to increase the secretion of urine.

potassium-sparing diuretic retains potassium and excretes other electrolytes.

potassium-wasting diuretic excretes potassium and other electrolytes.

diverticulum a sac or pouch in the wall of an organ.

dry weight normal body weight without excess water.

duodenal pertaining to the duodenum, which is the first part of the small intestine.

dyspnea a labored or difficult breathing.

edema an abnormal retention of fluid in the interstitial spaces.

dependent edema fluid present in the interstitial spaces due to gravity (frequency found in extremities after being in standing or sitting position).

nondependent edema fluid present in the interstitial spaces, but not necessarily due to gravity alone, e.g., cardiac, liver, or kidney dysfunction.

pitting edema depression in the edematous tissue.

pulmonary edema fluid throughout the lung tissue.

refractory edema fluid in the interstitial spaces that does not respond to diuretics.

e.g. for example.

electrolyte a substance that, when in solution, conducts an electric current.

endothelium flat cells that line the blood and lymphatic vessels.

enzyme a catalyst, capable of inducting chemical changes in other substances.

epidermis an outer layer of the skin.

erythrocytes red blood cells.

erythropoietin factor secreted by the kidneys that stimulates bone marrow to produce red blood cells.

exacerbation increase in the severity of a disease or any of its symptoms.

excess too much.

excretion an elimination of waste products from the body.

excretory pertaining to excretion.

expectorate coughing up or spitting out sputum or mucus from the lungs and airways.

extracellular fluid volume shift (ECF shift) shift of fluid within the ECF compartment from intravascular to interstitial spaces or from interstitial to intravascular spaces.

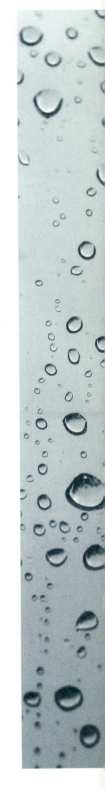

extract outside of.

extravasation the accumulation of vesicant or an irritant in the subcutaneous tissue.

febrile pertaining to a fever.

fatus gas in the alimentary tract.

forced expiratory volume the maximum volume of gas that can be exhaled over a specific time period.

forced vital capacity the volume of gas that can be exhaled as forcefully and rapidly as possible after a maximal inspiration.

fremitus a vibration palpated through the chest wall when an individual is speaking.

gastroenteritis an acute inflammation of the stomach and intestines associated with diarrhea and vomiting that is common in children. It may be caused by viral, bacterial, or parasitic infections.

generic name reflects the chemical family to which a drug belongs. The name never changes.

globulin a group of simple proteins.

glomerulus a capillary loop enclosed within the Bowman's capsule of the kidney.

glucose formed from carbohydrates during digestion and frequently called dextrose.

glycogen a stored form of sugar in the liver or muscle that can be converted to glucose.

glycosuria sugar in the urine.

gt abbreviation for drop.

gtt abbreviation for drops.

heart failure (HF) circulatory congestion related to pump failure.

hematocrit the volume of red blood cells or erythrocytes in a given volume of blood.

hemoconcentration increase in number of red blood cells and solutes and a decrease in plasma volume.

hemodilution an increase in the volume of blood plasma relative to red blood cells; decrease in red blood cell concentration in blood.

hemoglobin a protein conjugated with iron-containing pigment. It carries oxygen in red blood cells.

hemolysis destruction of red blood cells and causing release of hemoglobin into the serum.

heparin anticoagulant.

hepatic coma liver failure.

hernia a protrusion of an organ through the wall of a cavity.

inguinal protrusion of the intestine at the inguinal opening.

homeostasis uniformity or stability. State of equilibrium of the internal environment.

hormone a chemical substance originating in an organ or gland, which travels through the blood and is capable of increasing body activity or secretion.

ADH abbreviation for antidiuretic hormone; a hormone to lessen urine secretion.

hydrocephalus increased fluid retention in the ventricles of the brain.

hydrostatic pressure pressure of fluids at equilibrium.

hyperalimentation intravenous administration of a hyperosmolar solution of glucose, protein, vitamins, and electrolytes to promote tissue synthesis.

hyperbaric oxygenation oxygen under pressure carried in the plasma.

hypercalcemia a higher than normal calcium ion concentration in the blood.

hypercapnia a higher than normal carbon dioxide concentration in the blood.

hyperchloremia a higher than normal chloride ion concentration in the blood.

hyperglycemia a higher than normal glucose concentration in the blood.

hyperkalemia a higher than normal potassium ion concentration in the blood.

hypernatremia a higher than normal sodium ion concentration in the blood.

hyperosmotic increased number of osmols per solution. Increased solute concentration as compared to plasma, having a higher than normal osmolarity.

hyperplasia abnormal increase in the number of normal cells in tissue.

hyperresonance an exaggerated "empty barrel" sound heard over air-filled spaces when percussing the chest.

hypertension high blood pressure.

essential a high blood pressure that develops in the absence of kidney disease. It is also called primary hypertension.

hypertonic having a higher solute concentration than plasma, associated mainly with IV fluids.

hypertrophy increased thickening of a structure.

hyperventilation breathing at a rate greater than needed for body requirements.

hypervolemia a higher than normal blood volume.

hypocalcemia a lower than normal calcium ion concentration in the blood.

hypochloremia a lower than normal chloride ion concentration in the blood.

hypoglycemia a lower than normal glucose concentration in the blood.

hypokalemia a lower than normal potassium ion concentration in the blood.

hyponatremia a lower than normal sodium ion concentration in the blood.

hypo-osmolality condition where number for formed particles in the serum is decreased.

hypo-osmolar decreased number of osmols per solution. Decreased solute concentration as compared to plasma.

hypophysis the pituitary gland.

hypotension a low blood pressure.

hypotonic a lower solute concentration than plasma.

hypoventilation breathing at a rate lower than required to meet metabolic demands.

hypovolemia a lower than normal blood volume.

hypoxemia a lower than normal oxygen concentration in the blood. A decrease in PaO_2 that acts as a strong cerebral basodilator.

hypoxia decreased oxygen content in body tissue.

i.e. that is.

incarcerated constricted, as an irreducible hernia.

infusion an injection of a solution directly into a vein.

insensible perspiration water loss by diffusion through the skin.

inside-needle catheter (INC) an infusion device designed for short-term parenteral therapy (opposite of the over-needle catheter—ONC) that is constructed exactly opposite the ONC.

insulin a hormone secreted by the beta cells of the islets of Langerhans found in the pancreas. It is important in the oxidation and utilization of blood sugar (glucose).

inter between.

interstitial edema accumulation of excess fluid between cells; this is extracellular fluid.

intervention action.

intra within.

intracerebral edema accumulation of excess fluid within the brain tissue and structures.

intracerebral hypertension increased pressure within the brain structures.

intracranial pressure pressure exerted by fluid within the brain structures.

intrapleural within the pleura, the serous membrane surrounding the lungs and lining the thoracic cavity.

ion a particle carrying either a positive or negative charge.

ionization separation into ions.

ionizing separating into ions.

iso-osmolar having the same osmolarity as plasma.

isotonic same solute concentration as plasma.

jugular venous distention visible, abnormal dilation of the jugular veins as a result of fluid overload.

ketone bodies oxidation of fatty acids.

ketonuria excess ketones in urine.

Kussmaul breathing hyperactive, abnormally vigorous breathing.

kyphosis increased convexity of the curvature of the spine, hunchback.

lassitude weariness.

lethargy abnormally tired or drowsy, as in a stupor.

lidocaine also known as xylocaine. A drug used as a surface anesthetic. It also can be used to treat ventricular arrhythmias.

lymph interstitial fluid that has entered lymphatic vessels. Similar to plasma but with lower protein content; usually alkaline (pH = 7.4).

lymphatic system system of lymphatic vessels and lymph nodes that conveys interstitial fluid from the tissues to the veins.

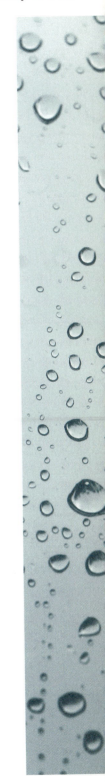

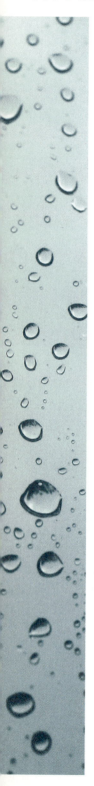

malaise uneasiness, ill feeling.

medulla the central portion of an organ, e.g., adrenal gland; also, the medulla oblongata of the brain stem.

membrane a layer of tissue that covers a surface or organ or separates a space; also, the outer surface of a cell.

mercurial diuretic a drug that affects the proximal tubules of the kidneys by inhibiting reabsorption of sodium.

metabolism the physical and chemical changes involved in the utilization of particular substances.

metabolites the by-products of cellular metabolism or catabolism.

midbrain connects the pons and cerebellum with the cerebral hemispheres.

milliequivalent the chemical activity of elements.

milligram measures the weight of ions.

milliosmol 1/1000th of an osmol. It involves the osmotic activity of a solution.

molar 1 gram molecular weight of a substance.

mucociliary pertaining to mucus and to the cilia in the airways.

myocardium the muscle of the heart.

narcotic a drug that depresses the central nervous system, relieves pain, and can induce sleep.

necrosis death of cells or tissue.

nephritis inflammation of the kidney.

nephrosis degenerative changes in the kidney.

neuromuscular pertaining to the nerve and muscle.

neuromuscular junction the innervation of the nerve with a muscle.

nondependent edema see edema.

nonvolatile acid fixed acid resulting from metabolic processes, excreted by the kidneys.

older age of 65 years or older.

oliguria a diminished amount of urine.

oral rehydration fluid oral fluids designed to replace fluid and electrolyte losses in patients (usually children) who are able to tolerate liquids. These fluids are made up of similar concentrations of glucose, sodium, potassium, chloride, and bicarbonate of soda. Examples include WHO, Hydra-lyte, Re-hydra-lyte, Lytren, ReSol, and Infalyte.

orthopnea difficulty breathing, unless in an upright position.

osmol a unit for measuring the number of dissolved particles in a solution.

osmolality the number of dissolved particles (osmols or milliosmols) per kilogram of solvent.

osmolarity the number of dissolved particles (osmols or milliosmols) per liter of solution.

osmosis the movement of a solvent (usually water) across a barrier (a membrane) from a solution of lower osmolality to a solution of higher osmolality.

osmotic pressure the pressure on water that develops when two solutions of different osmolalities are separated by a semipermeable membrane.

otorrhea drainage from the ear.

overhydration a state in which there is a saline overload or an extracellular volume overload, often associated with poor fluid management in children, which may result in water intoxication.

over-needle catheter an infusion device designed for short-term parenteral therapy (opposite of the INC).

oxygenation the combination of oxygen in tissues and blood.

oxyhemoglobin hemoglobin carrying oxygen.

packed cells red blood cells (RBCs).

pallor or pallid pale.

PAP abbreviation for pulmonary artery pressure. It measures the pressure in the pulmonary artery.

paracentesis the surgical puncture of a cavity, e.g., abdomen.

parathyroid an endocrine gland secreting the hormone parathormone, which regulates calcium and phosphorus metabolism.

parenchyma functional tissue of an organ.

parenteral therapy introduction of fluids into the body by means other than the alimentary tract.

parietal lobe lobe on the side of the brain lying under the parietal bone.

patency the state of being opened.

PCWP abbreviation for pulmonary capillary wedge pressure. Its reading indicates the pumping ability of the left ventricle. Left ventricular end-diastolic pressure (LVEDP) is the best indicator of ventricular function. PCWP reflects LVEDP.

perfusion passing of fluid through body space.

pericardial sac fibroserous sac enclosing the heart.

pericarditis inflammation of the pericardium or the membrane that encloses the heart.

peristalsis wavelike movement occurring with hollow tubes such as the intestine for the movement of contents.

peritoneal cavity a lining covering the abdominal organs with the exclusion of the kidneys.

permeability capability of fluids and/or other substances, e.g., ions, to diffuse through a human membrane.

phlebitis inflammation of the vein.

physiologic pertaining to body function.

pitting edema see edema.

plasma intravascular fluid composed of water, ions, and colloid. Plasma is frequently referred to as serum.

plasmanate commercially prepared protein product used in place of plasma.

pleural cavity the space between the two pleuras.

pleurisy inflammation of the pleura or the membranes that enclose the lung.

polycythemia increase in red blood cell mass.

polyionic many ions or ionic changes.

polyuria an excessive amount or discharge of urine.

pons part of the brain stem, between the medulla oblongata and the midbrain.

porosity the state of being porous.

portal circulation vessels carrying blood from the intestines to the liver.

postoperative following an operation.

potassium-sparing diuretics see diuretics.

potassium-wasting diuretics see diuretics.

prednisone synthetic hormonal drug resembling cortisone.

preload pressure of the blood that fills the left ventricle during diastole.

pressoreceptor see baroreceptor.

pressure gradient the difference in pressure that makes the fluid flow.

proprioception awareness of one's movement and position in space.

protein nitrogenous compounds essential to all living organisms.

plasma relates to albumin, globulin, and fibrinogen.

serum relates to albumin and globulin.

proteolytic splitting of proteins by hydrolysis of peptide bonds.

pruritis itching.

psychogenic polydipsia psychologic effect of drinking excessive amounts of water.

pulmonary artery pressure see PAP.

pulmonary capillary wedge pressure see PCWP.

pulmonary edema see edema.

pulse oximetry a device that measures oxygen saturation in the blood using a wave of infrared light and a sensor placed on an individual's finger, toe, nose, earlobe, or forehead.

pulse pressure the arithmetic difference between the systolic and diastolic blood pressure.

rationale the reason.

reabsorption the act of absorbing again an excreted substance.

refractory edema see edema.

retention retaining or holding back in the body.

reticular activating system alert awareness system of the brain formed from the thalamus, hypothalamus, and cortex.

rhinorrhea drainage from the nose.

sclerosis hardening of an organ or tissue.

selectively permeable membrane a membrane permeable to water and to some, but not all, solutes. The cell membrane is a good example.

semi-Fowler's position 45° elevation.

semipermeable membrane A membrane permeable to water but relatively impermeable to other solutes.

sensible perspiration the loss of water on the skin due to sweat gland activity.

serous cavity a cavity lined by a serous membrane.

serum consists of plasma minus the fibrinogen. It is the same as plasma except that after coagulation of blood, the fibrinogen is removed. Serum is frequently referred to as plasma.

serum albumin albumin in blood plasma or serum (as opposed to albumin in the interstitual fluid).

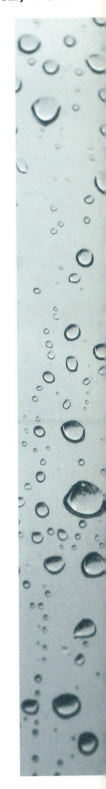

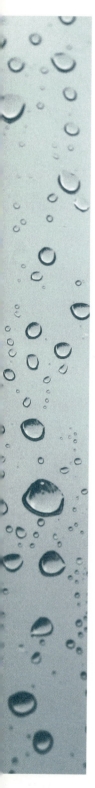

sign an objective indication of disease.

solute a substance dissolved in a solution.

solvent a liquid with a substance in solution.

specific gravity the density of a substance, e.g., urine, relative to that of distilled water. Water has a specific gravity of 1.000; the specific gravity of urine is higher.

steroids a large family of organic compounds having four hydrocarbon rings. Examples include cortisone, cholesterol, estrogen, and tetosterone.

stress effect of a harmful condition or disease(s) affecting the body.

stroke volume amount of blood ejected by the left ventricle with each contraction.

sympathetic nervous system a part of the autonomic nervous system. It can act in an emergency.

symptom subjective indication.

systolic dysfunction the inability of the left ventricle to pump enough blood to perfuse body tissues.

tachycardia a fast heart beat.

tachypnea rapid respirations.

TBSA abbreviation for total body surface area.

tenacious sticky, holding fast.

tetany a nervous affection characterized by tonic spasms of muscles.

thrombophlebitis inflammation of a vein with a thrombus or a blood clot.

tonicity effect of fluid on cellular volume, i.e., electrolytes, BUN, glucose.

total parenteral nutrition (TPN) also known as hyperalimentation.

trade name the name given to a drug by its manufacturer.

transudation the passage of fluid through the pores of a membrane.

trauma an injury.

urea the final product of protein metabolism that is normally excreted by the kidneys.

uremia a toxic condition due to the retention of nitrogenous substances (protein by-products), such as urea, which cannot be excreted by the kidneys.

Valsalva maneuver procedure in which individual takes deep breath and bears down to increase intrathoracic pressure for prevention of air injection. Forced exhalation closes the glottis.

vasoconstriction decrease in size of a blood vessel.

vasodilation increase in size of a blood vessel.

vasogenic originating within the blood vessels.

vasomotor pertaining to the nerves having a muscular contraction or relaxation control of the blood vessel walls.

vasopressors drugs given to contract muscles of the blood vessel walls to increase the blood pressure.

vein a vessel carrying unoxygenated blood to the heart.

ventilation the circulation of air.

pulmonary the inspiration and expiration of air from the lungs.

ventricles the lower chambers of the heart.

venules minute veins moving from capillaries.

vertigo dizziness.

volatile acid acid excreted as a gas by the lungs.

winged-tip infusion device see butterfly.

References/Bibliography

Acid-base tutorial. Tulane University School of Medicine, Department of Anesthesiology. (2006). Available at http://www.acid-base.com

Adams, M., & Pelter, M. (2004). Electrolyte imbalances. *American Journal of Critical Care, 13*(1), 85–86.

Adroque, H. J., & Madias, N. E. (2000). Hyponatremia. *New England Journal of Medicine, 342*(21), 1581–1589.

Allen, L., & O'Connor, C. (2007). Management of acute decompensated heart failure. *Canadian Medical Association Journal, 176*(6), 797–805.

Allison, S., & Lobo, D. (2004). Fluid and electrolytes in the elderly. *Current Opinion in Clinical Nutrition and Metabolic Care, 7,* 27–33.

American Academy of Pediatrics (AAP) & American College of Obstetricians and Gynecologists (ACOG). (2002). *Guidelines for perinatal care* (5th ed.). Washington, D.C.: Author.

American College of Surgeons Committee on Trauma. (2004). *Advanced trauma life support course.* 11th ed. Chicago: Author.

American College of Surgeons Committee on Trauma. (1999). *Resources for optimal care of the injured patient.* Chicago: Author.

American Diabetes Association. (2002). Hyperglycemic crises in patients with diabetes mellitus. *Diabetes Care, 25*(1), S100–S108.

American Nurses Association. (2004). *Standards of clinical nursing practice.* Kansas City: American Nurses Association.

American Thoracic Society. (2007). Standards for the diagnosis and care of patients with chronic obstructive pulmonary disease. American Thoracic Society (2007). *Standards for the diagnosis and treatment of patients with chronic obstructive pulmonary disease.* Retrieved August 7, 2007, from http://www.thoracic.org/sections/copd/for-health-professionals/introduction/index.html.

American Thoracic Society/European Respiratory Society Statement on pulmonary rehabilitation. (2005). Retrieved August 7, 2007, http://www.thoracic.org/sections/publications/statements/pages/respiratory-disease-adults/atserspr0606.html.

Baird, S. B., McCorkle, R., & Grant, M. (1996). *Cancer nursing: A comprehensive textbook.* Philadelphia: Saunders.

Balasubramanyam, A., Garza, G., Rodriguez, L. Hampe, C. S., Gaur, L., Lernmark, A., & Maldonado, M. R. (2006). Accuracy and predictive value of classification schemes for ketosis-prone diabetes. *Diabetes Care, 29,* 2575–2579.

Barnett, M. L. (1999). Hypercalcemia. *Seminars in Oncology Nursing, 15*(3), 190–201.

Barth, M., & Jensen, C. (2006). Postoperative nursing care of gastric bypass patients. *American Journal of Critical Care, 15*(4), 378–387.

Bartley, M. K., & Laskowski-Jones, L. (1995). Postsplenectomy sepsis syndrome. *American Journal of Nursing, 95*(1), 56A–56D.

Bayley, E., & Turke, S. (1999). *A comprehensive curriculum for trauma nursing.* Boston: Jones & Bartlett.

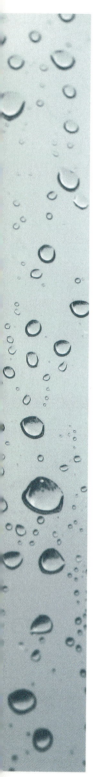

Behrman, R. E., Kliegman, R. M., & Arvin, A. M. (2000). *Nelson textbook of pediatrics* (16th ed.). Philadelphia: W. B. Saunders.

Black, J. M., & Matassarin-Jacobs, E. (2002). *Medical-surgical nursing* (6th ed.). Philadelphia: W. B. Saunders.

Bloch, A. S. (1990). *Nutrition management of the cancer patient*. Rockville, MD: Aspen.

Body, J. J. (2000). Current and future directions in medical therapy: Hypercalcemia. *Cancer, 88* (Suppl. 12), 3054–3058.

Bordow, R. A., Ries, A. L., & Morris, T. A. (2005). *Manual of clinical problems in pulmonary medicine* (6th ed.). Philadelphia: Lippincott, Williams & Wilkins.

Bove, L. A. (1994). How fluids and electrolytes shift after surgery. *Nursing 1994, 24*(8), 34–39.

Braman, S. S. (2006). Chronic cough due to chronic bronchitis: ACCP evidence-based clinical practice guideline. *Chest, 129,* 104S–115S.

Brownie, S. (2006). Why are elderly individuals at risk of nutritional deficiency? *International Journal of Nursing Practice, 12,* 110–118.

Burger, C. (2004). Emergency: hypokalemia. *American Journal of Nursing, 104*(11), 61–65.

Carleton, S. C. (1995). Cardiac problems associated with burns. *Cardiology Clinics, 13*(2), 257–262.

Carlstedt, F., & Lind, L. (2001). Hypocalcemic syndromes. *Critical Care Clinics, 17*(1), 139–153.

Carpentito, L. J. (2005). *Nursing diagnosis application to clinical practice* (9th ed.). Philadelphia: Lippincott.

Cawley, M. J. (May, 2007). Hypernatremia: current treatment strategies and the role of vasopressin antagonists. *Annual Pharmacotherapy, 41*(5), 840–850.

Celli, B. R., MacNee, W., American Thoracic Society/European Respiratory Society Task Force. (2004). Standards for the diagnosis and treatment of patients with COPD: A summary of the ATS/ERS position paper. *European Respiratory Journal, 23,* 932–946.

Clark, B. A., & Brown, R. S. (1995). Potassium homeostasis and hyperkalemic syndromes. *Endocrinology and Metabolism Clinics of North America, 24*(3), 573–591.

Copstead, L. C., & Banasik, J. L. (2005). *Pathophysiology.* Philadelphia: Saunders.

Cohn, J. N., Kowey, P. R., Whelton, P. K., & Prisant, M. (2000, Sept. 11). New guidelines for potassium replacement in clinical practice. *Archives of Internal Medicine, 160,* 2429–2436.

Cornell, S. (1997). Maintaining a fluid balance. *Advances for Nurse Practitioners, 5*(12), 43–44.

Cummins, R. O. (Ed.). (2005). *ACLS: Principles and practice.* Dallas: American Heart Association.

Daun, L. (2005). Don't assume dehydrated children always need IVs. *ED Nursing, 8*(6), 70–71.

Davidhizar, R., Dunn, C., & Hart, A. (2004). A review of the literature on how important water is to the world's elderly population. *International Nursing Review, 51,* 159–166.

Decaux, Guy (July, 2006). Is asymptomatic hyponatremia really asymptomatic? *The Journal of Medicine, 119*(7A), S79–S82.

Dechman, G., & Wilson, C. R. (2004). Evidence underlying breathing retraining in people with stable chronic obstructive pulmonary disease. *Physical Therapy, 84,* 1189–1197.

Des Jardins, T., & Burton, G. G. (2000). *Clinical manifestations and assessment of respiratory diseases* (4th ed.). St. Louis: Mosby.

Dunbar, S., Jacobson, L., & Deaton, C. (1998). Heart failure: Strategies to enhance patient self management. *AACN Clinical Issues in Advanced Practice and Critical Care Nursing, 9*(2), 244–256.

Ellis, D. A., Cunningham, P. B., Podolski, C. L., & Cakan, N. (2007). Multisystemic Therapy for adolescents with poorly-controlled type 1 diabetes: Stability of treatment Effects in a randomized controlled trial. *Journal of Consulting and Clinical Psychology, 73,* 168–175.

Emergency Nurses Association. (2000). *Trauma nursing core course* (5th ed.). Park Ridge, IL: Author.

Fall, P. J. (2000). Hyponatremia and hypernatremia. *Postgraduate Medicine, 107*(5), 75–82.

Figueroa, M., & Peters, J. (2006). Congestive heart failure: Diagnosis, pathophysiology, therapy, and implications for respiratory care. *Respiratory Care, 51*(4), 403–412.

Francis, J. (2001). ECG challenge-hypocalcemia. *Emergency Medicine, 33*(8), 41–42.

Gennan, F. J. (1998). Hypokalemia. *New England Journal of Medicine, 352,* 135–140.

Ginde, A. A., Pelletier, A. J., & Camargo, C. A. (2006). National study of U.S. emergency department visits with diabetic ketoacidosis, 1993–2003. *Diabetes Care, 29,* 2117–2119.

Glebish, G., Krapf, R., & Wagner, C. (2007). Renal and extrarenal regulation of potassium. *Kidney International, 72,* 397–410.

Global Initiative for Chronic Obstructive Lung Disease. (2006). *Pocket guide to COPD diagnosis, management, and prevention: A guide for health care professionals.* Retrieved August 7, 2007 from http://www.goldcopd.com/Guidelineitem.asp?l1=2&l2=1&intId=1116.

Global strategy for the diagnosis, management, and prevention of chronic obstructive pulmonary disease. (2001). NHLBI/WHO workshop report. Retrieved on March 29, 2002, from http://www.goldcopd.com/exec_summary/summary_2001

Gross, P. (2001). Correction of hyponatremia. *Seminars in Nephrology, 21*(3), 269–272.

Guell, R., Casan, P., Belda, J., Sangenis, M., Morante, F., Guyatt, G. H., et al. (2000). Long-term effects of outpatient rehabilitation of COPD: A randomized trial. *Chest, 117,* 976–983.

Gura, M. (2001). Heart failure: Pathophysiology, therapeutic strategies, and assessment of treatment outcomes. *Medscape Nursing.* Retrieved November 19, 2001, from http://nurses.medscape.com/Medscape/nurse/journal/2001/v01.no3/mns1105.01.gura.html

Guyton, A. C. (1995). *Textbook of medical physiology* (9th ed.). Philadelphia: W. B. Saunders.

Harding, L., Bellemare, S., Wiebe, N., Russell, K., Klassen, T. P., & Craig, W. (2007). Oral versus intravenous rehydration for treating dehydration due to gastroenteritis in children (review). *Evidence-Based Child Health: A Cochrane review journal, 2,* 163–218.

Held, J. L. (1995). Correcting fluid and electrolyte imbalance. *Nursing 1995, 25*(4), 71.

Hockenberry, M. (2005). *Wong's nursing care of children.* St. Louis: Mosby.

Hockenberry, M. J., Wilson, D., Winkelstein, M. L., & Kline, N. E. (2003). *Wong's nursing care of infants and children* (7th ed.). St. Louis: Mosby.

Hogg, J. (2004). Pathophysiology of airflow limitation in chronic obstructive pulmonary disease. *The Lancet, 364,* 703–721.

Iggulden, H. (1999). Dehydration and electrolyte disturbance. *Nursing Standard, 12*(19), 48–54.

Innerarity, S., & Stark, J. (2007). pp. 194–245. *Fluid and electrolytes.* Springhouse, PA: Springhouse.

Jones, A. M., Moseley, M. J., Halfmann, S. J., Health, A. H., & Henkelman, N. J. (1991). Fluid volume dynamics. *Critical Care Nurse, 11*(4), 74–76.

Jones, A., & Rowe, B. (2000). Bronchopulmonary hygiene physical therapy and chronic obstructive lung disease: A systematic review. *Heart and Lung, 29,* 125–135.

Kamel, K. S., Ethier, J. H., & Richardson, M. A. (1990). Urine electrolytes and osmolality: When and how to use them. *American Journal of Nephrology, 10*(2), 89–102.

Kaufman, J. S. (2007). Nursing management: Obstructive pulmonary diseases. In S. L. Lewis, M. M. Heitkemper, S. R. Dirksen, P. G. O'Brien, & L. Bucher (Eds.). *Medical-surgical nursing: Assessment and management of clinical problems* (7th ed., pp. 607–663). Philadelphia, PA: Mosby-Elsevier.

Kee, J. L. (2005). *Laboratory and diagnostic tests with nursing implications* (7th ed.). New Jersey: Prentice Hall Health.

King, C. K., Glass, R., Bresee, J. S., & Duggan, C. (2003). Managing acute gastroenteritis among children. *Centers for Disease Control—Morbidity and Mortality Weekly, 52* (RR16), 1–16.

Kitabchi, A. E., Umpierrez, G. E., Murphy, M. B., & Kreisberg, R. A. (2006). Hyperglycemic crises in adult patients with

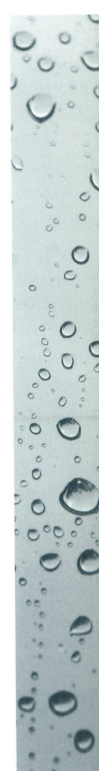

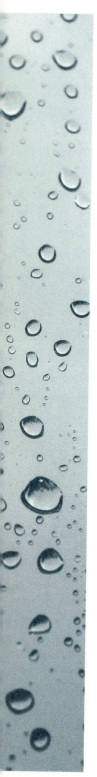

diabetes: A consensus statement from the American Diabetes Association. *Diabetes Care, 29,* 2739–2748.

Knebel, A. R., Bentz, E., & Barnes, P. (2000). Brief report. Dyspnea management of alpha-1 antitrypsin deficiency: Effect of oxygen administration. *Nursing Research, 49,* 333–338.

Kokko, J. P., & Tanner, R. L. (1995). *Fluids and electrolytes* (3rd ed.). Philadelphia: W. B. Saunders.

Laskowski-Jones, L., (2006a). Adult and Pediatric Emergency Drugs. In J. Kee, E. Hayes, & L. E. McCuistion (Eds.), *Pharmacology: A nursing process approach* (5th ed., pp. 906–923). St. Louis, MO: Saunders-Elsevier.

Laskowski-Jones, L. (2006b). Emergency! Responding to trauma—your priorities in the first hour. *Nursing 2006, 36*(9), 52–59.

Laskowski-Jones, L., (2006c). First aid for bleeding wounds. *Nursing 2006, 36*(9), 50–51.

Laskowski-Jones, L. (2007a). Nursing management: Acute intracranial problems. In S. L. Lewis, M. M. Heitkemper, S. R. Dirksen, P. G. O'Brien, & L. Bucher (Eds), *Medical-surgical nursing: Assessment and management of clinical problems* (7th ed., pp. 1467–1501). St. Louis: Mosby Elsevier.

Laskowski-Jones, L. (2007b). Nursing management: Peripheral nerve and spinal cord problems. In S. L. Lewis, M. M. Heitkemper, S. R. Dirksen, P. G. O'Brien, & L. Bucher, (Eds.), *Medical-surgical nursing: Assessment and management of clinical problems* (7th ed., pp. 1580–1613). St. Louis: Mosby Elsevier.

Laskowski-Jones, L., & Toulson, K. (2006). Emergency & Mass Casualty Nursing. In D. Ignatavicius, & M. L. Workman (Eds.), *Medical-surgical nursing: Critical thinking for collaborative care* (5th ed. pp. 156–172). Philadelphia: Elsevier Saunders.

London, M., Ladewig, P. W., Ball, J. W., & Bindler, R. (2007). *Maternal and child nursing care.* Upper Saddle River, N.J.: Prentice Hall.

Lewis, S., Heitkempe, M., & Dirksen, S. (2007). *Medical-surgical nursing assessment and management of clinical practice* (6th ed., pp. 314–333). Philadelphia: Mosby.

Lewis, S., Heitkemper, M., Dirksen, S. R., O'Brien, P. G., and Bucher, L., (2007). Medical-surgical nursing: Assessment and management of clinical problems 7th ed.

Luckey, A, & Parsa, C. (2003). Fluid and electrolytes in the aged. *Archives of Surgery, 138,* 1055–1060.

Lueckenotte, A. G. (1996). *Gerontologic nursing.* St. Louis: Mosby.

Mago, R., Bilker, W., Have, T., Harralson, T., Streim, J., Parmalee, P., & Katz, I. (2000). Clinical laboratory measures in relation to depression, disability, and cognitive impairment in elderly patients. *American Journal of Geriatric Psychiatry, 4*(4), 327–332.

Mandal, A. K. (1997). Hypokalemia and hyperkalemia. *Critical Care Clinics of North America, 81,* 611–639.

Mange, K., Matsuura, D., Cizman, B., Soto, H., Ziyadeh, F., Goldfarb, S., et al. (1997). Language guiding therapy: The case of dehydration versus volume depletion. *Annals of Internal Medicine, 127*(9), 848–853.

Martin, R. Y., & Schrier, R. W. (1995). Renal sodium excretion and edematous disorders. *Endocrinology and Metabolism Clinics of North America, 24*(3), 459–475.

Matheny, N. (1996). *Fluid and electrolyte balance* (3rd ed.). Philadelphia: Lippincott.

Matheny, N., Wehrle, M., Wierssema, L., & Clark, J. (1998). Testing feeding tube placement: Auscultation vs. pH method. *American Journal of Nursing, 98*(5), 37–42.

Mattox, K., Feliciano, D., & Moore, E. (2000). *Trauma* (4th ed.). Stamford, CT: Appleton & Lange.

McCool, F. D., & Rosen, M. J. (2006). Nonpharmacologic airway clearance therapies: ACCP evidence-based clinical practice guidelines. *CHEST, 129,* 250S–259S.

Meighan-Davies, J., & Parnell, H. (2000). Management of COPD. *Journal of Community Nursing, 14,* 10, 22, 24.

Munger, MA (Feb 2, 2007). New agents for managing hyponatremia in hospitalized patients. *American Journal of Health System Pharmacy, 64*(3), 253–265.

Murphy, R., Driscoll, P., & O'Driscoll, R. (2001). Emergency oxygen therapy for the COPD patient. *Emergency Medical Journal, 18,* 333–339.

NANDA. (2007). Nursing diagnoses: Definitions and classifications 2007–2008. Philadelphia: North American Nursing Diagnosis Association.

National Institute for Clinical Excellence (2004). *Quick reference guide: Chronic obstructive pulmonary disease: Management of chronic obstructive pulmonary disease in adults in primary and secondary care.* Retrieved August 7, 2007 from http://www.nice.org.uk/pdf/CG012quickrefguide.pdf.

National Kidney Foundation K/DOQI. (2002). Clinical practice guidelines for chronic kidney disease: evaluation, classification, and stratification. *American Journal of Kidney Diseases, 39*(Suppl. 1): S1–266.

Newman, S. P. (2005). Inhaler treatment options in COPD. *European Respiratory Review, 14,* 102–108.

Novartis Foundation Symposium. (2001). *Chronic obstructive pulmonary disease: Pathogenesis to treatment.* Chichester, UK: John Wiley & Sons.

Oren, R. M. (2005). Hyponatremia in congestive heart failure. *American Journal of Cardiology, 95*(Suppl), 2B–7B.

Oskvig, R. M. (1999). Special problems in the elderly. *Chest, 115*(5), 158–164.

Oster, J. R. Reston, R. A., & Materson, B. J. (1994). Fluid and electrolyte disorders in congestive heart failure. *Seminars in Nephrology, 14*(5), 485–505.

Perazella, M. A. (2000). Drug-induced hyperkalemia: Old culprits and new offenders. *American Journal of Medicine, 109*(9), 307–314.

Pereira, N., & Cooper, G. (2000). Systolic heart failure: Practical implementation of standard guidelines. *Clinical Cornerstone.* Retrieved July 16, 2001, from http://nurses.medscape.com/excerptaMed/clincornerstne/2000/v03.n02/clc03.02.pere.html

Popov, T. (2005). Review: Capillary refill time, abnormal skin turgor, and abdominal respiratory patterns are useful signs for detecting dehydration in children. *Evidence-Based Nursing, 8*(2), 57.

Porth, C. M. (2002). *Pathophysiology: Concepts of altered health states* (6th ed.). Philadelphia: Lippincott, Williams & Wilkins.

Powers, F. (1999). The role of chloride in acid-base balance. *Journal of Intravenous Nursing, 22*(5), 286–291.

Rabe, K. F., Beghe, B., Luppi, F., & Fabbri, L. M. (2007). Update in chronic obstructive pulmonary disease 2006. *American Journal of Respiratory and Critical Care Medicine, 175,* 1222–1234.

Ragland, G. (1990). Electrolyte abnormalities in the alcoholic patient. *Emergency Medicine Clinics of North America, 8*(4), 761–771.

Redden, M., & Wotton, K. (2001). Clinical decision making by nursing when faced with third-spacing fluid shift: How well do they fare? *Gastroenterology Nursing, 24*(4), 182–191.

Riera, H. S., Rubio, T. M., Ruiz, F. O., Ramos, P. J., Otero, D. D. C., Hernandez, T. E., et al. (2001). Inspiratory muscle training in patients with COPD. *Chest, 120,* 748–757.

Robertson, J., & Shilkofski, N. (2005). *The Harriet Lane Handbook: A manual for pediatric house officers* (17th ed.). Philadelphia: Elsevier Mosby.

Rose, B. D. (1997). *Clinical physiology of acid-base and electrolyte disorders* (5th ed.). New York: McGraw-Hill.

Rosenberger, K. (1998). Management of electrolyte abnormalities: Hypocalcemia, hypomagnesemia, and hypokalemia. *Journal of American Academy of Nurse Practitioners, 10*(5), 209–217.

Sadovsky, R. (2002). Managing dyspnea in patients with advanced COPD. *American Family Physician, 65,* 935.

Samann, A., Muhlhauser, I., Bener, R., Hunger-Dathe, W., Kloos, C., & Muller, U. A. (2006). Flexible intensive insulin therapy in adults with type 1 diabetes and high risk for severe hypoglycemia and diabetic ketoacidosis. *Diabetes Care, 29,* 2196–2199.

Schrier, R. W. (1997). *Renal and electrolyte disorders* (5th ed.). Boston: Little, Brown.

Selekman, J., Scofield, S., & Swenson-Brousell, C. (1999). Diabetes update in the pediatric population. *Pediatric Nursing, 25*(6), 666–669.

Shuey, K. M. (2004). Hypercalcemia of malignancy: part 1. *Clinical Journal of Oncology Nursing, 8*(2), 209–210.

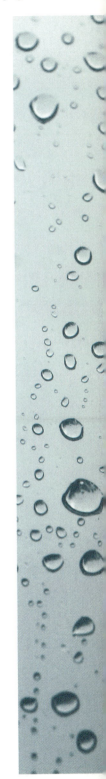

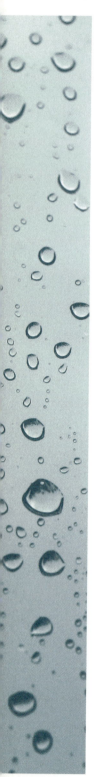

Simmons, P., & Simmons, M. (2004). Informed nursing practice: The administration of oxygen to patients with COPD. *MEDSURG Nursing, 13,* 82–86.

Singh, S, and Frances, S (2004). Management of hypercalcaemia. *Geriatric Medicine, 34*(5), 35–42.

Snow, V., Lascher, S., & Mottur-Pilson, C. (2001). The evidence base for management of acute exacerbations of COPD: Clinical practice guideline (Pt. 1). *Chest, 110,* 1185–1189.

Taccetta-Chapnick, M. (2002). Using Carvedilol to treat heart failure. *Critical Care Nurse, 22*(2), 36–58.

Terry, J. (1994). The major electrolytes. *Journal of Intravenous Nursing, 17*(5), 240–247.

The Merck manual. (2003). Acid-base balance (chap. 138). Available at http://www.merck.com/pubs/mmanual_home/sec 12/138.htm

Truesdell, S. (2000). Helping patients with COPD manage episodes of acute shortness of breath. *MEDSURG Nursing, 9,* 178–182.

Upadhyay, A, Jaber, B. L., and Madias, N. E. (2006). Incidence and prevalence of hyponatremia. *The American Journal of Medicine, 119*(7A), S30–S35.

Vriji, A., & Murr, M. (2006). Caring for patients after bariatric surgery. *American Family Physician, 73,* (1403–1408).

Waltman, N. L., Bergstrom, N., Armstrong, N., Norrell, K., & Braden, B. (1991). Nutritional status, pressure sores, and mortality in elderly patients with cancer. *Oncology Nursing Forum, 18,* 867–873.

Wang, J., Williams, D. E., Narayan, K. M. V., & Geiss, L. S. (2006). Declining death rates from hyperglycemic crisis among adults with diabetes, U.S., 1985–2002. *Diabetes Care, 29,* 2018–2022.

Watkins, S. L. (1995). The basics of fluid and electrolyte therapy. *Pediatric Annuals, 24*(1), 16–22.

Webster M., Brady, W., and Morris, F. (2002). Recognizing signs of danger: ECG changes resulting from an abnormal serum potassium concentration. *Emergency Medicine, 19*(1), 74–77.

Wolfsdoft, J., Glaser, N., & Sperling, M. A. (2006). Diabetic ketoacidosis in infants, children, and adolescents. *Diabetes Care, 29,* 1150–1159.

Wong, D. (1998). *Essentials of pediatric nursing* (4th ed.). Philadelphia: Mosby.

Wouters, E. F. M., Creutzberg, E. C., & Schols, A. M. W. J. (2002). Systemic effects in COPD. *Chest, 121,* 127S–130S.

Wu, C., Lee, Y. Y., Bain, K., & Wichaikhum, O. (2001). Coping behaviors of individuals with chronic obstructive pulmonary disease. *MEDSURG Nursing, 10,* 315–321.

Index

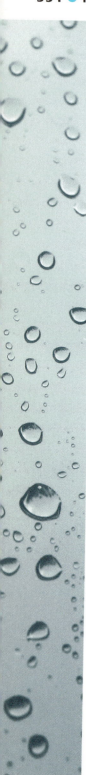

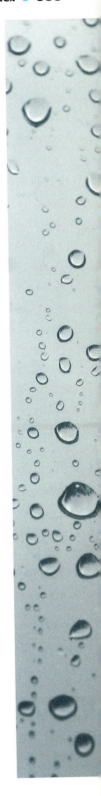

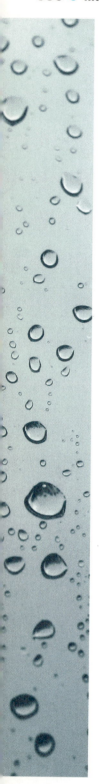

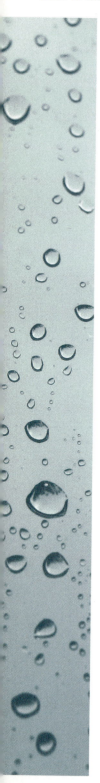

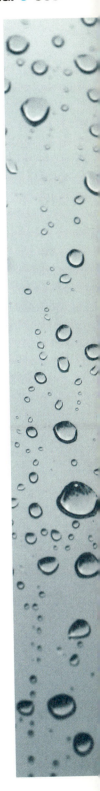

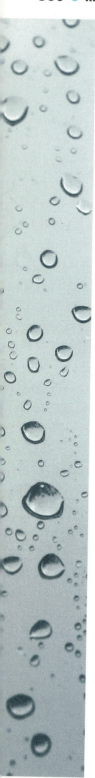

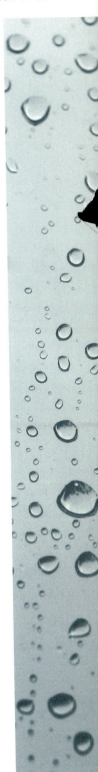

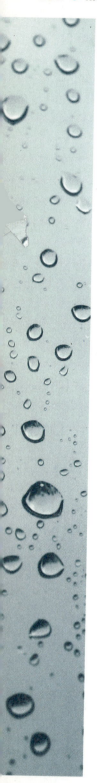

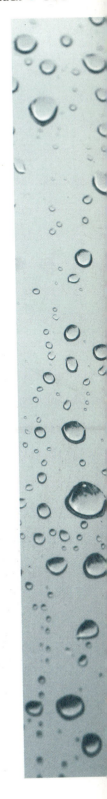

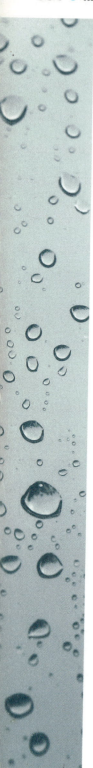